SIMPLE KITCHEN MAGIC

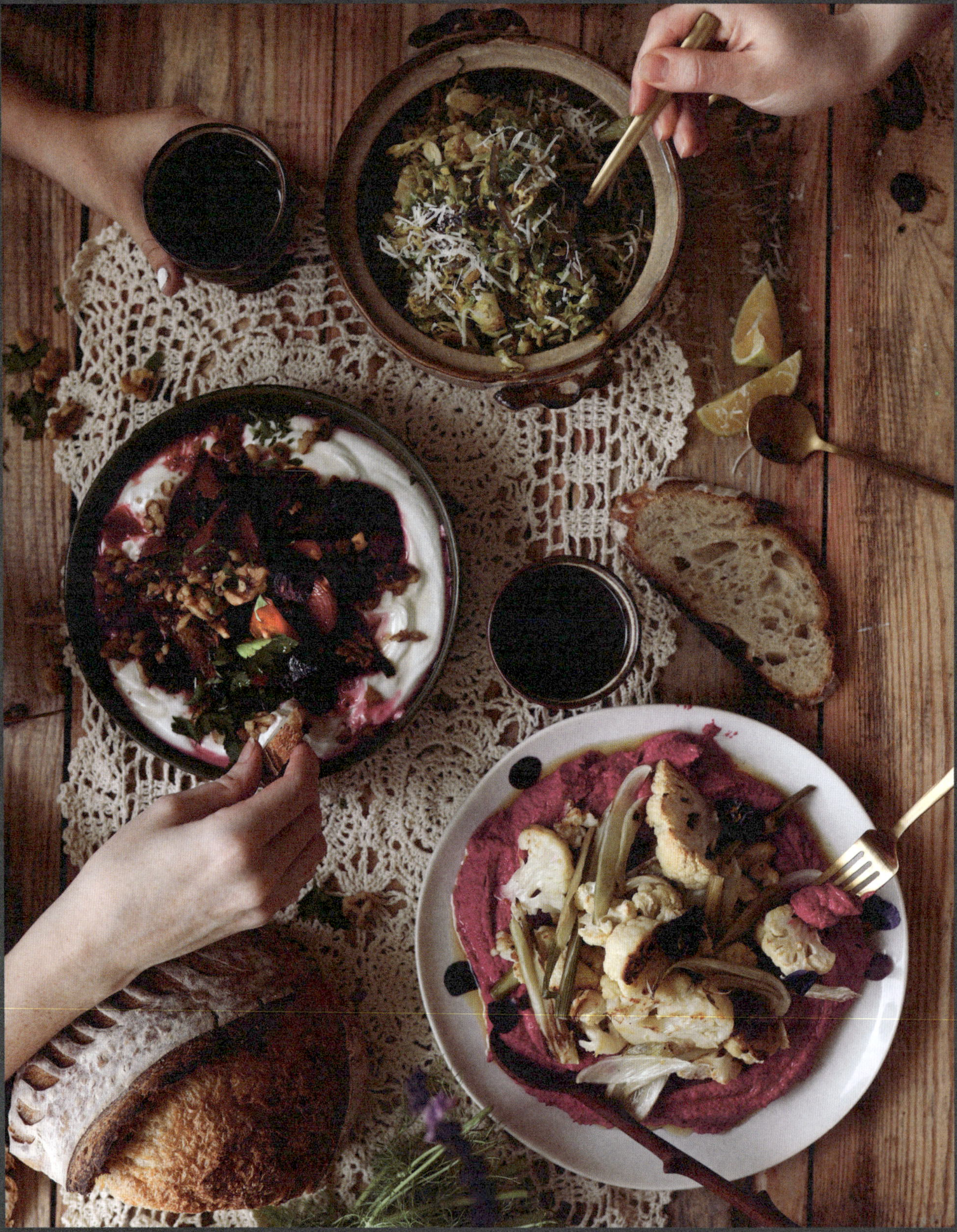

SIMPLE KITCHEN MAGIC

WHOLE-FOOD

RECIPES & REMEDIES

FOR A HOLISTIC LIFE

REBEKAH MOYER

DK

DK | Penguin Random House

Publisher Mike Sanders
Art & Design Director William Thomas
Editorial Director Ann Barton
Executive Editor Olivia Peluso
Designer Laura Palese
Editorial Assistant Resham Anand
Food Photographer Rebekah Moyer
Lifestyle Photographer Cadence Feeley
Illustrator Rebekah Moyer
Recipe Tester Molly Adams
Copyeditor Morgan Jefferson
Proofreaders Bianca Bosman & Taylor Plett
Indexer Celia McCoy

First American Edition, 2026
Published in the United States by DK Publishing
1745 Broadway, 20th Floor, New York, NY 10019

The authorized representative in the EEA is Dorling Kindersley Verlag GmbH.
Arnulfstr. 124, 80636 Munich, Germany

25 26 27 28 29 10 9 8 7 6 5 4 3 2 1
001–001-351041-Oct/2026

A catalog record for this book is available from the Library of Congress.
ISBN 978-0-5939-7153-6

Printed and bound in China

www.dk.com

FSC www.fsc.org MIX Paper FSC™ C018179

DEDICATION

TO THE GIRL WHO THOUGHT LIFE
HAD LOST ITS MAGIC AND ALL THE PEOPLE
WHO SHOWED HER IT HADN'T

Contents

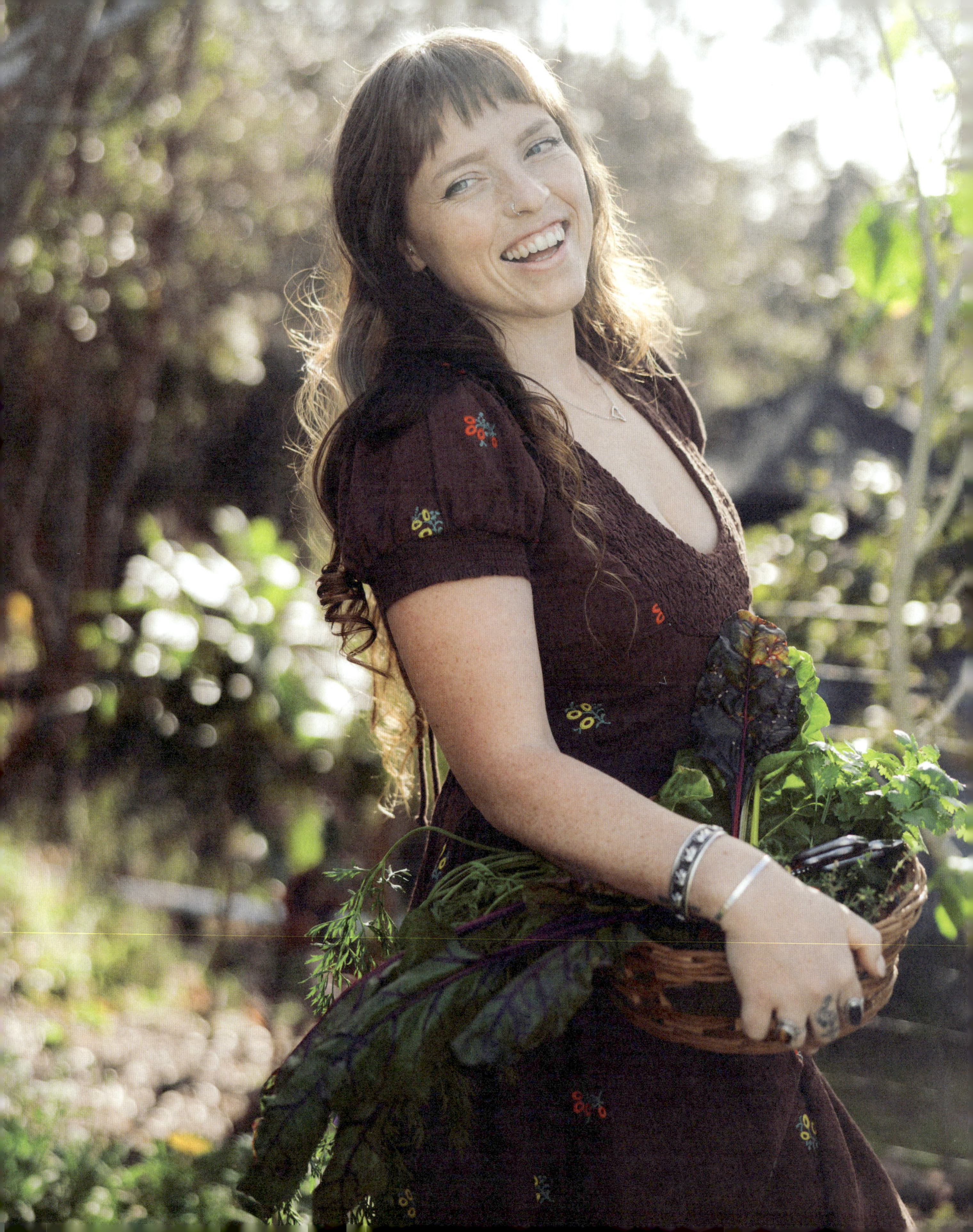

Food Is Magic

AND COOKING IS ALCHEMY. That's not even hyperbole: Every day, worldwide, billions of people work the land to produce food, taking that gift from the earth and transforming it through fire, water, air, and love into something that sustains life.

Food is the oldest medicine, and cooking has always been a spiritual process to me. I often daydream about the first humans who thought to put meat on a stick and cook it over the flames of those early fires. Who crafted a pot and was inspired to add water, roots, leaves, meat, and minerals to create a stew? Who, over time, tried this leaf, that bark, and those mushrooms, discovering what hurt and what healed? That something could be poisonous when raw but delicious and healing when cooked?

Honestly, it sounds like magic. But science makes the link: The evolution of cooking is directly linked to the development of modern humans. Cooking over a fire made food easier to digest, enabling early humans to absorb more nutrition in less time. This coincided with an increase in brain size, and thus humans and their food developed alongside one another. Without this relationship, we wouldn't be who we are today.

I imagine this experimental process was driven by deep intuition and even sparks of divine inspiration. Our ancestors lived and developed *with* the earth, connected to the beating heart of nature. We *were* nature: There was no separation between us and the ground beneath our bare feet. We were intimately attuned to the cycles of the earth.

Cooking became a part of that cycle, an alchemizing of the elements of nature. Picture this: Vegetables grow in the soil, sucking up minerals, turning them into specific nutrients, taking the literal earth and packaging it into a gift. We tended and gathered those gifts from the earth, used our human curiosity to cook and combine them, and they became even more powerful. When we eat and metabolize those gifts, a mystical (or very scientific, depending on how you choose to view it) exchange happens: Hundreds of earth's unique compounds disperse into our bodies to make us function. A beautiful, co-creating cycle.

Because of this, we developed a nutritional intuition. When we lacked something, our bodies craved it. When something was poisonous, we learned to avoid it. We ate foods when they were in season, and those foods served our needs best for that season. We gathered and formed community around harvests, hunts, and hearths. Food wasn't an afterthought; it was the goal. For thousands of years, we lived synergistically with the earth, and food was at the center of that relationship. Food was communal; it was sacred; it was simple. It was intuitive!

But over time, as humans have subdued nature rather than living as a part of it, many of

"For thousands of years, we lived synergistically with the earth, and food was at the center of that relationship."

us have become disconnected from that intuition. We built cities over fields; we industrialized food production and put everything into plastic. We added preservatives to keep food fresh and invented microwaves to heat it quickly. We no longer needed to get our fingers in the dirt to produce our life-sustaining fuel. We didn't need to live by the seasons, revel in the lengthy summer and its bounty, or store up harvests for winter. Food became a packaged afterthought. The food industry boomed, becoming a looming, sinister giant, with more concern for profit margins than nourishment. Along the way, food lost its magic. It became a poison rather than a potion.

And after years of this disconnect, we started to see the effects: disease, exhaustion, loss of community. We began to recognize the problems created by the processed food industry and to reeducate ourselves about food and its importance in the ecosystem of the body. Only this time, it became an obsession: *weight loss, calorie counting, low-fat, low-carb, fake sweeteners, bikini bodies, crash diets*—new buzzwords and diets to follow, to become our "healthiest" selves. Before long, capitalism capitalized, creating the "wellness industry." So much money has been made off of people's desire to find "health" that, in 2023, the the global wellness industry was valued at $6.3 trillion.

Health has become associated with wealth: If you can afford the best supplements, the highest quality food, the fanciest ingredients, and the best treatments, you might just have a shot at peak wellness. This means that healthy eating can feel inaccessible and complicated, like a secret formula just out of reach. Far from innate, it has become esoteric: To achieve "wellness," you have to pay to play.

In just a few generations, we've forgotten that intuitive wisdom: that we could listen to our bodies. We have become so familiar with our packaged, preserved reality that a berry plucked from the bush seems dirty and even dangerous.

Our grandparents lived in the boom of convenience but still knew where their food came from. Our parents were raised in a world where "artificial" foods were new and fun, and they paid for it with their health. They didn't teach many of us to grow, cook, and consume food mindfully, because they didn't know it was important. Now there is a whole generation of people who have lost the knowledge that our ancestors needed for basic survival. Many people haven't connected the food they eat with the way they feel because they were sold pills to cover up symptoms before they were ever asked about their diet. We have been duped into believing that we aren't smart enough to heal ourselves.

We forgot the magic.

But the magic has been there, all along, and it has been pulling us back in. The processed life, as much as it is convenient, is not sustainable. We have become *so* sick. And we realized what's been causing it: *It's the food.* And so a whole movement of people started going back to their roots—to dough kneaded by hand, patio-grown tomatoes, and foods made with fewer ingredients. In an uncertain world, people are gathering around the table again; the cool kids host potlucks, and it's increasingly *less* weird to offer a homemade ferment as a Christmas gift.

Of course, life is different now than it was for our great-great-grandparents. The world is far more chaotic, and community hearths and harvests seem distant when many of us are isolated in the day to day. We are trying to relearn this lost generational wisdom, but this can be so overwhelming in the information age. Who has time to sift through the info, work, parent, and perform, all while making and baking everything from scratch? What if you eat the wrong food? *I thought spinach was good for you!* you think in despair while watching a video about oxalates, and you cross another thing off your "safe to eat" list. But the intuition is still there, ready to be reawakened.

Remember the magic.

THE MAGIC RETURNS

In his groundbreaking book *In Defense of Food*, journalist and author Michael Pollan said it best: "Eat food. Not too much. Mostly plants." It's simple: Eat real food, in moderation, and don't stress about it too much. Don't be scared of it or obsess over it; honor it. It's hard to become truly unwell when you eat well-sourced food cooked at home. Think about it like this: You can absolutely eat chocolate cake. But if you commit to making the chocolate cake you eat, two things will happen: First, the ingredients in that cake will likely be higher quality and far simpler than those in any cake you buy at the store, with no fillers or preservatives, and less sugar. Second, because you will most likely not feel like making a whole chocolate cake very often, you won't eat it all the time. Making food yourself becomes this wonderful guidepost for balanced eating. You can take this as far as you'd like—even get a cow, churn your own butter, and make your own pasta, if you have the time and energy. But in general, the more precious and time-consuming something is to make, the less often you will eat it, and the more your snacks will look like whole, raw fruits and veggies, and your weekday meals like plates of simply cooked ingredients.

That is when the magic returns. When we prioritize simple, whole foods, we begin to heal just by eating with intention. Food is not just fuel; it is our source of life and wellbeing, our connection to the earth and our community. When we grasp this, the kitchen becomes the apothecary, and the pot on the stove a cauldron as we craft meals with that age-old intuition and care. The more we simplify our cooking, the more we're able to experiment. We begin to find not just joy in cooking, but also power—and a desire to invite others to the table.

This book is your guide to rediscovering the magic. In it, you will hopefully find empowerment and some foundational knowledge with which to build your own healing culinary practice. While the information in this book is all science-backed, this isn't a textbook or a protocol. This is simple, heartwarming food. It is basic nutritional science and biology. It is generational wisdom passed from my grandmother to my mother to me, as well as new research and my own experience.

I believe that knowledge is free and should be shared. I believe that healthy food should not be reserved for the wealthy. I believe that anyone can cook and everyone can be an expert in their own body.

Above all, when you plop this book on your countertop, I want you to feel like health is attainable, nutrition is simple, and cooking from scratch is doable. And as you begin to heal, I hope you sense, like I do, that food is magic.

HOW TO USE THIS BOOK

I'VE POURED MY HEART and soul into this book to make it informative, delightful, and delicious! Here are some notes for using these recipes.

- I love flavor. I like to season heavily, and I encourage you to flow with that, although there are places where I held myself back, as I'm aware not everyone wants eight cloves of garlic in their food all the time. So feel free to go hard—seasonings are where the most powerful medicine is!

- Sometimes salt is measured in these recipes; other times I say "salt, to taste," because personal taste does matter here. Be aware, though, that salt is so important for flavor, and many people undersalt their food. Don't go shoveling it in tablespoonfuls at a time, but don't be scared to really season things. Keep in mind that different types of salt have different levels of "saltiness." Avoid using table salt in recipes; it is super salty and low in nutrients. I almost always use fine sea salt in my recipes. A good pinch of salt should be at least ¼ teaspoon. So salt your food. Taste it. Season again.

- You'll also notice that I use soft, fresh herbs (like cilantro, parsley, and dill) a *lot*. This is partly for flavor and color, but also because they are so beneficial for digestive health and combating inflammation. Fresh herbs can get expensive, but thankfully they're super easy to grow, so I highly recommend you get a couple plants for your porch and keep them in rotation.

- There are a lot of repeated ingredients in this book—that is on purpose! My desire is that these recipes will be accessible, that you can predictably shop and stock your home with ingredients for which you will have multiple uses. Every now and then, you'll find a special, funky item. When I call for these items, it's for good reason, but you always have the power to adjust.

- I am not a good recipe follower. I am a *cook-with-my-heart, measure-in-pinches-and-plops* kind of girl. However, that doesn't really work for a cookbook. So while there are specifics in these recipes, I also encourage you to experiment, try different vegetable or herb combos, and discover what works for you. I want you to let your intuition guide you. That, after all, is the whole point—empowering your food journey, finding joy in the kitchen, and rediscovering the *magic*.

- Many recipes are labeled with cycle phases and contain ingredients to support hormones at those times. These aren't strict prescriptions; you won't cause harm by eating them "out of phase," and yes, men can eat them all, too! However, if you are experiencing hormone imbalance, you will be more sensitive to these nutritional specifications and will definitely notice a difference when you do "cycle sync" (see page 44). Recipes that aren't labeled (mostly sauces and drinks) are less specifically formulated.

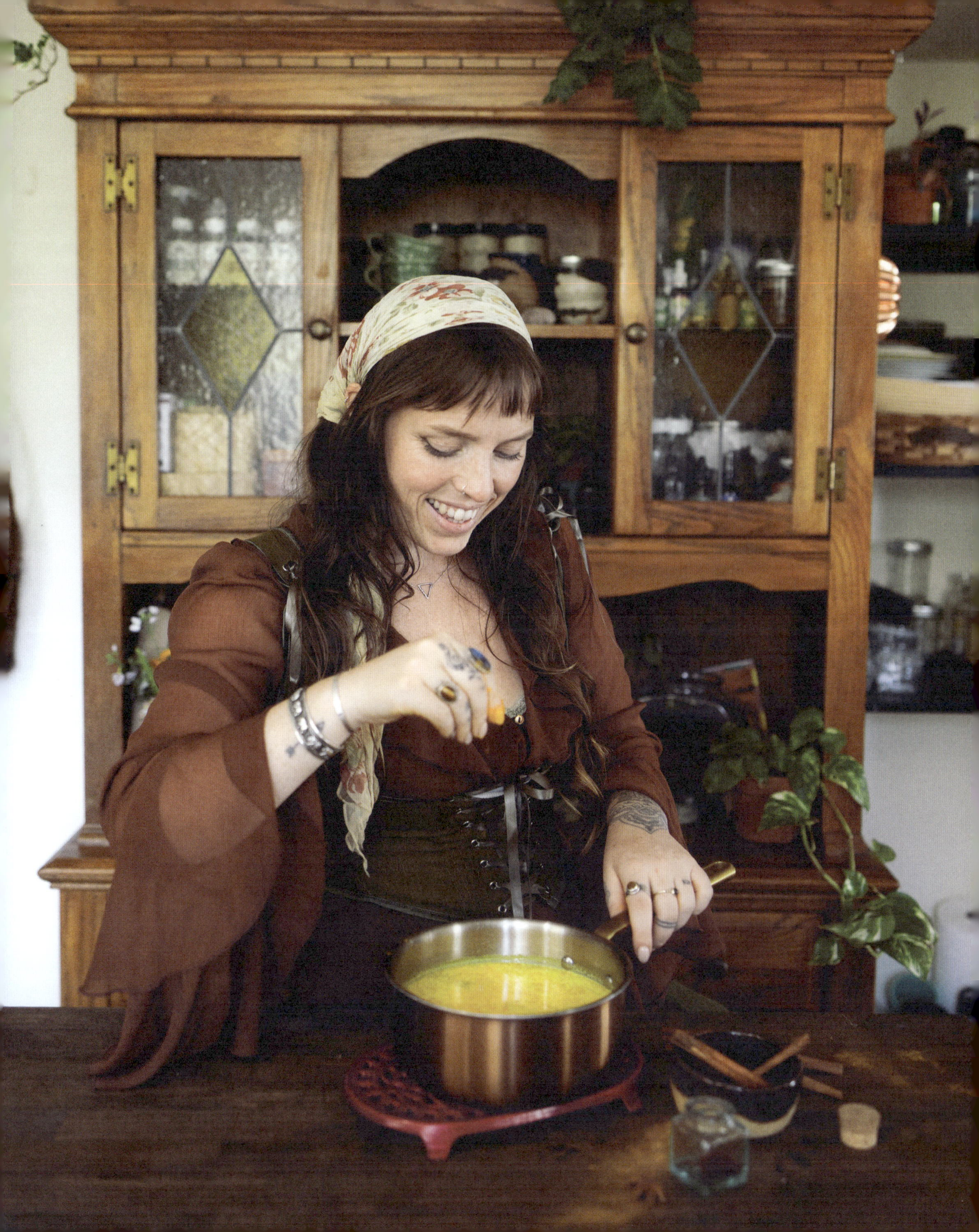

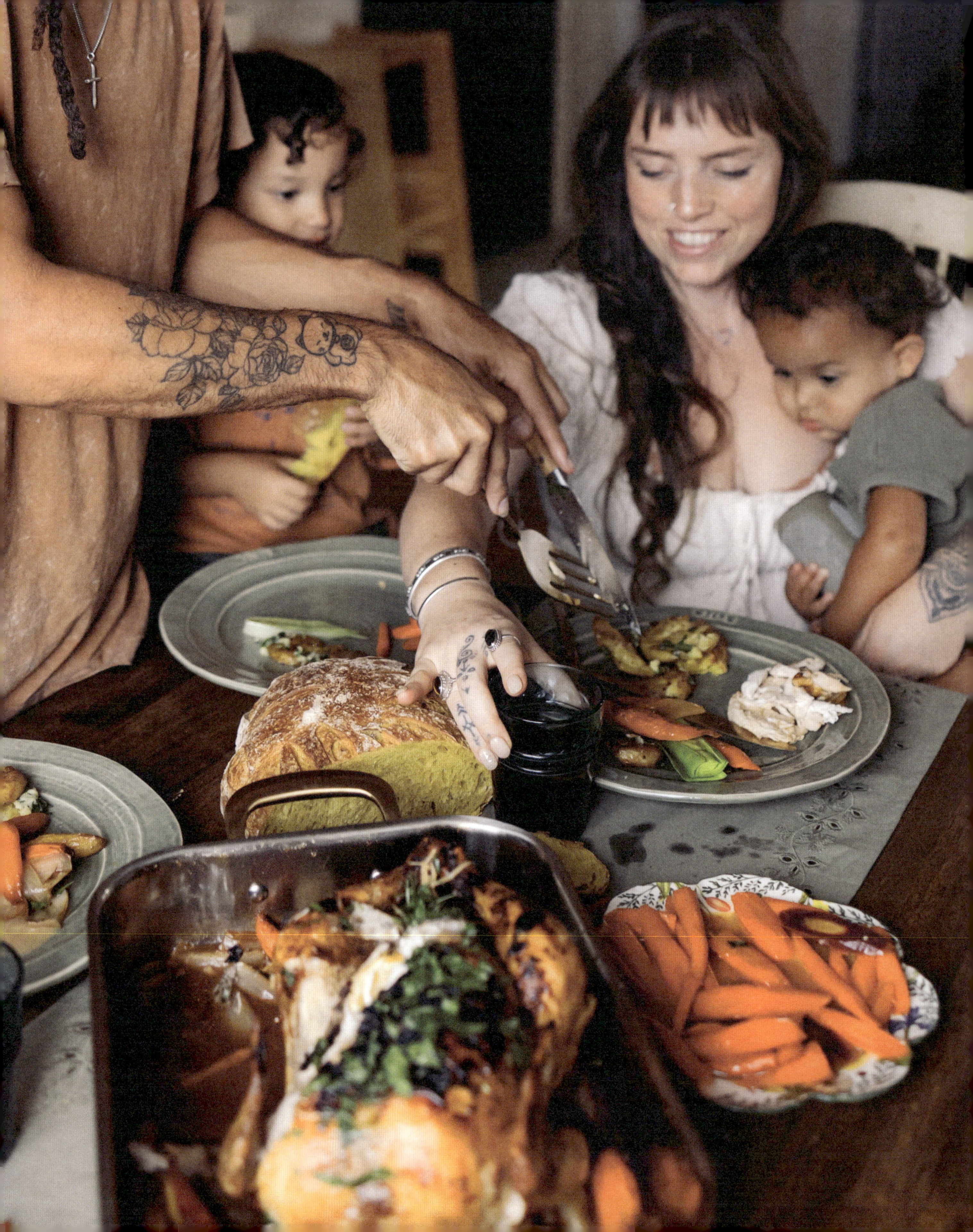

IT'S ALL CONNECTED:

THE IMPORTANCE OF FUNCTIONAL NUTRITION

MY RELATIONSHIP WITH FOOD has always been . . . interesting. I grew up in a healthy, frugal home with parents who loved to cook. Our table was always full of friends, family, laughter, and good conversation.

The food was nutritious and delicious, and everyone was fed even when we didn't have a lot. But I didn't always have a healthy relationship with food. I battled eating disorders for *years*. I wreaked havoc on my metabolic and hormone health by starving and binging, surviving on hummus and gin and pushing my body to its limits while fueling it with poison.

It wasn't until I was pregnant with my first baby that I really locked into healing, undoing the years of bad habits I had created. It took some time, but I saw results. I discovered cycle syncing, and my horrific periods and premenstrual dysphoric disorder (PMDD) shifted. I no longer dreaded my menstrual phase. I stopped vilifying whole food groups and fed myself real food and real calories, and my metabolism began to heal. Above all, I started to love myself, and to honor and listen to my body—and *that* made the biggest difference.

From then on, I began to experience firsthand the power of food, and it inspired me to learn like I hadn't in years. I began sharing my journey online, and it sparked a community of people like me who were hungry for change. The more I researched, the more the puzzle pieces fell into place as I realized: It really is all connected.

The foundation of all of this is functional nutrition, a science-based, holistic approach to nutrition that focuses on how food affects the body on a systemic, cellular, and individual level. Functional nutrition uses food as medicine to treat the causes, not just the symptoms, of a particular ailment or illness. This is all based in nutritional biochemistry, the study of how vitamins, minerals, and other nutrients are processed in the body. It also centers lifestyle medicine, an integrative approach to healing that looks at all areas of life, like how sleep or stress can affect hormone function.

"It is *so* much easier to be motivated to make changes and eat nourishing foods once you understand the magic those foods can create in your body."

Why does all of this matter? Because knowing the "why" is crucial for discovering the "how." It is *so* much easier to be motivated to make changes and eat nourishing foods once you understand the magic those foods can create in your body. Let's talk about some of these root causes, the things that have a domino effect on your physical and mental wellbeing. Increasingly, research points to two root causes of most of our ailments: inflammation and blood sugar imbalances.

INFLAMMATION

Inflammation is the body's natural response to injury, infection, or harmful stimuli. In the short term, it's protective; it helps the body heal. But when inflammation becomes chronic, it can slowly damage tissues, disrupt regular bodily function, and contribute to disease. Chronic inflammation often starts silently and builds over time due to poor diet, stress, lack of sleep, inactivity, and environmental toxins.

While not every outcome of inflammation can be reversed, we can reduce and control our inflammatory response by eating nourishing foods, moving our bodies every day, limiting our stress, reducing use of harsh chemicals, and getting adequate sleep. These habits address the root causes of chronic inflammation and help the body begin to heal.

Chronic Inflammation

Chronic inflammation has been linked to heart disease, type 2 diabetes, obesity, autoimmune diseases (like rheumatoid arthritis, lupus, and Hashimoto's disease), digestive disorders (like Crohn's disease, ulcerative colitis, and irritable bowel syndrome [IBS]), neurodegenerative diseases (like Alzheimer's disease and Parkinson's disease), cancer, depression and other mental health disorders, chronic fatigue and pain, skin conditions (like eczema, psoriasis, and acne), and more.

BLOOD SUGAR IMBALANCES

Blood sugar is the other major root cause of disease. It plays hand in hand with inflammation and doesn't just affect people with diabetes; everyone should pay attention to it. Blood sugar is your body's fuel. Food (especially carbohydrates) turns into sugar (glucose) in your blood, and the hormone insulin helps move it into your cells for energy. When this process works as intended, your energy, mood, hormones, and metabolic function remain steady and healthy. But frequent spikes and drops in blood sugar can cause inconsistent energy, mood swings, and more, which can lead to long-term issues, including hormonal conditions like polycystic ovary syndrome (PCOS), weight gain, heart disease, neurological conditions like dementia, and inflammation (yup, blood sugar can be at the root of inflammation, too!). Blood sugar spikes often come from the food we eat—most often highly processed sugars and carbs, particularly when eaten without sufficient protein and fiber to help them release more slowly into our bloodstream. It's the difference between eating an orange with 12 grams of sugar and a bunch of fiber to help it hit your system slowly and drinking a glass of orange juice with up to 50 grams of sugar and no fiber—a straight shot to your blood stream. High blood sugar can also be caused by inactivity, stress, and anxiety. Chronic stress causes elevated cortisol (the stress hormone produced by your adrenal glands), which triggers your fight-or-flight response, telling your body to release stored sugar into your bloodstream (in case you need energy to outrun a proverbial bear).

"It's. All. Connected.
The body is a finely tuned,
symbiotic community of cells,
hormones, and processes
that all affect each other."

INSULIN RESISTANCE

When we have prolonged high blood sugar, we can develop insulin resistance. This makes the body less sensitive to insulin, meaning it no longer easily recognizes glucose or properly metabolizes it. How does this happen? Frequent blood sugar spikes force the pancreas to pump out more and more insulin to carry that sugar where it needs to go. Eventually, our cells become desensitized to insulin, so our body can't transport the sugar very effectively. When this happens, all hell breaks loose: Sugar begins to build up in the blood, and since it's not reaching our cells to become energy, our bodies feel lacking and crave *more* sugar for quick energy. The more sugar we eat, the more our blood sugar spikes. And with nowhere to put it, the body stores it as fat, often visceral belly fat, which is hard to shift and releases inflammatory chemicals (adipokines and cytokines). This inflammation further damages our insulin receptors. The excess glucose also triggers the body to switch from burning fat to burning glucose as its primary energy source, making it harder to quell weight gain and further increasing that inflammation. We feel fatigued because we aren't getting the energy we need, making movement more challenging, increasing oxidative stress and inflammation, and triggering more sugar cravings. It's a vicious cycle.

HORMONES

The connecting piece to all of this? Hormones. Hormones are the chemical messengers of the body, essentially running all of our basic functions. They work in an interconnected web: If one hormone is pushed out of balance, best believe a bunch of others will be, too. Here's a little glimpse into how these threads all weave together, for better or for worse.

Surprise surprise, inflammation damages the hormone receptors in our bodies, causing cells to struggle to respond to the signals from hormones like estrogen, progesterone, cortisol, and insulin. When our bodies don't recognize insulin well, we struggle to balance blood sugar. Blood sugar swings trigger cortisol release, and chronic cortisol release keeps our bodies in stress mode, triggering adrenaline (our fight-or-flight hormone). This also raises blood sugar, contributing to insulin resistance, so our bodies produce excessive amounts of insulin to compensate. High insulin levels stimulate the ovaries to make more testosterone, which is a key driver of PCOS. Excessive insulin also sends a ton of mixed signals through the endocrine system, throwing sex hormones, stress hormones, appetite-regulating hormones, and thyroid hormones out of balance. This leads to further inflammation, stress, sugar cravings, mood swings, metabolic disruption, weight issues, menstrual issues . . . the list goes on.

"Every meal is a chance to reset.

It's. All. Connected. The body is a finely tuned, symbiotic community of cells, hormones, and processes that all affect each other. This can lead to illness and imbalance. To begin healing, all we need to do is interrupt the cycle of imbalance. Start by identifying one easy change to focus on. Inflammation and blood sugar issues are rooted in stress, and while there are many stressors that we cannot control, there are others that we can easily reduce or eliminate.

The simplest, most controllable stressor is food, which directly affects the state of our body and mind. We can view this as a burden *or* we can view it as a power. Every meal is a chance to reset. Thinking of one meal at a time, for immediate results rather than a lifetime of change, can feel less overwhelming. Over time, this turns into long-term, deep healing. This is how food becomes what it was always meant to be: our ally and a source of simple, life-giving delight.

THE BASIC "HEALTHY" DIET

"HEALTHY" MEANS DIFFERENT THINGS for different people. There are *so many* "healthy" diets that completely contradict one another. Are we supposed to be raw vegan or carnivore? Surely they both can't be right? I'm not going to tear down anyone's choices here, and I don't doubt that there are people who thrive on more extreme diets. But for most of us, there is a simple middle ground. There's a reason that diets like the Mediterranean diet, the Paleo diet, and the anti-inflammatory diet are popular: They all prioritize nutritious whole foods. It may sound boring, but trust me: I spent so long looking for the "secret sauce," the "magic pill" that would heal me, only to find that in general, an unprocessed, whole-food diet was the answer. These are the types of recipes you'll find in this book.

FOODS THAT HEAL

Choose whole, unprocessed foods, and you can't go wrong. But if you look more closely at the specific properties of foods, you can really harness their healing abilities. This is where our alchemy begins.

Macronutrients

Carbohydrates, proteins, and fats are the body's primary fuel and the foundational building blocks of our diet. A balanced diet should use them in proper proportions to stabilize blood sugar, fuel energy, and regulate hormones. The particular ratios may vary for targeted health needs, like weight loss or chronic illness management, but the average starting point is as follows.

- **CARBS** should make up 40 to 50 percent of your daily calories. They are not the enemy! Vegetables, fruits, whole grains, and legumes are all necessary fuel for your brain and body.
- **PROTEIN** should make up 20 to 25 percent of your calories. You probably don't eat enough protein. Lean animal proteins, including good-quality red meat, and plant proteins will keep you full longer, stabilize blood sugar, and support hormone health.
- **FATS** should make up 30 to 35 percent of your daily calories. Fat is also not the enemy; healthy fats do not cause health problems. In fact, they are essential for cellular health, brain function, nutrient absorption, and even weight loss. Minimally processed fats and natural fats (animal fats, olive oil, nuts, avocados, and fatty fish) are all great for you.

Notes

1. When I reference calories here, it's not because we are counting or restricting them; it's simply to give context for ratios. You should only be counting calories or eating in a deficit if you are on a weight-loss journey. Many of us (women particularly) eat too few calories. Restricting intake excessively without a proper balance of macronutrients can harm metabolic and blood sugar health.

2. To simplify things, many nutritional practitioners use color and variety as a litmus test for micronutrient balance; in other words, we should "eat the rainbow!"

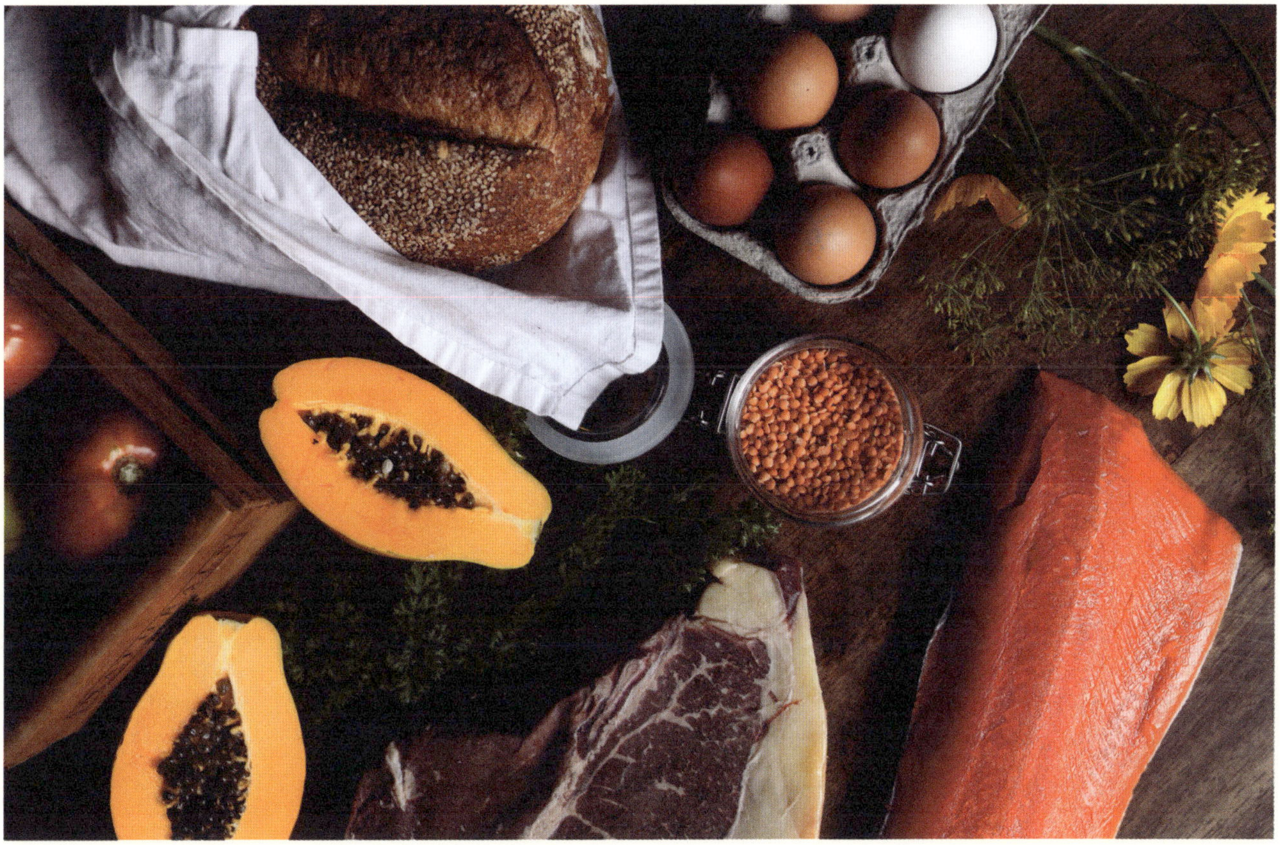

Micronutrients

Vitamins, minerals, and phytonutrients are where things get truly mystical. These are the chemical messengers that keep the body and its systems running. They fine-tune your hormones, metabolism, immune health, cell repair, and mental clarity. While you don't have to overthink them if you are eating a super varied diet, understanding micronutrients can help you leverage them to your advantage from day to day.

- **VITAMINS** fall into two categories: fat-soluble and water-soluble.
  - Fat-soluble vitamins (A, D, E, K) support vision, immunity, bone health, blood clotting, and hormone health.
  - Water-soluble vitamins (B-complex, C) support energy metabolism, the nervous system, stress response, detoxification, collagen production, and red blood cell count.
- **MINERALS** unlock the use of vitamins, enzymes, and tons of cellular functions.
  - Macrominerals (calcium, magnesium, potassium, phosphorus, and sodium) are needed in larger amounts for bodily fluid balance, bones, muscles, and nerves.
  - Trace minerals (copper, iodine, iron, manganese, selenium, and zinc) are needed in smaller amounts but are critical for immune health, thyroid function, oxygen transport, and enzyme function.
- **PHYTONUTRIENTS** (carotenoids, flavonoids, glucosinolates, polyphenols, and more) are plant compounds that support immune health, reduce inflammation, and provide so many additional health benefits.

FUNCTIONAL NUTRITION RAINBOW

YOU CAN CRAFT your plate according to specific needs, or just aim to eat the rainbow to unlock all of these benefits!

Red Foods

support hormone balance, energy, blood flow, and heart health

- **KEY NUTRIENTS:** antioxidants, vitamin C, folate, potassium
- **EXAMPLES:** beets, cherries, red cabbage, red peppers, strawberries, tomatoes

Orange & Yellow Foods

support hormone production and immune, skin, and eye health

- **KEY NUTRIENTS:** vitamin A (beta-carotene), vitamin C, potassium
- **EXAMPLES:** carrots, mangoes, pumpkin, sweet potatoes, yellow peppers

Green Foods

detoxify excess hormones; support PMS relief, liver function and cell health

- **KEY NUTRIENTS:** vitamin C, vitamin K, calcium, folate, magnesium
- **EXAMPLES:** peas, green herbs, bok choy, broccoli, brussels sprouts, kale, spinach

Blue & Purple Foods

support brain function and mood; reduce inflammation and cell damage

- **KEY NUTRIENTS:** vitamin C, manganese, fiber
- **EXAMPLES:** blackberries, blueberries, grapes, eggplant, red cabbage

White & Tan Foods

anti-inflammatory; support hormone elimination, liver function and blood pressure

- **KEY NUTRIENTS:** B vitamins, fiber, magnesium, potassium, selenium
- **EXAMPLES:** cauliflower, garlic, leeks, legumes, mushrooms, onions, parsnips, turnips

Brown Foods

support nervous system, mood, immunity, and hormone health

- **KEY NUTRIENTS:** vitamin E, magnesium, selenium, zinc
- **EXAMPLES:** almonds, brown rice, chickpeas, flaxseeds, pumpkin seeds, sesame seeds, walnuts, pumpkin seeds

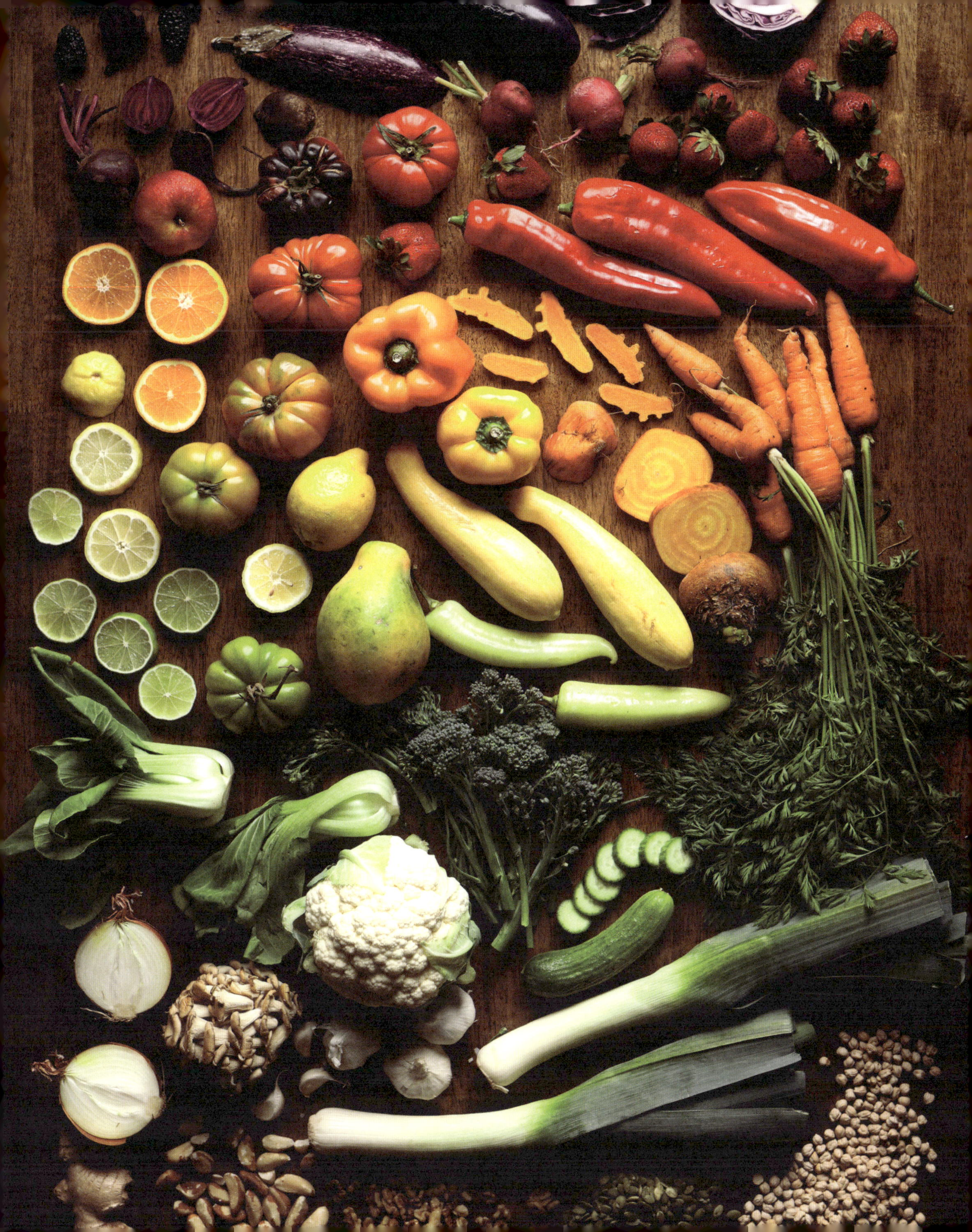

THE ENERGETICS OF FOOD

THERE IS A LOT of technical, scientific information here, but it's also worth leaning into the intuitive side of cooking and eating when selecting foods. Different foods hold different energies, and most of us automatically gravitate toward the ones that will serve us, especially as we increasingly tune into our bodies and notice how food makes us feel. This is particularly noticeable in cycle syncing, where foods align with the "season" of the menstrual cycle, and in seasonal eating, where you will find that it just *feels* right to eat gourds and root veggies in the fall and salads and uncooked veggies in the summer. There is no definitive list here, but I often think along these lines.

- **EARTHY, GROUNDING FOODS:** Deeply healing and nourishing foods, typically dark in color and rich in minerals. They often literally grow in or very close to the earth. Examples include mushrooms, beets, dark berries, dark grains, dark greens, and seaweed.
- **LIGHT, UPLIFTING FOODS:** Cleansing, fresh foods that aid elimination and offer hydration. Often vegetables that are bright in color, rich in vitamins A and C, and can be eaten raw. Examples include leafy greens, fresh herbs, bright berries and vegetables, lean meats, and eggs.
- **WARMING FOODS:** Energizing, expansive, high-fuel foods that boost metabolic function and support immunity. Often strongly flavored, they might make your nose run or aid digestion. Examples include warm spices like cinnamon and clove, hot peppers, roasted foods, and cooked meat.
- **COOLING FOODS:** Soothing, hydrating, slowing, and usually not calorie-dense. Often watery, crispy, lightly flavored, and anti-inflammatory. Examples include cucumber, melon, lettuce, green vegetables, citrus, and seafood.

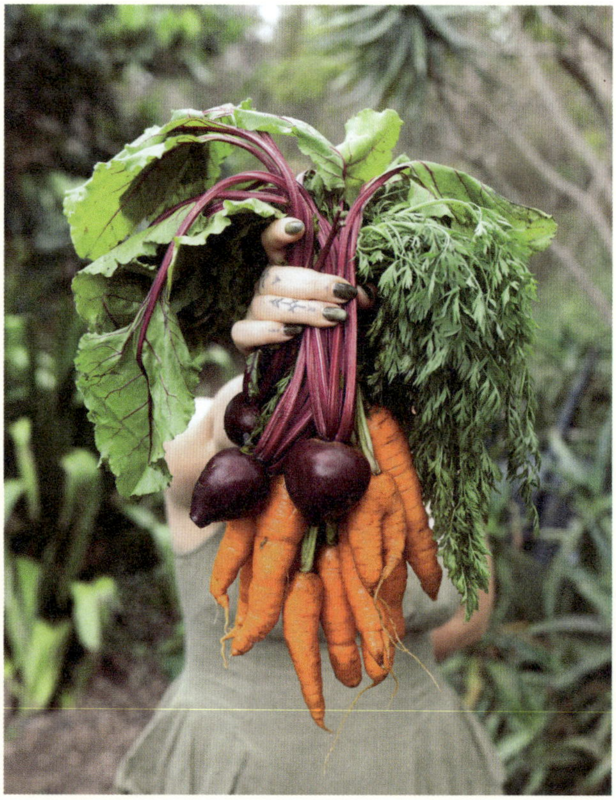

FOODS THAT HARM

MOST FOODS THAT ARE destructive to your health can be classified as inflammatory, but some more negatively affect hormone, gut, and metabolic health. Think of anything that you couldn't make easily at home, that is shelf-stable but probably shouldn't be, or that verges on addictive.

- **PROCESSED SUGAR:** candy, pastries, soda, sweetened foods
- **REFINED CARBOHYDRATES AND GRAINS:** processed white breads, pastas, baked goods
- **INDUSTRIALLY REFINED SEED OILS AND TRANS FATS:** hydrogenated vegetable oils, fried foods, margarine
- **HIGHLY PROCESSED AND PACKAGED FOODS:** ready-made meals, packaged snacks
- **PROCESSED MEATS OR LOW-QUALITY RED MEAT:** hot dogs, deli meats, bacon
- **EXCESSIVE AMOUNTS OF LOW-QUALITY DAIRY:** milk, cheese, dairy-based processed foods
- **EXCESSIVE ALCOHOL:** beer, wine, and liquor consumed in quantities greater than one or two drinks per week
- **ARTIFICIAL ADDITIVES, SWEETENERS, AND FILLERS:** aspartame, sucralose, preservatives, stabilizers

"The most sustainable way to make change is little by little."

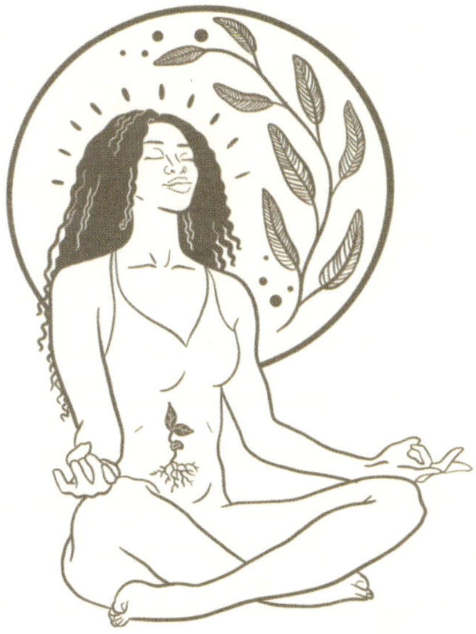

Avoiding these foods seems pretty simple—and it is, in theory! Still, our modern Western diet has been so hijacked that it can be quite challenging to return to real food. So if this feels overwhelming, don't stress. The most sustainable way to make change is little by little. If your diet contains a lot of these harmful foods, don't throw the entire contents of your cupboard into the trash and drop hundreds of dollars at the health food store just yet. Make easy swaps first, slowly add new recipes and practices into your lifestyle, and give yourself time to grow. Slow and steady. You can do this!

SETTING UP YOUR SANCTUM:

KITCHEN ESSENTIALS

IF YOU'RE GOING TO make culinary magic, you need to have a kitchen that is set up for the job. The right tools make all the difference.

POTS AND PANS

When choosing cookware, avoid nonstick pots and pans at all costs. Teflon cookware, or even cheaper "ceramic" versions, contain PFAS (perfluoroalkyl and polyfluoroalkyl substances) and other harmful "forever" chemicals that break down at high heat, enter your food, and accumulate in the body. They are associated with hormone issues as well as developmental, immune, liver, and thyroid complications.

Instead, look for stainless steel or cast-iron pots and pans. They are affordable to buy new but you can often find them thrifted, and since they are built to last and don't get damanged by heat or scratching, they are usually in great condition. There is a learning curve to cooking with them, but once you get it down, it's so easy.

- **STOCKPOT:** If you are going to be making homemade stocks and broths (which I highly recommend, since it is easy, reduces food waste, and is cheaper than buying them from the store), it's worth having a big pot around.

- **DUTCH OVEN:** A Dutch oven is a heavy-duty, usually cast-iron pot with a heavy, oven-safe lid. It's great for soups, stews, braises, and bread.

How to Cook with Cast Iron and Stainless Steel

Cast iron builds up a "seasoning," a nonstick layer, over time. To create and protect this, wash your pan without soap and dry it completely with a kitchen towel. Place it on the stovetop over low heat to fully dry and then add a teaspoon-ish of fat or oil (animal fats like lard or clean bacon grease work best, but avocado or flaxseed oil are great, too) to the pan and use a kitchen towel to rub it around. Do this after each use.

Stainless steel doesn't build up a nonstick layer; instead, you prepare it for each use. Heat the pan over medium heat until hot. (You can check if it is hot enough by flicking a droplet of water into the pan; if it bounces around instead of evaporating, it's hot enough.) Add some high-smoke-point oil (I use avocado); it should immediately spread across the pan like water. Swirl to fully coat and then adjust the temperature as needed, and you will have a nonstick and completely toxin-free pan!

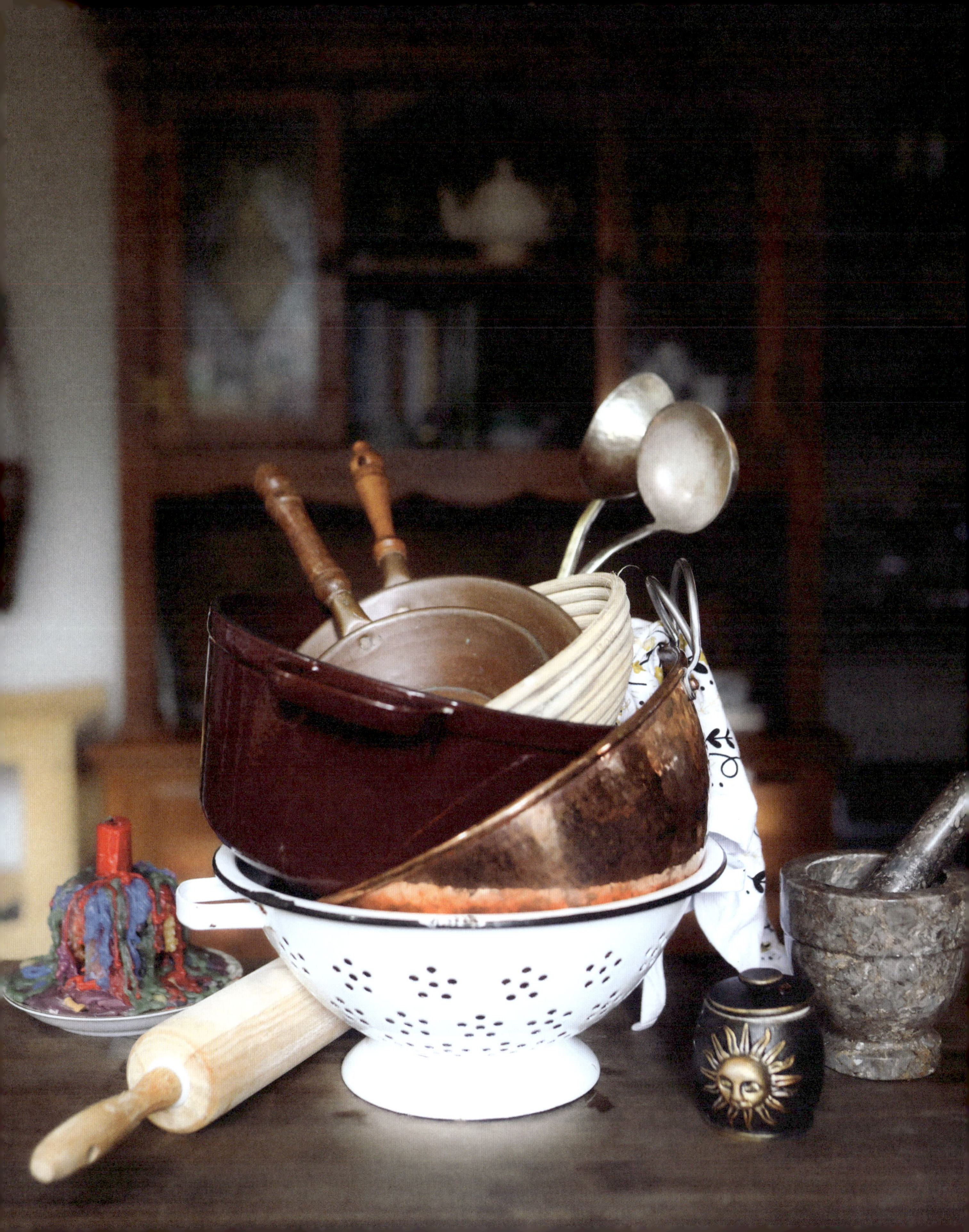

TOOLS

- **KNIVES:** Good knives can make or break your kitchen experience—dull knives make for a horrible time. Not only is it safer to use a properly honed, sharp knife, but it's also faster and more efficient. You don't have to spend a fortune, and you can also get these secondhand. Avoid "ever-sharp" knives that have a micro-serrated edge; instead, get a stainless steel knife set and a sharpener and learn how to use it!

- **MICROPLANE:** A microplane is a special grater that grates things basically into a pulp. It's fast, efficient, easy to clean, and the best $10 I waited way too long to spend. If you use a lot of aromatics in the kitchen (garlic, ginger, turmeric)—which, baby, I do and you are about to, too—this is *by far* the easiest way to prepare them. When I reference "crushed garlic" in recipes, I am always using my microplane to "crush" it.

- **PEELER:** Get a good peeler. It's another $10 investment that will save you incredible amounts of prep time.

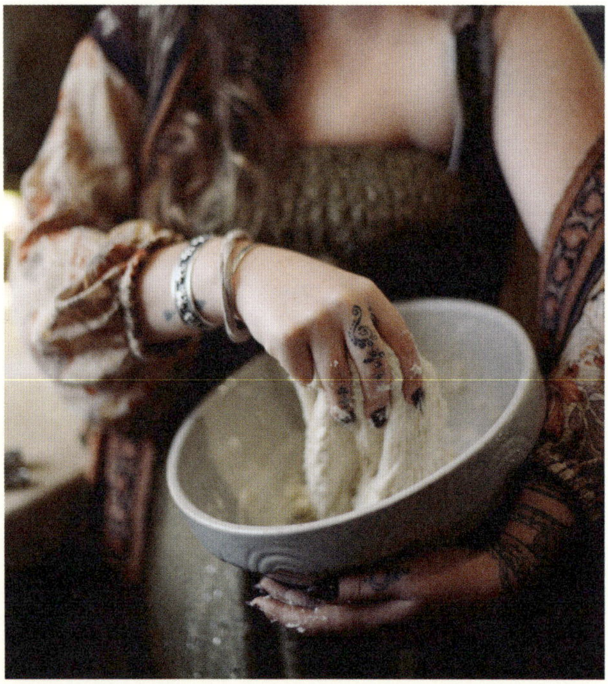

BREAD MAKING

You may want to wait until you know you're into sourdough baking before purchasing these, but they are really helpful in the process.

- **BANNETONS:** These little wooden baskets are made specifically for resting bread in before baking. They're lightweight and pretty cheap.

- **RAZOR:** You will need one of these for scoring bread dough so it doesn't explode into weird shapes when baking (trust me, a knife won't cut it; *pun intended*). You can just get a pack of straight razor blades, but it's nice to have a holder for your razor. It's easier to use and keep track of.

- **SCALE:** A kitchen scale is helpful for measuring ingredients when making sourdough and other baked goods. It's also essential for ferments.

APPLIANCES

I don't have an appliance-heavy kitchen, but these are my favorite kitchen appliances, in order of non-negotiable to nice-to-have.

- **IMMERSION BLENDER:** Immersion blenders are small, portable, and powerful, and you can use them to make homemade sauces—like mayo—right in the jar. They're incredible for pureeing soups, sauces, and baby food, and can be used for frothing and whisking.

- **UPRIGHT BLENDER:** An upright blender is great for making smoothies, of course, but a good quality one can even grind grain or make ice cream. It can do many of the mixing and chopping things that a food processor can do, so if you can only get one of the two, I would invest in a blender. I thrifted my KitchenAid blender for $5, and it's still going strong after five years.

- **INSTANT POT:** I know this sounds like a splurge, but my Instant Pot has paid for itself a hundred times over. It's a pressure cooker and slow cooker all in one. I have used it to defrost and cook a chicken and then make stock all within an afternoon, and that is so valuable to me, because time is of the essence!

- **HAND MIXER:** If you don't plan on baking, scoot this lower down the list. But before you drop cash on a pretty red stand mixer, know that a basic handheld will get you really far. Even budget-friendly options will be a big improvement from a hand whisk.

- **RICE COOKER:** A plug-in rice cooker saves stovetop space when making big meals and cooks rice perfectly with zero effort. You can also use it to cook quinoa and other grains. We got our first one from the thrift store, again, for $5 and replaced it eventually with a new one that cost a whopping $20. So simple and so effective.

- **FOOD PROCESSOR:** A food processor is helpful for food prepping and baking. I use it to grate large quantities of veggies for fermenting or slice cabbage for sauerkraut or coleslaw. It's also great for baking, particularly because lots of processed-sugar–free recipes use dates, which need to be chopped and blended into things (it's nearly impossible to make a bliss ball without a food processor).

- **WATER FILTER:** Clean water is an often-overlooked aspect of a holistic kitchen, largely because, in the developed world, we assume that our water is clean enough. While most tap water in the US meets official safety standards, much of it can still contain PFAS, lead from old pipes, chemical byproducts, pesticides, and even pharmaceuticals. It's also often cleaned with chlorine, which itself can be harmful to health with long-term exposure.

Getting a good water filter is the ideal solution; it's a one-time purchase, and it filters out organic and chemical contaminants. The best types of filters are reverse osmosis, UV, or activated carbon composite gravity filters.

FERMENTING

- **MASON JARS:** Even if you aren't canning, mason jars deserve a spot in every kitchen. We use them for everything from drinking water to storing leftovers or holding flowers. They're a great way to reduce plastic use, and they last forever. If you are canning or fermenting, you will definitely need them.

- **FERMENTING WEIGHTS:** These aren't absolutely necessary, but they're useful for fermentation and worth having around. They help prevent mold during the fermentation process by keeping your produce submerged.

- **FUNNEL:** Having one decent wide-mouth funnel and another narrower one will help you get all your goodies into your jars, whether for fermentation or storage. Extra points if you can find stainless steel ones!

- **FERMENTING LIDS:** You can definitely get by without these, but they make fermenting much more hands off! These special lid attachments release gasses while keeping jars sealed.

EXTRA MAGIC

- **MORTAR AND PESTLE:** Essential for grinding the freshest herbs and spices. Look for solid granite or stone with a rough surface.

- **CANDLES:** Lighting a candle makes anything a ceremony. I keep colored beeswax taper candles just for my kitchen. When I light them, I'm reminded to center myself and slow down.

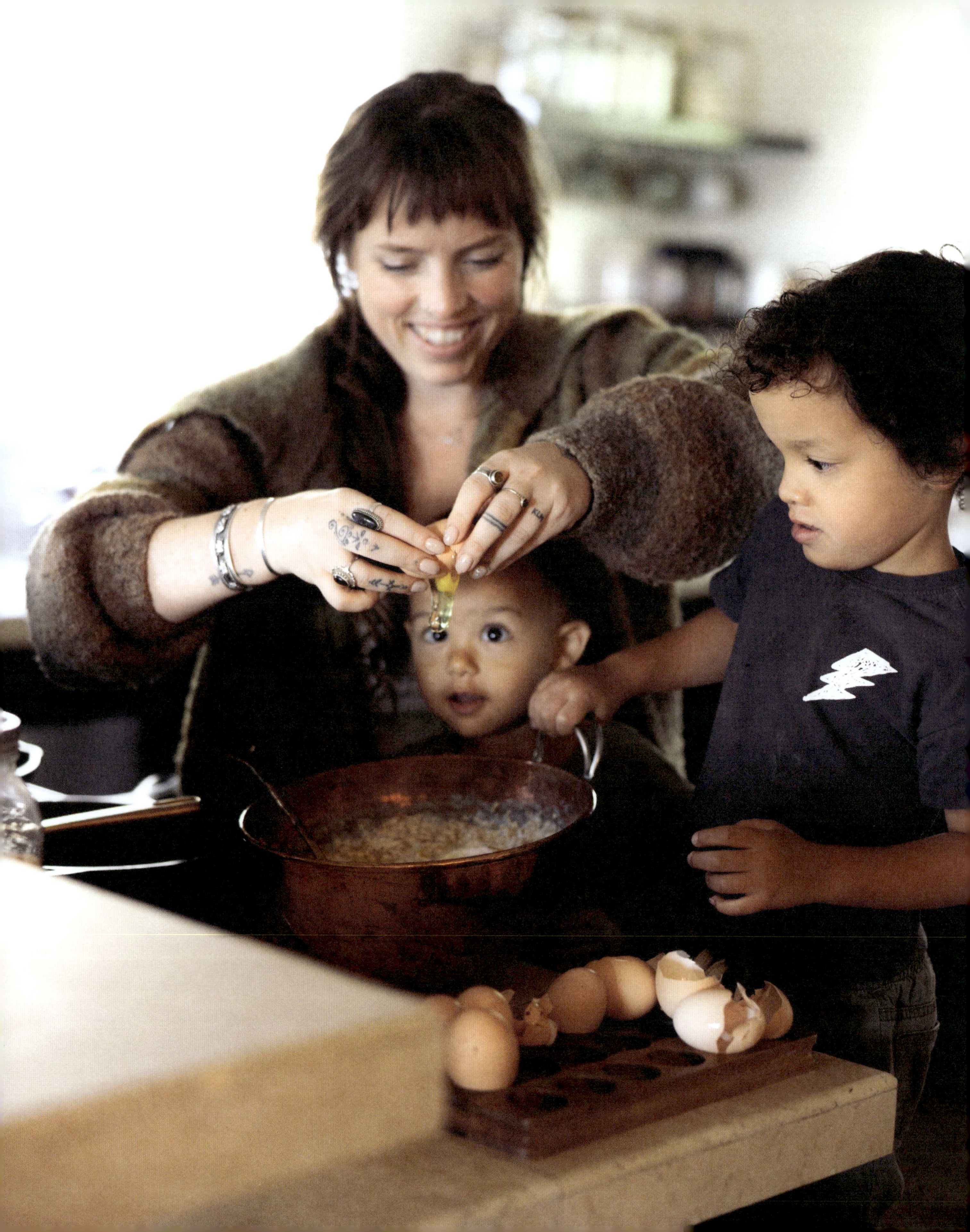

GATHERING YOUR STORES:

PANTRY ESSENTIALS

STOCKING YOUR KITCHEN like a little fairy readying for winter makes cooking from scratch *so* much easier. Instead of planning and shopping for each meal, buy basic ingredients in bulk, store as much as you can, and shop your kitchen. Then you can intentionally shop for fresh and special ingredients based on what's in season, what's on sale, or even what phase of your menstrual cycle you're in. There are many days when our fridge (or bank account) is running on empty, and I can pull together a stellar meal from only our pantry shelves and freezer stores. So here's my big list: These are all the things that I try to keep stocked, along with a few extras.

CARBS

- **OATS** (organic): Quick oats and rolled oats are both staples in our home. Look for organic, glyphosate-free oats specifically.
- **PASTA:** If you handle gluten well, look for quality pasta brands without fillers. If you don't handle gluten well, some brands with great gluten-free options are Barilla, Banza, and Ancient Harvest.
- **POPCORN KERNELS:** Cheaper and cleaner than traditional popcorn! It's so easy to make in a big, lidded pot.
- **QUINOA:** Quinoa is one of the rare complete plant proteins that is fiber- and micronutrient-dense. It's nutritionally superior to rice, but it does take a little more finesse to get a good flavor!
- **RICE AND RICE NOODLES** (white and brown): There's actually not a major health difference between brown and white rice. If you are struggling with digestion, go for white. If you are struggling with blood sugar control, go for brown. If you're struggling with both, try quinoa instead. Precooked wild rice packs are great to keep on hand for last-minute dinners.
- **SOBA NOODLES** (buckwheat): Another complete plant protein (although it has less protein per serving than quinoa), buckwheat is naturally gluten free!
- **TORTILLAS OR TORTILLA CHIPS:** If you can make your own—awesome. Otherwise, I love the Siete brand; they are made with high-quality, simple ingredients. I usually keep their almond flour tortillas in stock, and I love their chips: They have grain-free options as well as traditional corn chips made with avocado oil.

DRY-GOOD PROTEINS

- **BEANS:** Adzuki beans are known for their blood sugar benefits. Black beans are high in minerals. Chickpeas are essential for hummus and salads and are rich in folate and fiber.

- **NUTS:** Nuts are full of omega-3s, healthy fats, vitamins, and minerals. I usually keep almonds and walnuts on hand and buy other types of nuts on sale or in small amounts as I want or need them. Brazil nuts are great for hormone health!

- **SEEDS:** I love to sprinkle seeds on anything to add an extra layer of targeted nutrition. Hemp and chia seeds are great for protein and omega-3s, and if you're seed cycling for hormone health, you'll need sunflower, flax, pumpkin, and sesame seeds (more on this on page 230).

BAKING GOODS

- **BAKING POWDER AND BAKING SODA:** These are essential leavening agents for most baked goods.

- **CHOCOLATE CHIPS:** A little chocolate never hurt anyone, no matter the brand. Some great healthier brands are Enjoy Life and Taza. There are also sugar-free options like Pascha or stevia-sweetened chocolate like Lily's.

- **COCOA OR CACAO POWDER:** Cacao is minimally processed and not roasted, so it retains many more minerals and antioxidants. Cocoa is roasted at high heat, losing much of its nutritional value but creating a smoother flavor. Either one is a necessity in my book, because we need a good chocolate treat here and there.

- **CORNSTARCH:** This is a useful thickener for sauces and baked goods.

- **SUGAR:** Yep, I do stock sugar! I don't use it often (I prefer honey or maple syrup), and when I do, it's most often brown, but I also keep granulated on hand for specific baking projects.

- **VANILLA EXTRACT:** So much flavor! Look for pure extract (Simply Organic is great) or make your own with vanilla pods and alcohol.

- **WARM SPICES:** Cinnamon, nutmeg, and pumpkin spice are great for baked goods—and, if you're like me, coffee.

- **WHITE AND WHEAT FLOUR:** Buy organic and unbleached flour, especially for sourdough (to ensure the dough ferments properly).

DRIED FRUITS

- **DATES:** Dates are super sweet but don't negatively affect blood sugar—a secret weapon! They're great as a healthy treat and for baking.

- **MANGOES AND OTHER DRIED FRUIT:** Check the ingredients for added sugar. The only ingredient should be dried fruit.

- **RAISINS:** Raisins are the cheapest dried fruit you can buy. They make great snacks and are easy toppings for granola and oatmeal.

- **SHREDDED COCONUT:** A standard for granola, oatmeal, muffins, and other baked goods. Look for coconut with no fillers or added sugar. The only ingredient should be coconut.

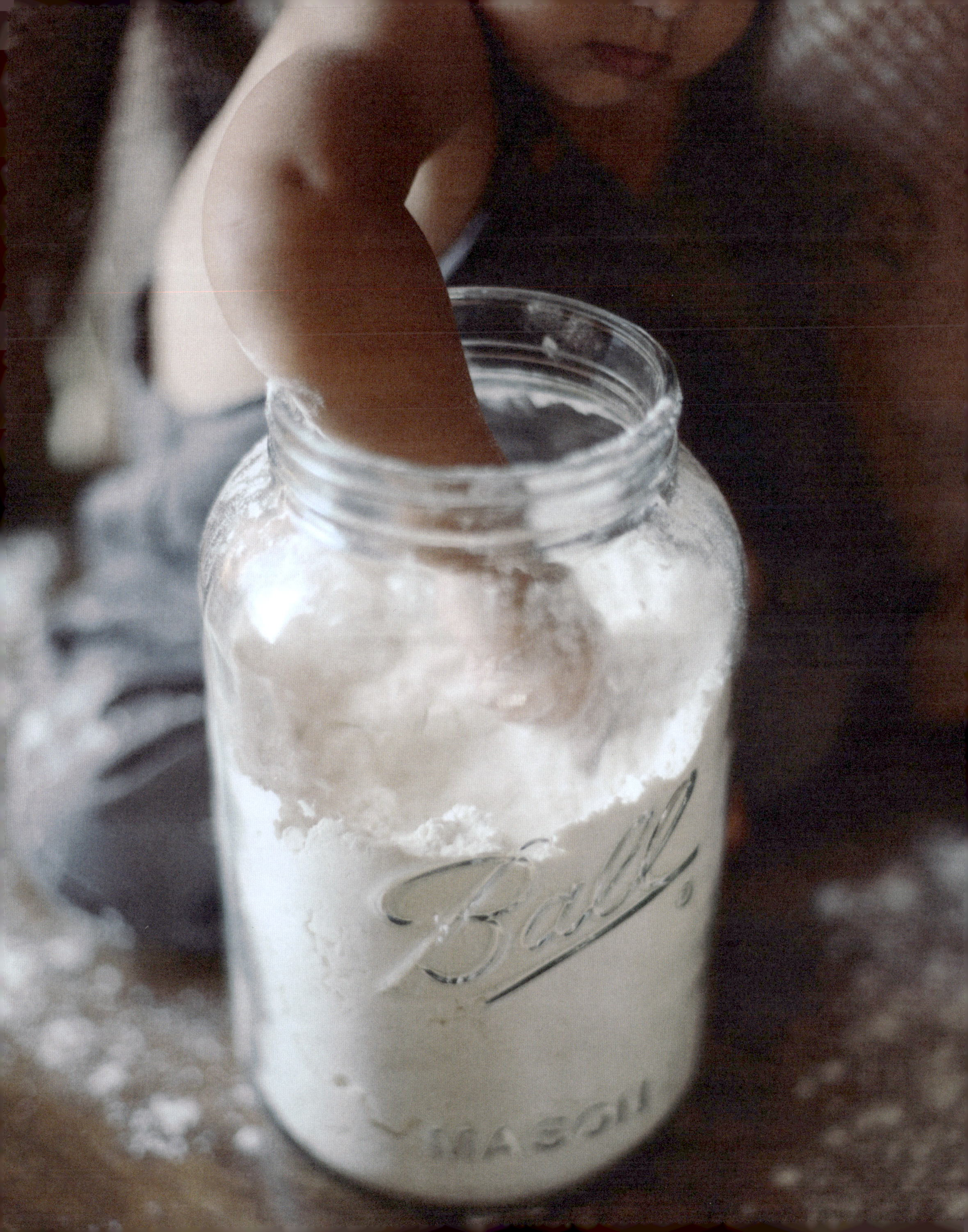
Ball
MASON

CANNED GOODS

- **BEANS:** Buy canned whole or refried beans for when you don't have time to soak dried beans.
- **COCONUT MILK:** I use this mostly for curries, smoothies, and breakfast things. Look for full-fat coconut milk with no added sugar or fillers.
- **FISH:** I like tuna and sardines, but you can buy any kind of fish you like. Look for wild-caught fish (Fishwife, Wild Planet, and Safe Catch are great brands). Tuna can contain higher levels of heavy metals than other fish; albacore and white tuna have the highest levels, while skipjack typically contains the lowest. Neither should be a problem as long as they aren't consumed more than a few times a week.
- **SALSA:** Keep salsa on deck for snacks. It's also a good flavor addition to chili, soups, and Mexican-inspired meals.
- **TOMATO PRODUCTS:** I buy canned crushed and diced tomatoes, tomato paste, and basic premade marinara sauce.

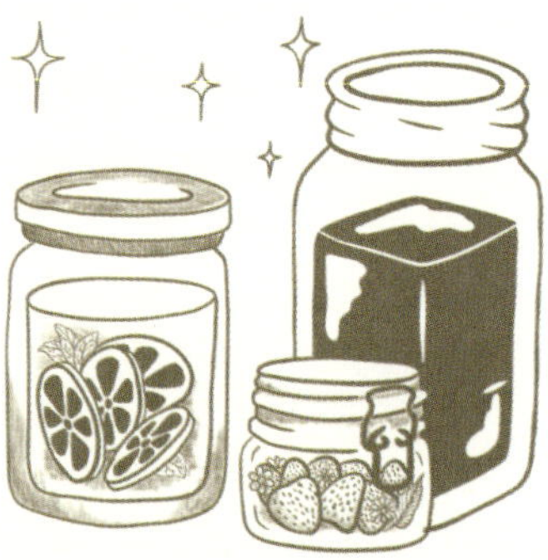

OILS

Oils deserve extra attention, as different oils can have major health benefits or negative effects.

Always avoid hydrogenated or partially hydrogenated oils. These are liquid vegetable oils that have been altered to be firm and spreadable. They pose a known cardiovascular risk. Margarine, shortening, nondairy creamers, packaged baked goods, frostings, and processed snack foods almost always contain them.

Cooking oils are a little more complicated. Americans have long been advised to use lots of processed polyunsaturated vegetable oils like canola and sunflower, all the while experiencing declining health and increased heart disease, cancer, and diabetes. Worldwide, many of the healthiest communities use unprocessed or very minimally processed saturated fats, like lard, butter, tallow, ghee, and coconut oil. Saturated fats are far more stable than polyunsaturated fats, meaning heat and chemical interactions don't cause them to produce toxic byproducts.

On the other hand, processed vegetable fats oxidize at high heat, increasing the risk for free radicals (cancer-causing compounds) in your body. And while the oils themselves contain compounds that are good for you, they pose a much bigger health risk after they are processed and cooked. There are a few exceptions: Avocado oil is generally considered very stable for high-heat cooking due to its very low polyunsaturated fat content and high smoke point. Some cold-pressed seed oils, like pumpkin, sesame, and hempseed, have different fatty acid profiles and more health benefits than standard seed oils but still should not be heated to high temperatures.

Cooking technique matters a lot here. Olive oil is so great for you but ideally should not be heated to super high temperatures. Some seed oils have health benefits, but the refining process poses a problem. Cold-pressed, virgin seed oils are best used cold or added after high heat. For deep frying, the absolute best oils you can use are saturated fats: tallow, lard, ghee, and refined (but not hydrogenated) coconut oil.

Avoid at All Costs

- Hydrogenated oil
- Margarine
- Partially hydrogenated oil
- Shortening

Best Avoided

- Canola (rapeseed) oil
- Corn oil
- Cottonseed oil
- Grapeseed oil
- Rice bran oil
- Safflower oil
- Soybean oil
- Sunflower oil

Mid-Range Oils

High-heat oils (400 to 475°F/205 to 245°C)
Work for high-heat cooking where large amounts are needed, like deep frying. Not incredibly toxic, but still best largely avoided.

- High-oleic canola, safflower, and sunflower oils
- Peanut oil

Top-Tier Oils

Low-heat oils (under 325°F/160°C)
Best for salad dressings, drizzling, and dips. Avoid sautéing, frying, and roasting with them.

- Flaxseed oil
- Pumpkin seed oil
- Walnut oil

Medium-heat oils (325 to 375°F/160 to 190°C)
Best for sautéing, light stir-frying, and roasting veggies at or below 325°F/160°C. Use medium-low stovetop settings.

- Butter (~300 to 350°F/150 to 175°C)
- Extra virgin olive oil (~325 to 375°F/160 to 190°C, varies by quality)
- Unrefined sesame oil (~350°F/175°C)

Medium-high-heat oils (375 to 425°F/190 to 220°C)
Best for pan-frying, stir-frying, baking, and oven-roasting up to 425°F/220°C. Use medium to medium-high stovetop settings.

- Unrefined, cold-pressed coconut oil (~375°F/190°C)
- Unrefined avocado oil (~375 to 400°F/190 to 205°C)
- Refined sesame oil (~410°F/210°C)
- Duck fat and lard (~410°F/210°C)

High-heat oils (425 to 450°F/220 to 230°C)
Best for deep-fat frying, high-heat searing, wok cooking, and oven-roasting at 425°F+ (220°C+). Use high stovetop burner settings.

- Ghee (clarified butter) (~450°F/230°C)
- Refined/light olive oil (~465°F/240°C)
- Refined coconut oil (~450°F/230°C)
- Refined avocado oil (~480 to 520°F/250 to 270°C, very high)

The Oils I Keep on Hand and Use the Most

✴ **AVOCADO OIL:** For low- to high-heat cooking. Choose a naturally refined and high-quality brand, like Chosen Foods or Nutiva. This is the oil I use most for daily cooking.

✴ **COCONUT OIL** (unrefined, cold-pressed): For low- to mid-heat cooking or using fresh. Great for baking, pancakes, curries, and personal care.

✴ **GHEE** (clarified butter): For high-heat cooking. Ghee is super anti-inflammatory and nutrient-rich, used for thousands of years in ayurvedic cooking. It can be pricey but it's worth it; it's great for curries and roasting veggies.

✴ **HEMP OIL:** For dressings and cold preparations. Hemp oil is a fancy extra that I use more as a supplement to increase omega-3 intake, particularly for kids.

- **OLIVE OIL:** For eating in cold preparations or cooking over low heat. Choose extra virgin olive oil and buy the best quality you can afford. Use for salads and dressings, for low-heat, slow-simmer sauces like marinara, or for health tonics.

- **TALLOW** (rendered beef fat): For high-heat cooking. Similar to ghee, tallow is full of incredible fat-soluble nutrients and healthy fats. Great for roasting veggies and frying.

VINEGARS & FLAVOR BOMBS

- **APPLE CIDER VINEGAR** (with the mother): "The mother" is the murky substance present in fermented apple cider vinegar. It's a mixture of yeast and good bacteria that signals the vinegar is full of gut-healthy probiotics. This vinegar is ideal for use in dressings and sauces or as a tonic for digestion, blood sugar control, and immune health. It's also great for personal care.

- **BALSAMIC VINEGAR:** For dressings, sauces, and salads. I will eat any fresh veggie with a good glug of balsamic.

- **GOCHUJANG:** Korean fermented chile paste, an incredible flavor bomb any time you want a little spice and umami flavor.

- **RICE VINEGAR:** So essential for East and Southeast Asian dishes.

- **SOY SAUCE OR LIQUID AMINOS:** Liquid aminos are a milder, gluten-free alternative to soy sauce, used for sauces and adding rich flavor to savory dishes.

- **WORCESTERSHIRE SAUCE:** A vinegar base with a blend of potent flavors that brings depth to gravies and stews. I love it on grilled cheese.

OTHER PANTRY ITEMS

- **MAPLE SYRUP:** I buy this in bulk from Costco and keep it around for coffee and baking. It's a more mineral- and vitamin-rich choice than refined sugar.

- **PEANUT BUTTER:** Always, on everything. I use this for snacks, baking, breakfasts, and more. Go for an organic peanut butter with one simple ingredient: peanuts. It will come with a layer of oil on top that should be stirred in before using, to prevent the very bottom of the jar from becoming hard and dry.

- **RAW HONEY:** I use this mostly in fresh preparations, as it contains so many antioxidants, minerals, and vitamins that can be damaged by the cooking process.

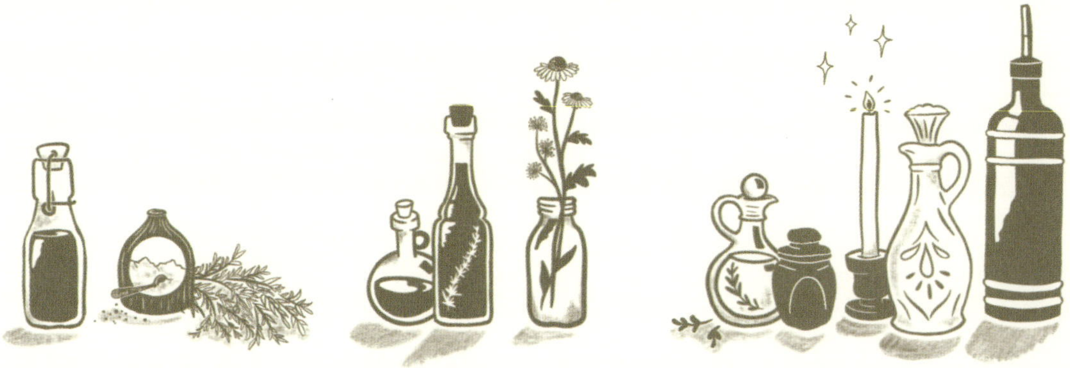

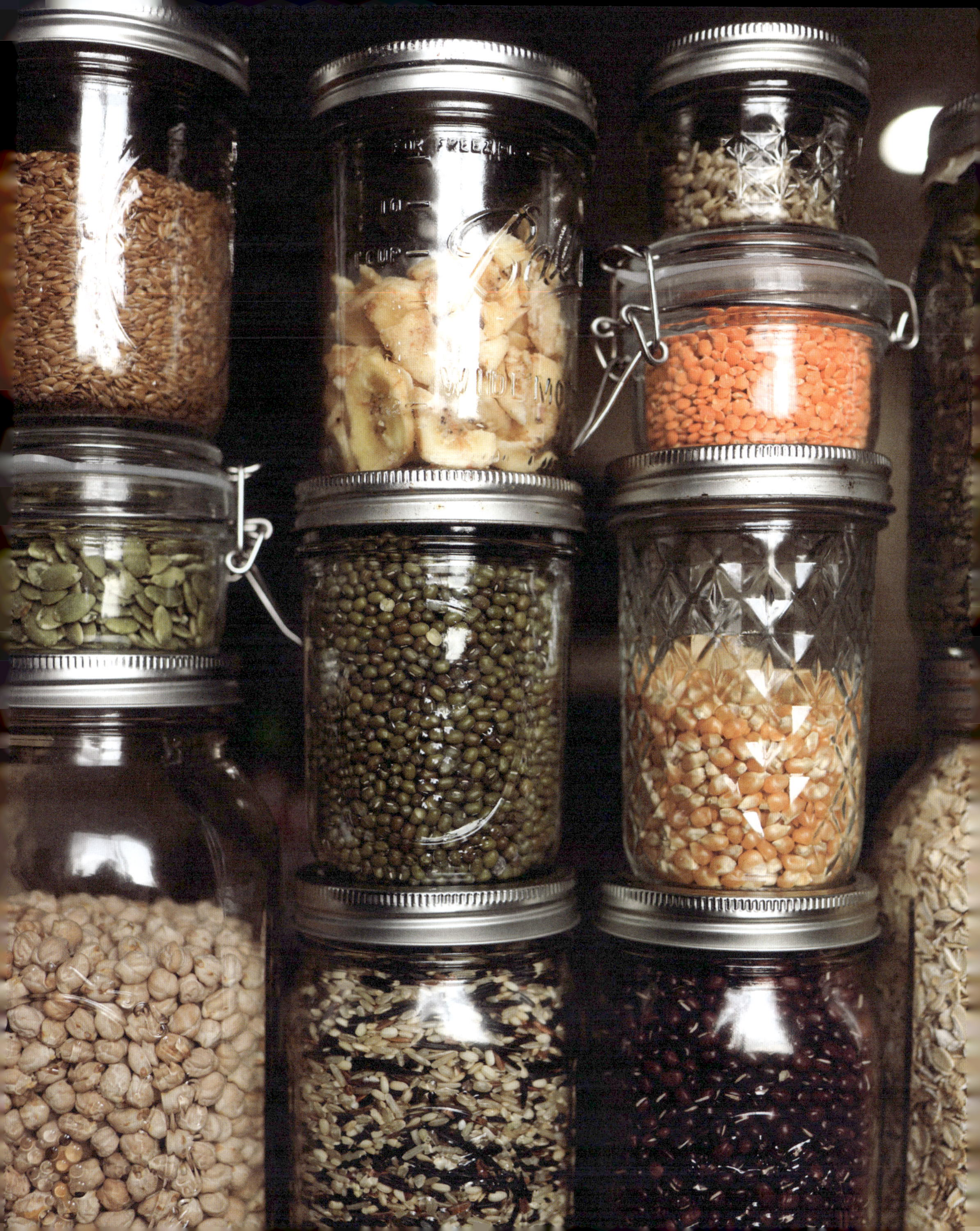

DAIRY

Dairy gets mixed press: Some claim it's inflammatory and hard to digest, while others claim it contains essential fat-soluble nutrients. Where I land is that you should do your best to get good-quality dairy and don't overuse it. Spend a little more to get grass-fed dairy products wherever possible, and use them sparingly.

- **FULL-FAT GREEK YOGURT:** A great source of protein and healthy fats, and full of probiotics.

- **GRASS-FED BUTTER:** Contains vitamin A, vitamin K2, and healthy cholesterol. I use grass-fed butter pretty liberally, as it doesn't carry the same digestion difficulties as other dairy. Good butter is truly a healthy fat, supplying vitamins that can be somewhat hard to find and are essential for brain, eye, immune, and reproductive health. Note: grass-fed butter is especially great for toddlers and little kids, who need to eat way more fat than adults. They need fat-soluble vitamins (A, D, E, and K) for proper growth and development. Cholesterol is super important for their brain and nerve function and is a building block for cell membranes, which is extra necessary during rapid growth.

- **GRASS-FED MATURE CHEDDAR:** I'm a big fan of cheese. But higher quality cheeses can be pricey. I have learned that I can use it sparingly and still have it almost every day. Mature cheddar has a stronger flavor than other cheeses, so you can use less of it per serving.

- **WHOLE MILK:** I always advocate for whole, full-fat dairy. It's a healthy fat that contains important nutrients like vitamins A, D, E, and K, omega-3s, and so much more—particularly if you buy grass-fed milk. It also keeps you satiated. However, milk is completely unfermented, straight-up dairy. Not everyone can handle a whole glass of it, although some might find A2 whole milk easier to digest.

EGGS

Eggs are of the most nutrient-dense foods; they are super quick and easy to cook. They contain the fat-soluble vitamins A, D, E, and K2, as well as tons of micronutrients and protein. *Don't* skip the yolk; it contains choline, which is essential for brain health and development! They can also help raise your good cholesterol levels.

> ### Note
> Research suggests pregnant women should eat two to four eggs per day to help meet their nutritional needs. All those nutrients in the yolk promote fetal brain development!

ROOTS & VEGGIES

- **CABBAGE:** Cabbage lasts forever and is *so* cheap. If you want to make Sauerkraut (page 70), stock up!

- **CARROTS:** Carrots are *magic.* They're versatile, they last forever, and they're super cheap. They contain both soluble fiber (which dissolves in the body to help digestion) and insoluble fiber (which doesn't dissolve in the body and feeds beneficial bacteria), which makes them amazing for hormones and gut health.

- **CELERY:** An important base for soups, stocks, and stews, celery contributes lots of flavor and tons of fiber.

- **FRESH LEAFY GREENS:** Kale, spinach, and Swiss chard are in our weekly rotation. If you can grow your own, even better!

- **FROZEN BROCCOLI:** Frozen veggies have as much as or more nutritional value than fresh! I keep them on hand for last-minute dinners.

- **FROZEN GREENS:** Whenever I'm not able to use my fresh greens in time, I chop them up and throw them into the freezer, then pull them out to add to smoothies, soups, and sautés.

- **FROZEN MIXED VEGGIES, PEAS, OR GREEN BEANS:** Classic. Easy peasy. These are all high-fiber veggies, and storing them frozen makes it so easy to throw them into dishes!

- **GARLIC:** One of the most medicinal ingredients in the kitchen cupboard for everything from colds and flus to heart health. I put it in almost everything.

- **GINGER:** Fresh ginger is far superior to powdered, and it's a medicinal powerhouse. Ginger is really helpful for digestion and worth having on hand for curries and warming recipes as well as treating colds and nausea.

- **ONIONS:** I keep both yellow and red stocked; almost all of my meals start with them.

- **POTATOES:** Potatoes are a great source of nutrient-dense carbohydrates, and they're lower in calories and higher in fiber than rice and many other refined grains. Red potatoes are the most nutrient-dense, but they're all great.

- **SWEET POTATOES:** Sweet potatoes are a good choice for those with inflammatory conditions who are bothered by nightshades (which includes potatoes), as they don't belong to the nightshade family. They are high in fiber, vitamin A, and beta-carotene.

FRUIT

There are so many fun fruits, but they can be expensive. Stick to the basics or buy whatever's local and in season, and get the others on sale or when you can.

- **APPLES:** An apple a day might actually keep the doctor away. They're cheap, they last forever, and they're great for gut health, especially when cooked!

- **BANANAS:** Eat them as is, or freeze them for smoothies if they start to turn.

- **FROZEN BERRIES:** Buy blueberries and/or mixed berries for smoothies, desserts, oatmeal, and snacks.

- **ORANGES:** Keep that scurvy at bay, especially if you're an adrenal cocktail baddie (see page 244).

MEAT

When buying meat, I shop the sales as much as possible. I love to get steaks, lamb, turkey, salmon—all that good stuff—but here's what I always have (often bought in bulk and placed in the freezer for later use).

- **CHICKEN:** Buy whole chickens (you'll need those bones for broth; see page 156!), chicken thighs (the cheapest option), and chicken tenders (these thaw *so* quickly if, like me, you tend to forget to take things out of the freezer).

- **CHICKEN SAUSAGE:** We keep this around for a quick-fix lunch or dinner.

- **GROUND BEEF:** Buy the best-quality beef you can afford, and look for grass-fed and finished beef if possible.

HERBS & SPICES

Never underestimate the power of herbs and spices in the kitchen. Herbs are the fresh, leafy parts of plants, and spices are seeds, roots, bark, and dried fruits. These are what elevate your cooking from just edible food to an experience, offering complex flavor and deeply medicinal properties. Almost any time I cook, I pause to consider if there's an herb or spice I don't usually use that could complement the dish. You can intentionally customize the herbs you use according to how you're feeling or what your body needs, or you can throw them in just because they match the flavor profile of your dish. Either way, using herbs and spices gives you some extra healing juju! Here is a list of common herbs and spices along with their medicinal properties.

- **SEA SALT:** Not technically an herb or spice, but an integral flavor component that provides valuable nutrients. Sea salt contains essential minerals and electrolytes like potassium and magnesium. I love celtic salt like Eden or Redmond, but pink Himalayan salt is also great.

Herbs

- **BASIL:** Provides digestive support for nausea, cramps, and colic. Traditionally used for stress relief and rest. Also antiparasitic and supportive of breastmilk production.
- **CILANTRO:** Stimulates digestion and supports metabolism, aiding in the elimination of metabolic waste (detoxifying) and easing digestive spasms.
- **DILL:** Traditionally used as a digestive aid and a remedy for intestinal upset and colic. It's also helpful for colds, cough, and flu. Can increase milk production and help manage cholesterol, diabetes, and osteoarthritis.
- **LEMON PEEL:** Helps eliminate toxins, aids digestion and bile production, and boosts immune and skin health. A natural astringent.
- **MINT:** One of the best digestive relief herbs, helping with heartburn, gas, nausea, bloating, cramping, vomiting, morning sickness, and IBS. Relieves congestion and headaches. Supports mood and mental clarity, and eases anxiety symptoms.
- **ONION:** A classic cough and cold cure due to its expectorant properties. Used for respiratory distress, digestive issues, wound healing, and hair loss. Can also help regulate blood sugar and lower blood pressure.
- **OREGANO:** A powerful herb that's highly antimicrobial against many pathogens, viruses, and infections. Relieves gastrointestinal distress and cramping, supports microbial health, clears the airways, and aids in eliminating metabolic waste.
- **PARSLEY:** Relaxes the nervous system, particularly within the digestive tract. Stimulates the urinary tract and kidneys and supports immune function.

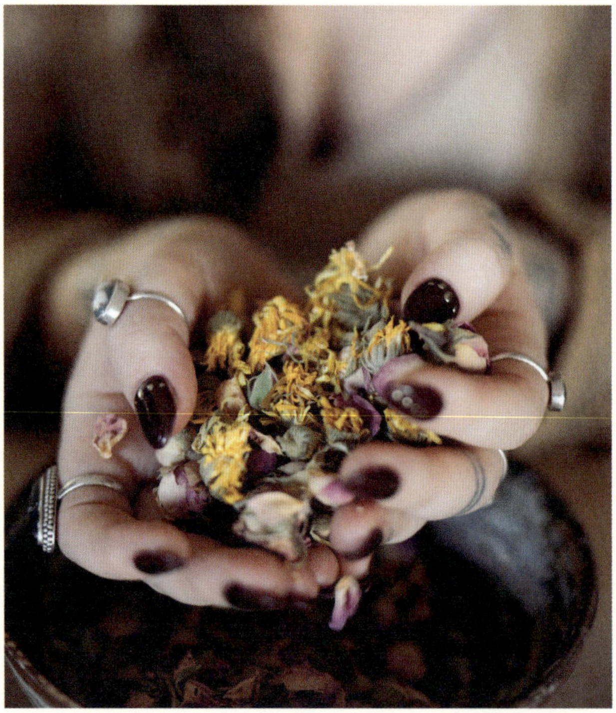

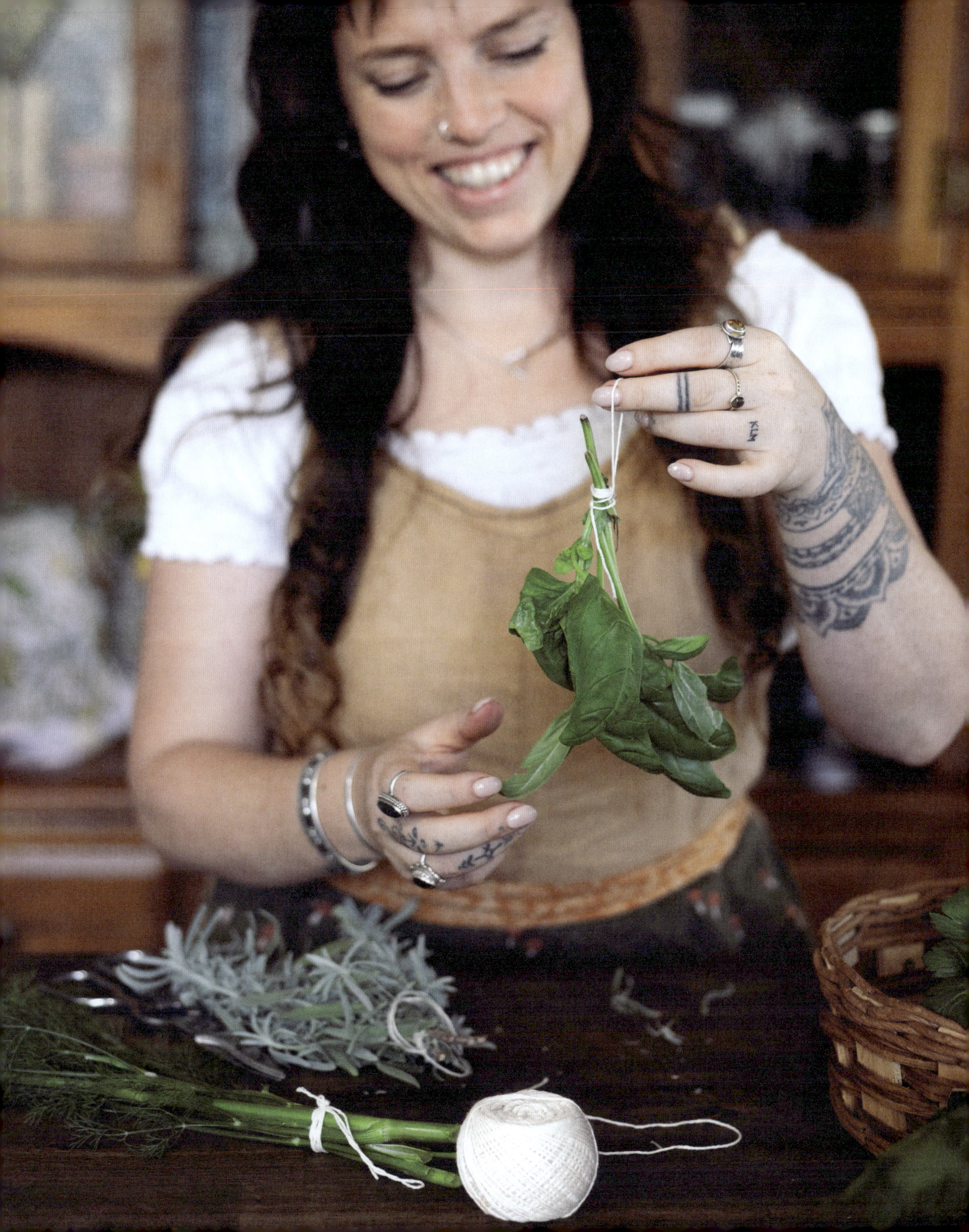

- **ROSEMARY:** Boosts brain function, increases mental clarity and focus, and reduces stress and inflammation. Also supports digestion, fights free radicals, and improves immune response.

- **SAGE:** A nootropic herb that supports memory and cognitive functions. Excellent for digestive function, improves assimilation of fats, and treats heartburn, gas, and bloating. Relieves excessive sweating. Helpful for mouth sores, tonsillitis, gingivitis, and other oral issues, as well as colds, coughs, and infections.

Spices

- **ALLSPICE:** Helps with inflammatory conditions, muscle aches and pains, and tooth and joint aches—while also preventing cellular damage, supporting immune function, and digestion. Inhibits the growth of bacteria and can treat infections.

- **BLACK PEPPER:** Enhances the absorption of many phytochemicals (like the curcumin in turmeric); stimulates the liver and digestion, and may improve circulation and relieve mild pain. Helps expel parasites.

- **CARDAMOM:** Provides digestive relief (especially for bloating and gas), is antispasmodic, and helps heal ulcers. A warming expectorant for coughs, colds, and asthma relief, and a mild diuretic that lowers blood pressure.

- **CAYENNE:** Can increase metabolic rate, stimulate digestive circulation, warm the body, and loosen congestion. Can also help break a fever and relieve pain if applied topically.

- **CINNAMON:** Historically used to improve digestion and circulation, cinnamon may also have benefits for blood sugar regulation, insulin sensitivity, and cholesterol. Antimicrobial and useful for food preservation.

- **CLOVE:** A powerful antioxidant and anti-inflammatory that stimulates circulation. Historically used to treat toothaches and oral infections. Also provides digestive support and relief from nausea and bloating. Has antimicrobial properties for food preservation.

- **CORIANDER** (cilantro seed): Stimulates digestion; can reduce bloating and gas. Mildly antimicrobial. Used for detox and may help bind heavy metals. Has blood sugar benefits.

- **CUMIN:** A digestive and metabolic aid that relieves gas, diarrhea, and colic. Stimulates metabolic rate, aids nutrient absorption (particularly iron), and supports liver function and bile production. Good for bone health.

- **FENNEL SEED:** Good for sore throats, coughs, respiratory distress, and digestive health. Helpful for menstrual cramps and breastmilk production. May fight cancer, heart disease, and arthritis and help prevent mental decline.

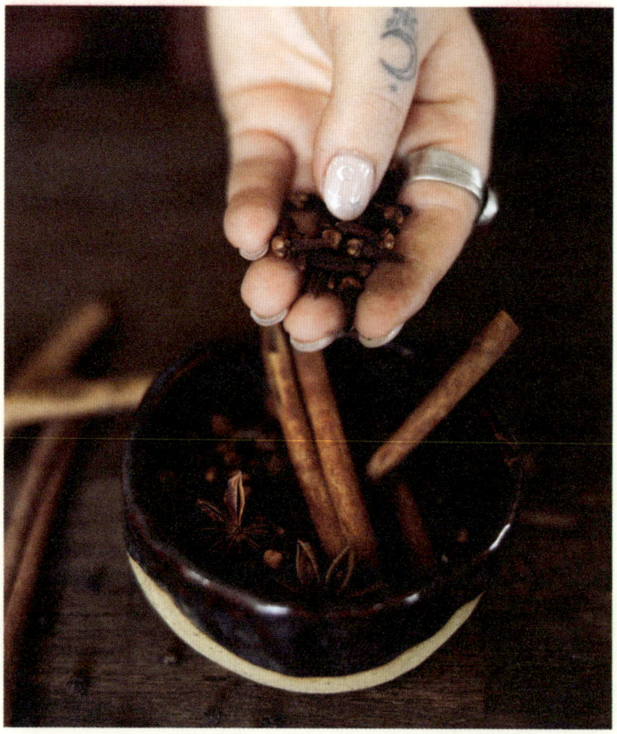

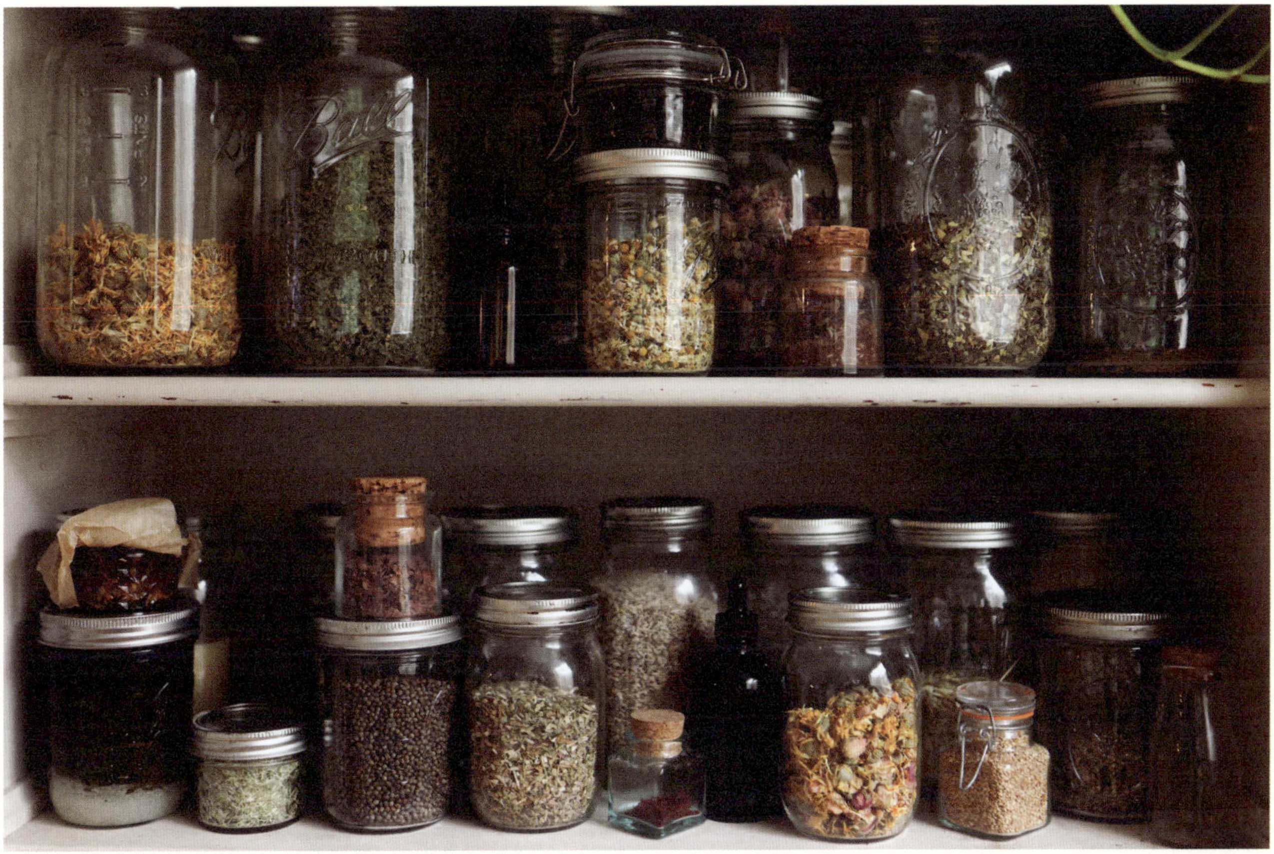

✶ **GARLIC:** Great for everything: cardiovascular, respiratory, immune, and digestive health. Has strong antibacterial qualities, regulates blood sugar, and lowers cholesterol. A go-to cure for colds, chest infections, and coughs. A prebiotic that increases microbiome diversity and aids the liver in waste elimination.

✶ **GINGER:** Widely used for nausea and vomiting, digestion, metabolic stimulation, and bloating. Especially good for colds, congestion, and fever. Stimulates circulation to soothe muscles, and cramping, and is magic for migraines, cholesterol, arthritis, and morning sickness.

✶ **NUTMEG:** Good for gastrointestinal pain, bloating, and indigestion. Calming for the nervous system, anxiety, and physical tension. Also helpful for urinary tract and reproductive health and said to be an aphrodisiac.

✶ **SAFFRON:** Supports the nervous system; good for depression, anxiety, and brain health. Can promote menstrual health—reducing pain, headaches, and low mood. Supports gastrointestinal health, stimulates circulation, and aids in reducing high blood pressure and age-related degeneration.

✶ **STAR ANISE:** Great for digestive support (bloating, colic, and gas). Supports the immune system and is a powerful flu and infection fighter, often used for colds, coughs, sinus congestion, and phlegm. May help with insomnia.

✶ **TURMERIC:** A powerful spice with adaptogenic properties, it can restore a dysfunctional immune system, treat chronic inflammation, and aid in recovery and gut restoration. Stimulates bile flow, soothes mucous membranes, and offers relief for menstrual dysfunction. Basically, it does everything.

FOOD PREP

COOKING FROM SCRATCH can be time-consuming, so anything you can make ahead is going to be a game changer—especially if you are cycle syncing (matching the food you eat to the phase of your cycle; see page 44) or have a health need that requires very specific food attention. Note that this section is about "food prep," not "meal prep." Meal prep is what you think of when you see fitness baddies pre-making and portioning out individual meals for the week. Food prep is preparing ingredients, sides, baked goods, and other aspects of your food. Meal prep involves a lot more planning; it never works for me, because I will not eat something if I'm not in the mood. Food prep gives you freedom to be flexible. Each season of life has different needs and different energy, so whatever you do for prep, it should serve you.

WAYS TO PREP

There are two ways I approach food prep.

- **BUST IT OUT:** Take one afternoon (or often a whole day) each week to prep. It makes the week so much easier, especially during busy seasons or if you're cycle syncing (see page 44)!

- **BATCH IT UP:** If you find yourself without large chunks of time, practice making extra food anytime you cook. It only takes a little more time, and the extra food can be used that week or put in the freezer. You can double the quantity of a whole meal, or just a component, like sautéed onions or roasted sweet potatoes. Then, rather than spending a whole day prepping, you can spread it throughout the week and maybe even find time to whip up a batch of granola or bread to round things out.

WHAT TO PREP

Here's what I usually like to prep.

- **A BREAKFAST ITEM:** Getting the day started is sometimes the biggest challenge! I like to make Egg Bites (page 90), pancakes (see pages 81 and 82), or Power Muffins (page 234). For grain bowls (see page 92), you can soak and cook the grain ahead of time and prep a vegetable to add.

- **A BAKED GOOD:** Most often, I make a loaf or two of sourdough bread (see page 62), but I also try to add a snack item of some kind as well: Cycle Syncing Buckwheat Granola (page 233), Seed Cycling Bliss Balls (page 237), or Sourdough Discard Crackers (page 66).

- **A COOKED VEGETABLE:** Roasting a big tray of something-or-other is so easy and a great way to have a quick side for dinner or something to throw under eggs at breakfast. You'll find a few of my go-to sheet-pan veggies on page 134.

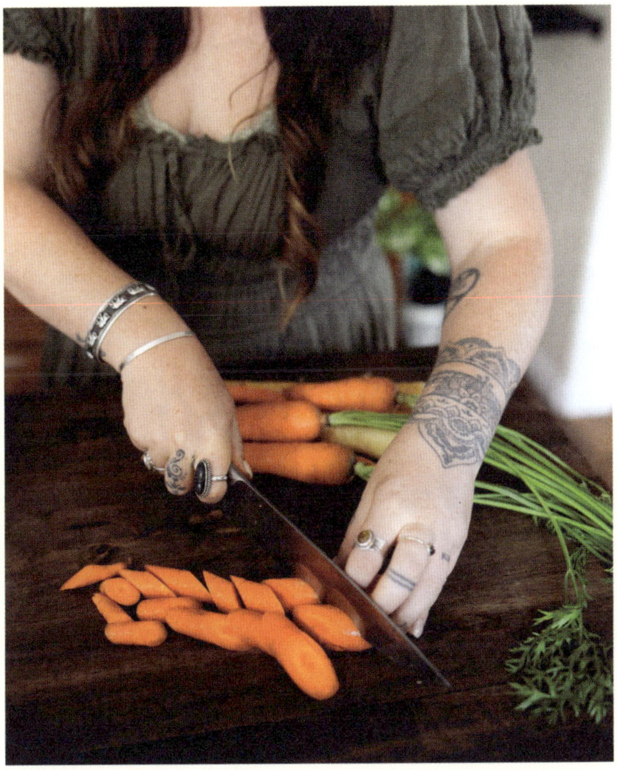

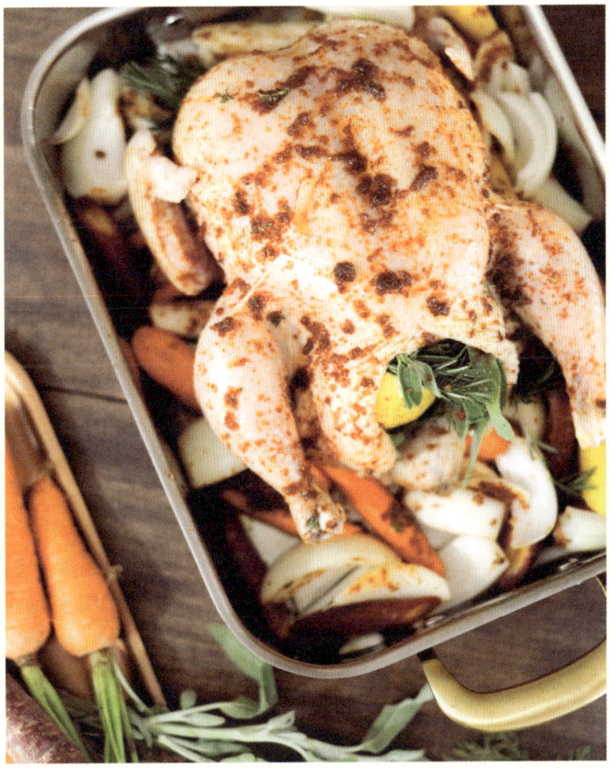

* **A FRESH VEGETABLE OR SALAD:** Sometimes this is as simple as the rubbed kale from my Rubbed Kale and Acorn Squash Salad (page 108) or carrot salad (see page 120). Other times, I make a coleslaw (see page 111) or bean salad (see page 116). Just remember, if prepping a salad ahead of time, either choose things that won't wilt (like cabbage or kale, which actually get easier to digest as they soften) or don't pre-dress your salad.

* **A PROTEIN:** I usually make a protein with quick lunches in mind. Chicken strips, like the ones in my Honey Mustard Chicken Salad (page 104), Smoky Salmon Bites (page 192), and tuna salad are some of my favorites! Roasting a whole chicken (see page 200) is also surprisingly easy, and as my mom always said, you might as well fill up the oven if you're gonna turn it on. You can eat some roast chicken for dinner, make leftovers into a chicken salad or fajitas, and then use the bones for broth (see page 159).

* **SOUP** (sometimes): Soup is a great way to use up scraps and leftovers, and it's a great quick meal. I eat soup for breakfast, especially in colder months; starting the day with a substantial, protein- and fiber-rich meal is so good for our blood sugar and hormone health! If you make a big batch, it will usually last for a couple of dinners and still give you enough to heat up for a quick lunch, or freeze if you're tired of it! There's a whole chapter of soups on page 154.

* **A SWEET TREAT:** This often overlaps with a baked good, but especially in the second half of my cycle and as I approach the menstrual phase, I try to plan ahead for sweet cravings! I love Black Bean Brownies (page 223) or my Coconut "Caramel" Cookies (page 238). In the summer, I make sure there is fruit in the freezer for when the inevitable watermelon sorbet (see page 228) cravings hit!

CYCLE SYNCING

IF "HORMONES" SOUNDS LIKE a dirty word to you, welcome—you are not alone. Many people associate hormones with a mysterious internal goblin that makes women moody once a month and gets in the way of life. In actuality, hormones are the essential messengers of our bodies, and when we learn to support them, we can better connect to ourselves. If you are a woman and have ever felt at odds with your own body, I invite you gently into this practice of cycle syncing: aligning your food and lifestyle with the monthly flow of your hormones. Let's circle back to hormone health. It is estimated that up to 80 percent of women and up to 50 percent of men struggle with hormone-related health issues at some point in their lives, and the wild part is that food and lifestyle changes can resolve most of them. If you aren't sure whether this applies to you, have a look at this list of symptoms. If any of them are familiar for you, read on.

METABOLIC & STRESS SYMPTOMS

Carb cravings or binging
Sugar and chocolate cravings
Reliance on coffee, soda, or energy drinks
Consuming more than three alcoholic beverages per week
Skipping meals
Anxiety
Insomnia
Waking during sleep
Headaches
Low libido
Excess facial or body hair
Weight gain
Hypothyroidism
Metabolic syndrome
Diabetes

ELIMINATION SYMPTOMS

Irritable bowel syndrome (IBS)
Oily skin
Bloating and water retention
Acne or cystic acne
Dandruff
Eczema
Hair loss
Constipation
Diarrhea or loose stools
Body odor
Night sweats

CYCLE SYMPTOMS

Mood swings
Premenstrual syndrome (PMS) or premenstrual dysphoric disorder (PMDD)
Irregular cycles
Fibroids
Ovarian cysts
Cystic breasts
Breast tenderness
Polycystic ovary syndrome (PCOS)
Unexplained infertility
Cramps
Heavy periods
Painful periods
Missing periods
Migraines
Depression

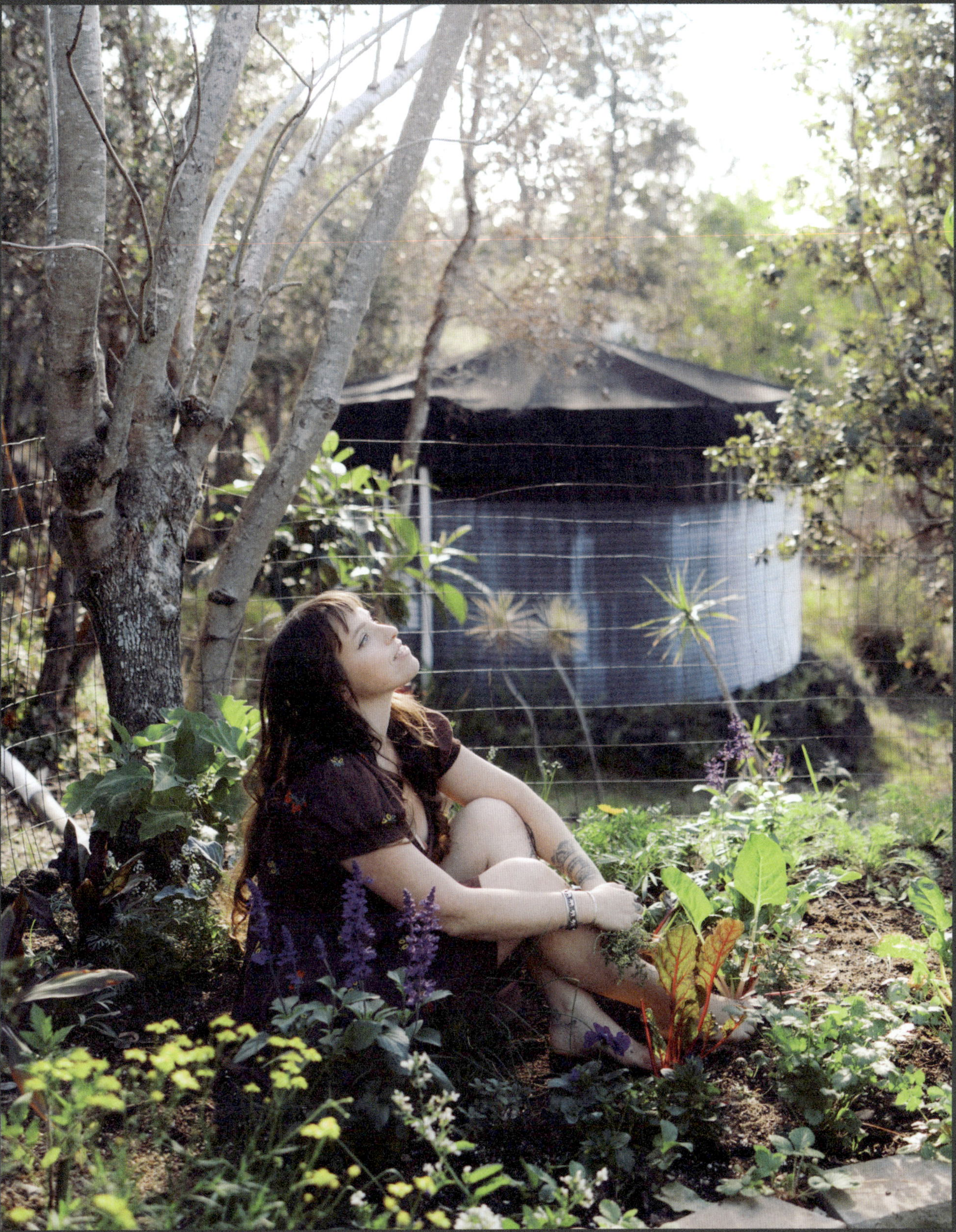

CYCLE PHASE FOODS

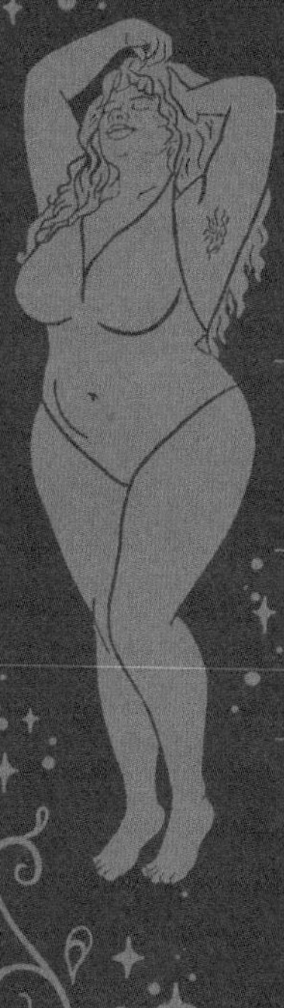

	MENSTRUAL	FOLLICULAR	OVULATION	LUTEAL
FRUIT	Blackberries Blueberries Concord Grapes Watermelon	Citrus Plums Pomegranates Sour Cherries	Cantaloupe Figs Persimmons Red Berries	Apples Dates Raisins Stone Fruits
VEGETABLES	Beets Collard Greens Kale Mushrooms Seaweeds Sweet Potatoes	Avocados Broccoli Carrots Green Beans Peas Zucchini	Asparagus Brussels Sprouts Eggplant Spinach Swiss Chard Tomatoes	Cabbage Cauliflower Leeks Pumpkin Radishes Root Vegetables
GRAINS & PULSES	Adzuki Beans Buckwheat Kidney Beans Wild Rice	Barley Black-eyed Peas Oats Green Lentils	Amaranth Black Beans Quinoa Red Lentils	Brown Rice Chickpeas Farro Navy Beans
NUTS & SEEDS	Chestnuts Flaxseeds Pumpkin Seeds	Cashews Flaxseeds Pumpkin Seeds	Almonds Sesame Seeds Sunflower Seeds	Sesame Seeds Sunflower Seeds Walnuts
ANIMAL PROTEINS	Beef Pork Shellfish	Chicken Eggs Trout	Lamb Salmon Shrimp	Beef Cod Turkey
EXTRAS	Ginger Nettle Raspberry Leaf	Dill Parsley Sauerkraut	Cilantro Dandelion Turmeric	Garlic Lemon Balm Spearmint

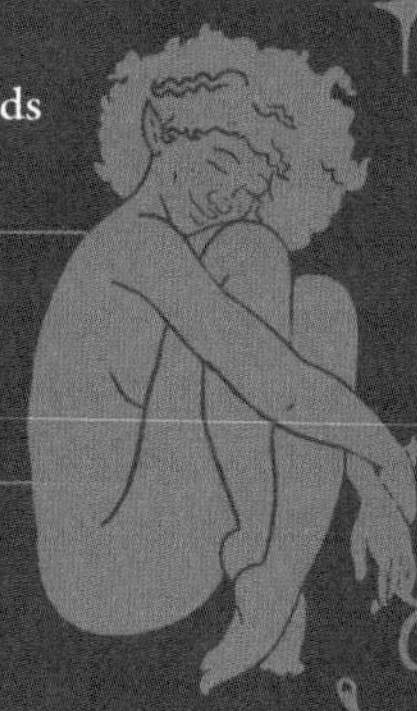

So many of these symptoms are things women write off as normal, when in fact they point to an underlying imbalance that is fixable and problematic if left unchecked. Hormone imbalances, while inconvenient in one phase of life, can be devastating in another, leading to infertility, long-term health issues, and an early and difficult menopause.

At the heart of the hormone health epidemic are generations of women who have not been taught about their hormone cycle. Most of us were given the cursory period chat and left to our own devices. It's no wonder we have no idea what's going on in our own bodies.

Hormones are connected to every function of the body and can be disrupted by anything from stress to food to environmental toxins. The major impactors are blood sugar, food, adrenal overexertion (chronic stress), poor elimination causing a buildup of hormonal waste, and hormone-disrupting chemicals (PFAS, artificial fragrances, and forever chemicals).

For many women, these imbalances make the menstrual cycle more challenging than it should be, causing mood swings, irritability, and heavy, painful, inconsistent periods. The good news? Hormones are directly affected by food and lifestyle!

Women have a roughly 28-day hormone cycle, meaning our hormones move through a long, varied pattern. We are not meant to feel the same and have the same energy every day! When we understand this, we can live in sync with this flow and start to see the benefits.

By adjusting your lifestyle to serve your changing hormonal needs throughout the month, you will absolutely see a difference in symptoms of imbalance. This practice is called cycle syncing, developed by renowned hormone health practitionier Alisa Vitti (her book *WomanCode* should be required reading for every woman).

This is not a prescription; it's a guideline to help map the journey. Start by tracking your cycle, noticing how you feel through the month. Slowly adjust your lifestyle to plan more rest on your period and more big events during ovulation. Make food choices to provide the specific nutritional needs that support your hormones through the month, or just focus on a diverse, whole-food diet.

Lean into the energetics of foods: Eat grounding "winter" foods in your menstrual phase and cooling "summer" foods during ovulation. Your hormone story is unique, so you have to find what works for you. If you have an inconsistent or non-existent cycle, simply look for any time you menstruate or ovulate and begin cycle syncing from there. Move through the phases until you notice menstruation or ovulation, and then start again. You will likely begin to see more consistency in time. If you really can't find a rhythm, use the moon to create your cycle, starting with the "menstrual" phase on the full moon or new moon.

"Hormones are connected to every function of the body."

If you are on hormonal birth control, the medication will override your food choices when it comes to hormones. But I truly believe every woman benefits from living in a cyclical flow. It's in our nature! It does something on a spiritual level, I swear. You may notice that you feel less burned out and more in tune with your own rhythms.

Your cycle can be broken down into four phases: the menstrual phase (day 1 to approximately day 6), the follicular phase (approximately days 7 to 14), the ovulation phase (approximately days 15 to 17), and the luteal phase (approximately days 18 to 28). These days will vary from person to person and depending on your hormone health.

If this all sounds a bit overwhelming, I felt that way, too. Truly the most transformational thing is to begin shifting your mindset towards your body's hormone cycle. When I was in peak hormone imbalance and at my unhealthiest, I was constantly fighting against this natural flow. When I stopped trying to force my body into submission and consistency and started looking at it with grace, things shifted. I stopped feeling embarrassed by my period and instead began honoring the cycle I was made to live in.

If you are ready to take it a step further and eat in tune with your hormonal needs (which you will find especially helpful if you do struggle with PMDD or PCOS, or if you're concerned about fertility or other reproductive health issues), the chart on page 46 will help guide you towards the right foods for each phase.

THE FOUR PHASES

THE PHASES are often categorized as seasons, an easy way to generalize how your lifestyle and food choices should align for each phase. Every woman's cycle varies slightly, but the average "healthy" hormonal flow looks like this.

MENSTRUAL PHASE

(Winter)

3 TO 7 DAYS

(day 1 of bleeding through the end of bleeding)

Estrogen and progesterone drop from their peak to their lowest, triggering the shedding of the uterine lining and the start of a new cycle. This process cleanses the uterus if an egg isn't fertilized.

- **PHYSICALLY**, this phase is marked by lower energy, lower libido, and greater rest needs. Menstrual symptoms should be mild and short-lived, but strong symptoms like heavy bleeding, intense cramping, and nausea can be signals of hormone imbalance.
- **EMOTIONALLY**, this is an introspective phase. Research suggests increased communication between the brain hemispheres, making this a good time for journaling and planning with balanced intuition.
- **LIFESTYLE-WISE**, gentle movement is best, as gentle stretching and walking can help bloating and cramps, but take it easy otherwise. Your focus should be sleep, relaxation, stress reduction, mindfulness, and decreased physical workload if possible.
- **CHOOSE** cooked, easily digestible foods like soups, stews, and roast veggies, with healing iron- and mineral-rich ingredients, like dark, leafy greens, mushrooms, seaweed, and beets.

FOLLICULAR PHASE

(Spring)

7 TO 10 DAYS

(end of bleed until beginning of ovulation)

Estrogen progressively increases to thicken uterine lining, while follicle-stimulating hormone prepares follicles to release an egg.

- **PHYSICALLY**, energy returns and increases to almost your peak. You'll likely notice improved skin and better digestive function.
- **EMOTIONALLY**, this phase is marked by more optimism, creativity, and motivation, along with increased social and mental drive.
- **LIFESTYLE-WISE**, that creative drive makes this a good time to pursue new goals, increase workload, network, or tackle creative projects. Now is the time for high-intensity workouts.
- **CHOOSE** fresh, fibrous, lightly cooked foods to aid elimination and support your energy. Lean protein, healthy fats, and complex carbs will fuel your adventures. Estrogen is at its lowest, so it's a good time to eat phytoestrogens (foods with estrogen mimicking properties), like oats, soy, and flaxseeds.

OVULATION PHASE

(Summer)

3 TO 4 DAYS

(short peak fertile window)

Testosterone surges; follicle-stimulating hormone and luteinizing hormone rise suddenly to release an egg Estrogen and progesterone continue to rise.

- **PHYSICALLY**, you'll notice increased discharge and sometimes brief, slight pain when the egg releases. Libido and energy peak and circulation improves.
- **EMOTIONALLY**, almost everyone feels their most confident and outgoing during this phase, along with more assertiveness and better communication skills.
- **LIFESTYLE-WISE**, your social battery is high so it's a good time for trying new things, meeting people, and getting out and about. That confidence makes it a perfect chance to increase productivity, make money moves, and take risks. Try pushing your limits with new or higher intensity exercise.
- **CHOOSE** light, nutrient-dense, fresh foods. Your energy is high, so eat lower carb foods that won't slow you down. Go for antioxidant-rich, hydrating foods like salads, smoothies, and lightly cooked or raw veggies with tons of fiber to eliminate excess estrogen.

LUTEAL PHASE

(Fall)

10 TO 14 DAYS

(ovulation until the next bleed)

Progesterone and estrogen rise continually, falling quickly a few days before menstruation if the egg is not fertilized.

- **PHYSICALLY**, energy decreases, digestion slows, and hormones suddenly shift as you near menstruation, causing premenstrual symptoms. Extreme symptoms like PMDD (premenstrual dysphoric disorder) or excessive physical discomfort can be a sign of hormone imbalance.
- **EMOTIONALLY**, you may notice lower stress tolerance and higher sensitivity—this isn't always a bad thing. I think of it as an intuitive time where your bullshit-ometer is at peak performance.
- **LIFESTYLE-WISE**, it's time to begin reining in your energy, shifting focus to yourself and your nest. You may feel called to home projects, organization, and self-care, so use this time to shore up for the menstrual phase and month ahead. Find gentler, lower-intensity workouts like yoga or moderate strength training, and increase your sleep.
- **CHOOSE** comforting, nourishing foods and complex carbs with lots of B vitamins to satisfy sugar cravings. Think "fall" with root vegetables, squashes, and roasted warm foods with lots of fiber. Avoid excessive sugar, alcohol, and caffeine, which can exacerbate PMS symptoms.

CYCLE SYNCING MEAL PLANS

MENSTRUAL PHASE

FOOD PREP

Roast beets from Honey Roast Beets with Labneh (page 141), kale salad from Rubbed Kale and Acorn Squash Salad (page 108), soaked buckwheat from Buckwheat Breakfast Bowl (page 92)

BREAKFAST

Beet-Berry Chia Pudding (page 77), Chocolate Cherry Overnight Baked Oatmeal (page 85), Buckwheat Breakfast Bowl (page 92)

LUNCH

Beet and Farro Salad (page 138) (use buckwheat instead of farro), Quick Ramen (page 169), Kale Pesto Pasta (page 173)

DINNER

Adzuki Bean Salad (page 116), Korean-Style BBQ Beef Bowls (page 196), Spiced Beef Stew (page 160), Honey Roast Beets with Labneh (page 141)

TREAT

Black Bean Brownies (page 223), Bone Broth Hot Cocoa (page 254)

FOLLICULAR PHASE

FOOD PREP

Teriyaki Roast Broccoli (page 134), The Carrot Salad (page 120), Herbaceous Green Dressing (page 210)

BREAKFAST

Mama Tessa's Overnight Oat Pancakes (page 81), Egg Bites (page 90), Savory Oats Breakfast Bowl (page 92)

LUNCH

Honey Mustard Chicken Salad (page 104), Excessively Green Salad (page 115)

DINNER

Magic Zucchini Pasta (page 174), Cast Iron Chicken with Saffron Rice (page 186), Smoky Salmon Bites with Coconut Rice (page 192), Half-Smashed Peas with Lemon and Dill (page 145)

TREAT

Berry Crumble (page 227)

OVULATION PHASE

FOOD PREP

Quinoa from Quinoa Salad (page 107), Food Prep Roast Veggies (page 134), Tahini Dressing (page 208)

BREAKFAST

Quinoa Breakfast Bowl (page 93), Shakshuka (page 86), Gluten-Free Banana Pancakes (page 82)

LUNCH

Quinoa Salad (page 107), Ovulation Phase Jar Salad (page 103)

DINNER

Lentil Dal (page 179), Kofta-Style Meatloaf with Tzatziki (page 199), Quinoa Salad (page 107) or Excessively Green Salad (page 115), Harissa Baked Eggplant (page 146)

TREAT

Watermelon Mint Sorbet (page 228)

LUTEAL PHASE

FOOD PREP

Smoked Paprika Sweet Potatoes (page 134), soaked farro from Beet and Farro Salad (page 138), Good Gut Coleslaw (page 111)

BREAKFAST

Farro Breakfast Bowl (page 93), Roast Tomato and Goat Cheese Frittata (page 97), Chorizo Sweet Potato Hash (page 89)

LUNCH

Rubbed Kale and Acorn Squash Salad (page 108), Chipotle Steak Bowls (page 205) (use farro instead of rice), Coconut-Crusted Fish Tacos (page 190)

DINNER

Easy Peasy Roasty Squash Soup (page 163), Sunday Roast Chicken (page 200) with Roast Cauliflower and Fennel (page 130), Butternut Sage Risotto (page 180), Pan-Seared Sea Bass with Lemon Butter Sauce (page 189)

TREAT

Baked Apple Crumbles (page 224)

CHAPTER ONE

FERMENTS

FERMENTED FOODS ARE THE OG PROBIOTIC.

Fermentation occurs when the microorganisms that are naturally present on fruit and vegetables transform these foods into probiotic preserves. Under the correct conditions, these microorganisms or "good" bacteria are able to thrive and multiply. The bacteria feed upon sugars in the food, fermenting it and preventing it from rotting. Traditionally, fermentation was used as a way to preserve foods. It's one of those processes that is so mystical to me—how brave people discovered a way to turn simple foods into nutritional powerhouses and preserve them for years without molding. Wild!

But many ferments are actually super simple to do. Once you learn the basics, you will be so inspired and empowered to see what else you can ferment! The most common ferment is sourdough, which requires a specific "starter" bacteria; if you haven't embarked on the obsessive sourdough journey yet, I've got all the info you need to begin on page 59. Other ferments like yogurt's gutsier cousin Kefir (page 69) also require a starter, but once you have that starter, you just feed it what it wants to eat, and you're set. And then there are lacto-fermented vegetables like Sauerkraut (page 70) that just need the right amount of salt and a few days to themselves to become a powerful probiotic. Read on to get all the juicy details and prepare your supplies, or skip ahead to the recipes to get straight down to business.

GUT LOVE

In recent years, "gut health" has become so buzzy that I think it's lost all meaning. In reality, the health of your gut—your digestive system—is *foundational* to not only your digestive function, but also your wellbeing as a whole.

When we chat about the gut, we mean your digestive system: mouth, stomach, intestines, and colon. Gut *health* is most often referring to the state of your gut microbiome, the community of trillions of bacteria and microorganisms living within your digestive system. Imagine it like a community: Some of its residents are actively working for you, helping your body break down and process nutrients (fuel), some of which your body cannot physically process without these specific bacteria. Some residents are pretty neutral, just hanging out, and a few are disease-carrying bad guys, out to attack your system. Most of us have developed strong enough immune systems that those bad guys don't really affect us, so don't freak out.

What's wild is that our gut microbiome is in direct and constant communication with our brain. Our central nervous system (connected to the brain) and our enteric nervous system (connected to the gut) have a two-way communication system called the "gut-brain axis." As our gut microbes feed on the food we eat, they produce metabolites that contact our central nervous system, informing our brain function. Even hormones and essential vitamins are created or converted by our gut microbiome. So if your gut microbiome is substantially off-kilter or lacking, it has a direct impact on the messaging systems in your body; this can lead to neurological symptoms like anxiety, depression, poor sleep, and even Alzheimer's disease.

So how do you create or sustain a healthy gut microbiome? Your microbiome begins in utero and is further established during birth, so your mom plays a big part in the initial development. But food and lifestyle are the biggest factors. Processed foods full of simple sugars, fillers, and unhealthy fats will wreak havoc on your gut, since they are difficult to process, offer little food for your bacteria, and cause inflammation.

You can improve and strengthen your gut bacteria by eating lots of prebiotic- and probiotic-rich foods. *Pre*biotic foods are high in insoluble fiber, which is fiber that the body itself doesn't digest but your bacterial community *loves*. Most vegetables are prebiotic, but carrots, cabbage, broccoli, legumes, and whole grains are especially prebiotic-rich. *Pro*biotics are fermented foods rich in good bacteria that actively introduce more and new strains of bacteria into your microbiome, increasing its diversity and workforce.

You can take probiotics in pill form, but the general consensus is that it is *far* better to get them from fermented foods. Most probiotic pills are not high enough quality to contain living bacteria, and even if they do, many of those bacteria won't actually make it to your gut alive.

Fermented foods are quite readily accessible and, especially if you make them at home, pretty cheap. Foods like yogurt—or even better, kefir—sauerkraut, kimchi, and other fermented vegetables, along with drinks like kombucha should all be in the daily rotation to support your gut health and, ultimately, your overall health.

It can feel a bit daunting initially. Like, I'm really just going to let this food sit out and . . . get funky, and then eat it? But while there are

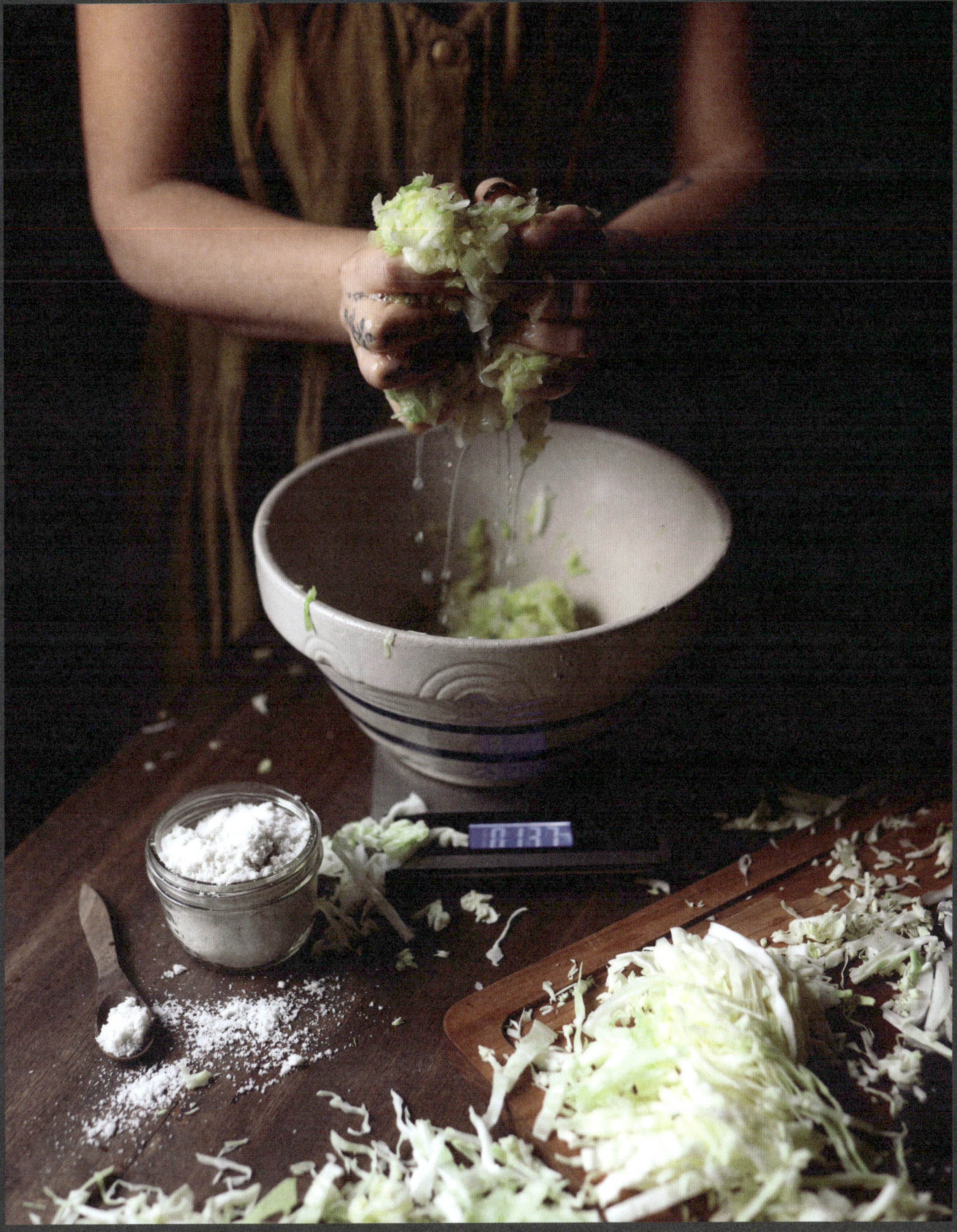

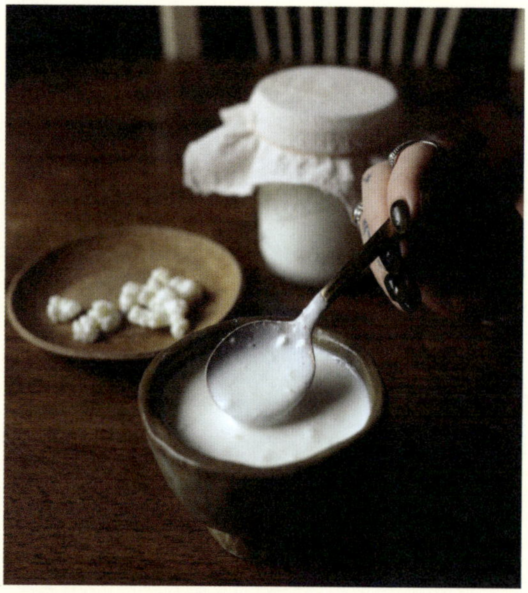

some wild and truly funky ferments out there (I unfortunately don't have a recipe for hákarl, Icelandic fermented shark), many ferments are incredibly simple and near-foolproof. Sourdough just needs a starter, which takes some babying but, once established, is indestructible. Kombucha and kefir need their particular SCOBY (symbiotic culture of bacteria and yeast) and a base of tea or milk, respectively.

For fermenting vegetables, the most common method is also the simplest: lacto-fermentation. It makes use of the lactic acid bacteria that are already present in most vegetables to get things started. There are a couple of essential components and simple formulas to follow. Once you learn them, and how to recognize a good ferment vs. spoiled food, you're off and away and can experiment with fermenting all kinds of veggies!

CULTURE

Every ferment needs a microbial culture to begin. Spontaneous cultures (like in lacto-fermentation) come from the vegetable itself. Backslopping is the use of a previously fermented product to begin the process, like adding some sauerkraut juice to a new batch of cabbage.

SALT

Salt pulls water and sugars from vegetables for microorganisms to use. It helps prevent the growth of harmful bacteria and preserves the product during the fermenting process.

The amount of salt used in a ferment is key, and it varies for different vegetables. You can easily look up suggested salt amounts if you get a sudden urge to ferment some celery or pickle a pear. The amount will be a percentage of the total weight of whatever you are fermenting.

Salt can be added directly or "dry" into vegetables, enabling them to release water and create their own brine (this is how sauerkraut is made), or it can be added by creating a brine with water that is poured over the vegetables: This is typically the best route for veggies with lower water content, like carrots.

The type of salt matters, too: It should be pure, high-quality, and without additives. Anti-caking agents, iodine, low-sodium salt, or impurities found in some natural salts can all impede the fermentation process. You can use canning or pickling salt, or just a high-quality, very clean, finely ground sea salt (I use Eden or Redmond sea salt).

VEGETABLES

Choose produce that is free of damage, mold, or disease. Make sure to thoroughly clean it and remove any "bad" parts.

CONTAINER

You can get a ceramic fermenting crock, made specifically for this process. It will have a heavy weighted lid, and the ceramic will completely block out light, which is ideal for fermentation. *But* you can totally just use a glass mason jar. Make sure it's free of cracks or chips, and be sure to put it in a dark cupboard away from the light. You can purchase fermenting weights, which keep the produce from sticking out into the air above the brine (this can cause mold), but you can also make homemade weights: marbles or rocks in a ziplock bag works great!

Once you have your supplies, produce, and salt, the process is pretty simple. Figure out the salt percentage needed for your ferment, then decide on a brine or a dry salt method. Make sure all your tools, your workspace, your jar, and your hands are clean; no need to sterilize, but wash everything.

Always ensure your produce is fully submerged in brine, and always store in a cool, dry place. For more details and to start your own ferment, turn to the Sauerkraut recipe on page 70.

Different vegetables will take different amounts of time to ferment, and the timing is also dependent on your personal taste. Once fermentation begins, you can taste your ferment every day or two. When it's tangy and pickle-ish to your taste, remove the weight and shove it in the fridge! A refrigerated ferment will keep almost indefinitely as long as you always use a clean utensil in the jar!

Troubleshooting: DID IT GO BAD?

If you follow all of the above, usually things will turn out right. But sometimes, even the most experienced fermenters get a dud batch! Here are the signs to look out for—and which ones mean a batch should go in the compost bin.

- **MY FERMENT HAS A WHITE FILM ON TOP:** If the film is flat, filmy, and plain white, it is **KAHM YEAST**, a harmless substance. Skim it off the top and proceed.
- **MY FERMENT HAS FUZZY, RAISED GREEN, BLACK, RED, OR PINK SPOTS:** These are mold. A lot of old-school ladies will say to skim off the top layer and keep on truckin'. However, the safest option is to discard and start again. Make sure your jar, hands, and weight are nice and clean next time!
- **MY FERMENT SMELLS WEIRD:** Use your nose! Does your ferment smell like something you want to eat? If not, don't eat it. If it smells pickled and slightly like whatever vegetable it is, and if mold isn't present, give it a taste. Taste good? You're good.
- **WHAT ABOUT BOTULISM?** It's not really as common as you might think, but if you are concerned, there is a simple way to rule it out. Get some pH testing strips and dip a strip in your ferment. If the pH is below 4.6, botulism *cannot* be present.

Armed with this info, you are ready to embark on your fermenting journey. It's so fun! Once you get the hang of the basics, it's really easy and super rewarding. Just don't take it too seriously at first and know you may have a few duds along the way. I've included some of the simplest, near-foolproof ferments here so that you can start making your own probiotics without much room for error.

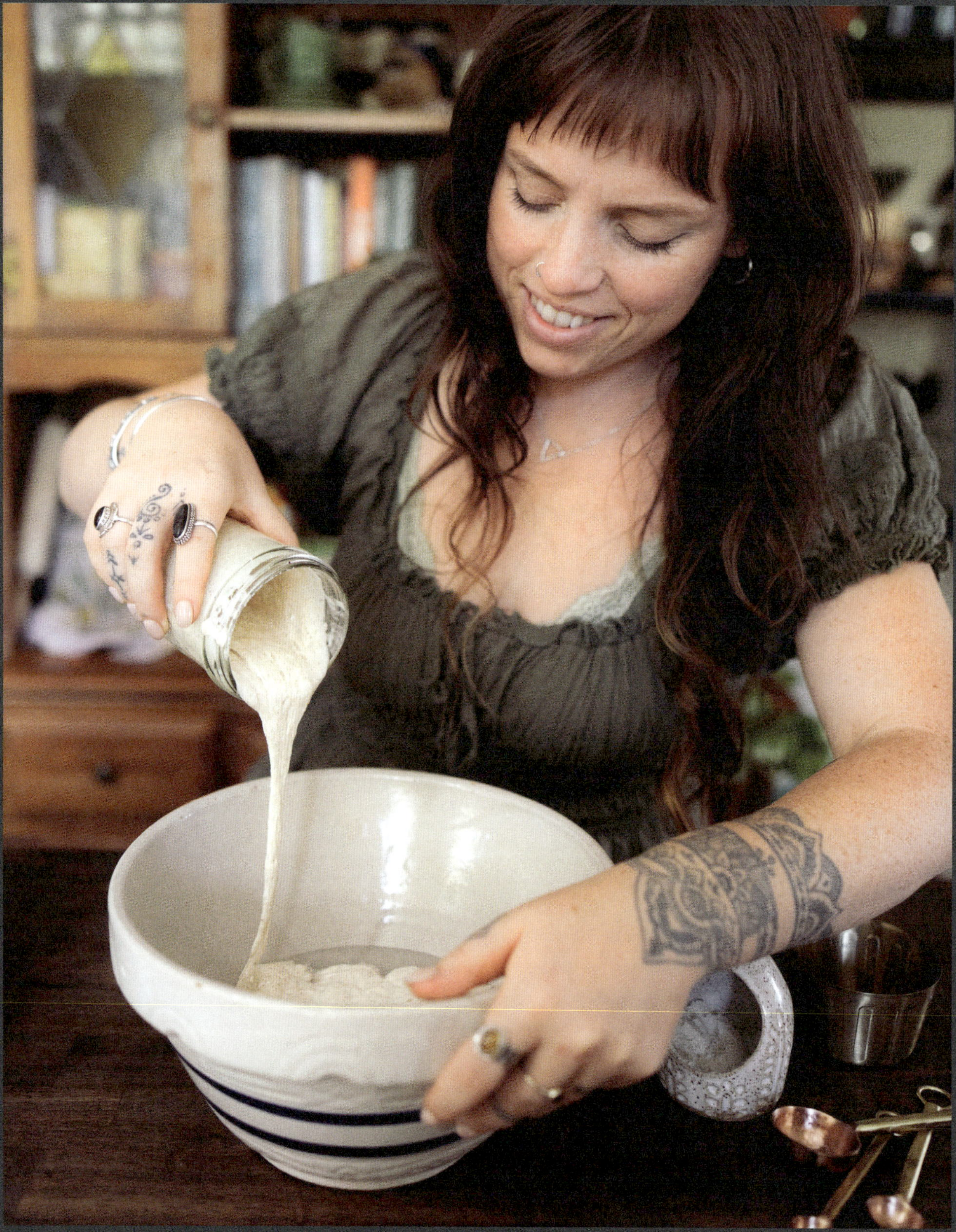

SOURDOUGH

Bread making is a distinctly human experience; it's the simplest form of alchemy, using our synergy with earth, air, and fire to turn three simple ingredients—flour, salt, and water—into sustenance. It's *magic*, in my opinion. And sourdough bread is the epitome of that magic: Without requiring yeast or a long, drawn-out kneading process, anyone can make bread. And sourdough is deeply nutritious. Fermentation breaks down compounds in wheat like phytic acid, which impedes mineral absorption. This makes the bread easier to digest and increases its antioxidant content.

Sourdough has a lower glycemic index than regular yeast bread, and, as with any bread made at home, will not have any of the added sugars or fillers that many store-bought breads contain. Some people who are gluten intolerant even find that sourdough doesn't bother them (but since it still contains gluten, it's still not good for those with celiac disease).

Sourdough seems complex but it is a really basic ferment; you can start making it at home and become a pro in no time. But I will warn you: It is addictive! Making sourdough can be precise and scientific, but it becomes even easier once you learn the *feel* of it: the texture, the signs to look out for, the rhythm of making a loaf. Once you learn this rhythm, you won't even need a recipe!

To get started, you first need a sourdough starter. You can get one from a friend or make it yourself, and honestly, it's the most involved part of the whole process. You will need to baby your fledgling starter for a week or more, twice a day. Once it is established, though, that baby is resilient. You can keep it in the fridge for a week or more at a time (I've left mine in there for months) and remove and feed it when you are ready to make a loaf. If you left it alone for quite a while, you may need to feed it twice before using, but really, your starter is pretty independent.

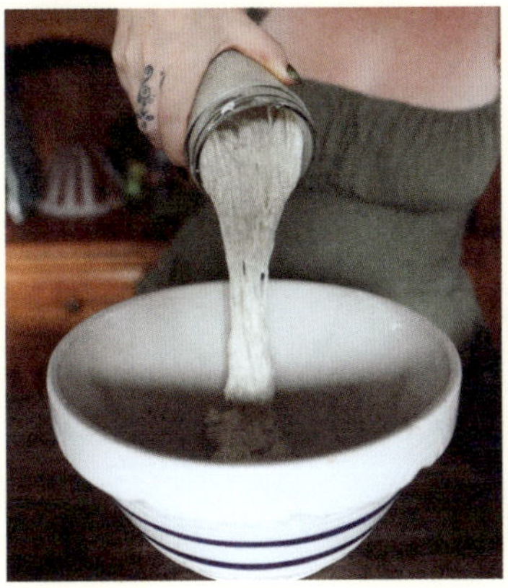

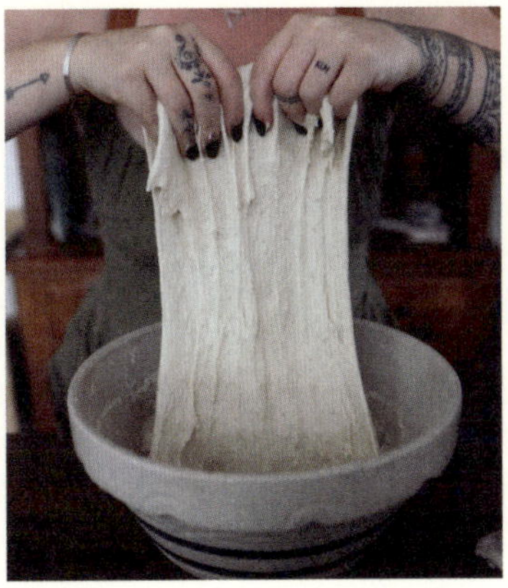

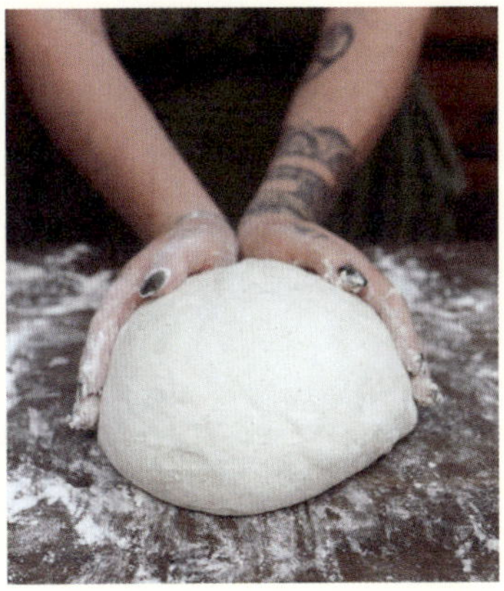

How to Make a Sourdough Starter

Prepare to baby your starter for 6 to 9 days, depending on the temperature of your home and a ton of other minute environmental details (even elevation makes a difference).

YOU WILL NEED

- One or two 16-ounce (480 ml) wide-mouth mason jars
- Bread flour (unbleached, ideally organic) or all-purpose flour
- Rye flour (organic)
- Water (filtered or purified, without chlorine or contaminants)

DAY 1

1. Place ¼ cup plus 2 tablespoons (about 45 g) bread flour and 2 tablespoons (about 15 g) rye flour (½ cup/60 g total) in the mason jar.

2. Pour in ½ cup (120 ml) water.

3. Mix thoroughly, ideally using a nonmetal utensil. I like to use wooden chopsticks, but a small silicone spatula works well, too.

4. Cover lightly. I use a flat mason jar lid without the ring or a small square of muslin secured with a rubber band.

5. Leave on the countertop in a warm area of your kitchen for 24 hours.

6. Name your starter. Not only is this a cute thing to do, but it will also help you remember to check on it every day. I named mine Rebreadkah, because she is my daughter.

DAY 2

1. Check on your starter baby! Give it a stir, note any activity, and encourage it with a kind word.

2. Feed the starter exactly as you did yesterday: ½ cup (60 g) flour mixture and ½ cup (120 ml) water. Stir well.

3. Place the jar on a small plate just in case it bubbles over.

4. Return the light cover and leave for 24 hours.

DAY 3

1. Check on your baby. Depending on the temperature of your kitchen, you might see a lot of activity between days 2 and 4. Don't get too excited—it'll likely stop doing anything for the next couple of days. This is normal, so be patient.

2. Discard: Pour ½ cup (about 120 g) of the starter into a fresh, clean jar—or pour out all but ½ cup (about 120 g)—and compost the rest. (While you can use the discard from an established starter in recipes, you can't use this discard yet!)

3. Feed the starter as normal: ½ cup (60 g) flour mixture and ½ cup (120 ml) water.

4. Stir thoroughly, cover lightly, and leave for 24 hours.

DAY 4

1. Check on the starter baby! If she seems flat and dead, don't fret. She's saving her energy for later.

2. Discard, feed, and stir as you did yesterday.

3. Cover and leave for 12 hours. From now on, you will discard and feed your starter every 12 hours until it is active and ready to use.

4. You don't need to get a new jar every time—just refresh it if it gets sticky and gunky.

DAYS 5 TO 9+

1. Continue discarding and feeding your starter twice a day, exactly as you did on day 4, until it begins to double in size after each feed.

2. Once it begins doubling in size, give it a couple more feeds for good measure and you should be ready to bake with it!

3. To double-check that the starter is active and ready, try the float test: When the starter is at *peak* (its most active point, after doubling in size following a feed), drop a little glob of it in a glass of water. If she floats, even a little, she should be good to go!

4. A mature starter should have complex, large bubbles—so many of them that if you wiggle it around at peak (most expanded), it should look like some kind of living organism or something from the Upside Down. Yours may not quite be at organism status yet, but it should have lots of large bubbles!

FEEDING YOUR STARTER

To make sure your starter is strong and ready to bake with, I like to feed it once with a different ratio. I usually use about 2 tablespoons of starter, about ½ cup (60 g) bread flour, ¼ cup (30 g) rye flour, and *just* enough water to mix it all together, creating a very thick batter consistency. Leave it on the counter, lightly covered, for around 12 hours, or until doubled in size (again, this will vary depending on your kitchen temperature), and then you're ready to bake!

STARTER MAINTENANCE

Looking after your established starter is easy. Just be sure to leave a couple tablespoons in the jar after using it so that you can keep it alive for the next bake. Feed the starter as normal, then place it immediately in the fridge. This will slow down the fermentation process, allowing the starter to sit longer between feedings. It is ideal to feed it once a week to keep it ready to go. During busy seasons, I only bake bread once a week, so refrigeration works great at those times.

If possible, pull your starter from the fridge a full 24 hours before you are ready to use it. Give it a feed and cover. Once it peaks, discard the excess and feed it a second time before using. This will fire up your starter and bring back some of its "sour" tang. You can save the discarded starter in the fridge to use in recipes like the Sourdough Discard Crackers (page 66).

If you plan to bake a lot and want to keep your starter active, save and feed a much smaller ratio of starter daily. For instance, you could save 1 teaspoon of starter and feed it 2 to 4 teaspoons of both flour and water. This way you don't waste lots of flour and your starter stays really strong and ready to use. Make sure to feed it more when you are ready to bake with it, though, so you have enough active starter for your chosen recipe.

A NOTE ON RATIOS

Once you get the hang of things, you'll notice talk of different feeding ratios. A common beginner ratio is 1:1:1, meaning equal parts of starter, flour, and water. This means the starter doesn't have a lot of flour to eat through, and it will come to peak much faster: usually in 4 to 6 hours. I use about a 1:6:3 ratio: a little starter, a lot of flour, and less water. This gives the starter a lot of food and makes it nice and strong, but it takes longer to come to "peak" (12 to 16 hours, which works well for my schedule). Experiment and discover what works for you, your kitchen, and your schedule!

BASIC B SOURDOUGH

There are so many different sourdough recipes out there that I've come to believe almost anything goes. A good loaf depends on a combination of factors—the starter, the flour, the ratios, the rise time, your home's temperature, the baking process... But once you get the feel, you can adjust as you go and find your own perfect recipe every time. To begin with, though (or to ensure you get consistent outcomes), a basic recipe is helpful. This is my go-to. You can measure the ingredients in cups, but I've always had more success with a scale. I've included average timings in the method, since that part can be confusing when starting out, but those times will vary depending on the conditions in your kitchen.

MAKES 1 LOAF

Rest: ***24 hours***
Prep: ***30 minutes***
Cook: ***50 minutes***

Anti-Inflammatory
Gut Healthy
Low FODMAP

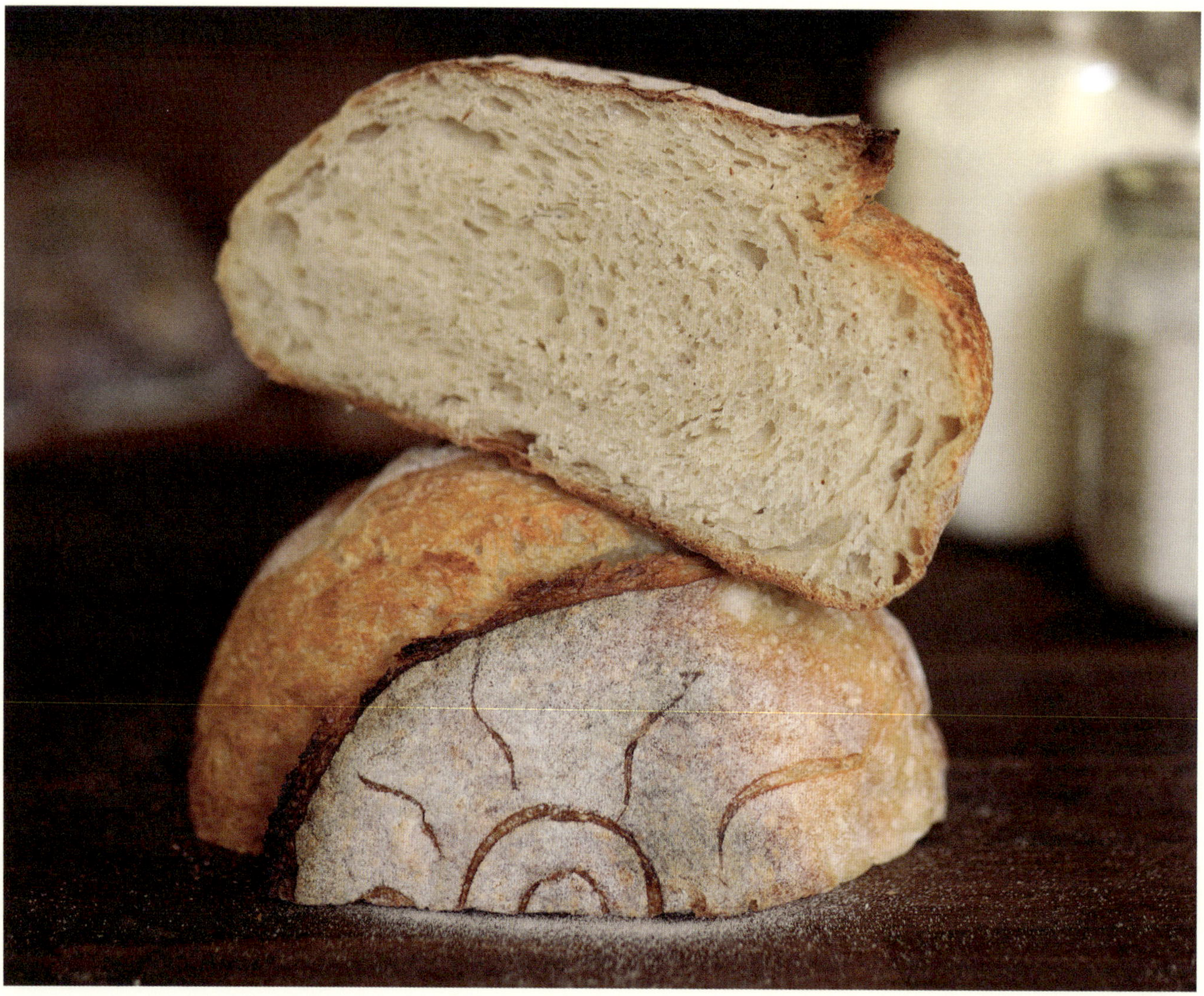

100 grams (½ cup) active starter (see page 60)
414 milliliters (1¾ cups) filtered water, at room temperature
500 grams (4 cups) organic unbleached bread flour or all-purpose flour, plus more for dusting
9 to 12 grams (1½ to 2½ teaspoons) sea salt
Rice flour, for dusting
Butter, for serving (optional)

- **8:00 PM:** *Feed your starter* 8 to 12 hours before you plan on using it.
- **8:00 AM:** *Mix the dough.* Once the starter is peaked and just starting to fall (see Tip 1), pour it into a large bowl with the filtered water. Mix well. Add the flour and salt and mix into a rough, shaggy dough. Try to incorporate all the flour, but it doesn't have to be perfect. Cover with a damp kitchen towel or plate and let rest somewhere warm for about 20 minutes. Feed your remaining starter and return it to the fridge.
- **8:30 AM:** *Stretch and fold.* Remove the covering. Wet your hands with cold water and grab the dough on one side of the bowl with both hands. Pull upward, gently shaking the dough as it stretches out. Fold it down to meet the opposite side of the bowl and gently press on it. Rotate the bowl a quarter turn and repeat, stretching and folding on all four "sides." Cover and let rest for 20 minutes. Repeat four more times, stretching and folding five times altogether, over the course of about 90 minutes.
- **10:00 AM:** *Bulk rise.* Cover the dough again and allow it to rise until it doubles in size. This timing can vary a lot depending on the conditions, and it can be hard to tell. You can use a high-sided clear container for your bulk rise, or you can put a spoonful of dough in a shot glass, set it next to your bowl, and use that as an easier marker of doubling. This can take 3 to 12 hours.
- **6:00 PM:** *Shape the dough.* Once your dough is domed, is pulling slightly away from the sides of the bowl, has visible bubbles, and has doubled in size, gently dump it onto a floured surface. Pull the dough into a rough, large rectangle. Fold it into thirds (like a letter) by folding the left side over the center and then the right side on top of the left. Roll it up from bottom to top so you have a little round loaf. Gently spin and pull the dough toward you along the countertop diagonally, using both hands. It should stay right side up, but the tension created when the dough sticks to the countertop will push more bubbles up through your bread and give it a nice round shape. Let rest for 20 minutes.
- **6:45 PM:** *Proof and second rise.* Dust a banneton or large bowl lined with a cotton cloth liberally with rice flour. Lightly dust your dough with rice flour and then quickly scoop it up and flip it upside down into your banneton as gently as possible. I like to use a bench scraper for this. Give the dough a final shape by grabbing it from opposite sides of the bottom and pinching in the middle. Cover and put in the fridge overnight or for 12 to 18 hours.
- **8:00 AM:** Preheat your oven as high as possible, 500°F (260°C) or above. If you're using a Dutch oven, preheat it in the oven for at least 30 but ideally 60 minutes (see Tip 2).
- **9:00 AM:** *Score the dough.* Remove the loaf from the fridge. Cover the banneton with a large square of parchment paper, flip it onto the counter, and lift it to release the dough. Score with a razor blade or very sharp knife (see Tip 3).
- **9:15 AM:** *Bake.* Reduce the heat to 450°F (230°C). Carefully remove your Dutch oven from the oven and plop the loaf (parchment and all) down inside. Cover with the lid. Place an empty baking sheet on a rack just below the one your bread will be baking on (this will help prevent a burned bottom). Bake for 20 minutes.
- **9:35 AM:** Remove the Dutch oven from the oven and remove the lid. Return to the oven and bake uncovered for another 30 minutes, until the loaf is deep golden brown, sounds hollow when knocked, and has an internal temperature between 200 and 210°F (93 and 99°C).
- **10:25 AM:** I'm supposed to say that you should let the bread fully cool before slicing it so the crumb can develop and the bread will hold its shape—but you could also cut a thick slice of your fresh-baked bread, smother it in butter, and enjoy the spoils of your victory.

* TIPS *

1. The starter is at peak when it has doubled in size, is slightly domed on top, and is laced with giant bubbles. I usually use it when it's just past peak and has started to fall again, as then it will be hungry and ready to do its thing.

2. If you don't have a Dutch oven, you can absolutely use any oven-safe pan. You may not get quite as full of an oven rise, but it will still do fine! If you're using a pan without a lid, add a shallow pan of water to the oven on a rack below the bread, to add extra steam and keep it from drying out. You may need to cover the bread with foil during the final 30 minutes of baking to keep it from burning.

3. Scoring is so much fun once you get the hang of it! Cut deeper than you would think for your main score line, and use long, smooth strokes. I like to make either a crescent-shaped score or a crisscross. Then, use shallower cuts to make it pretty.

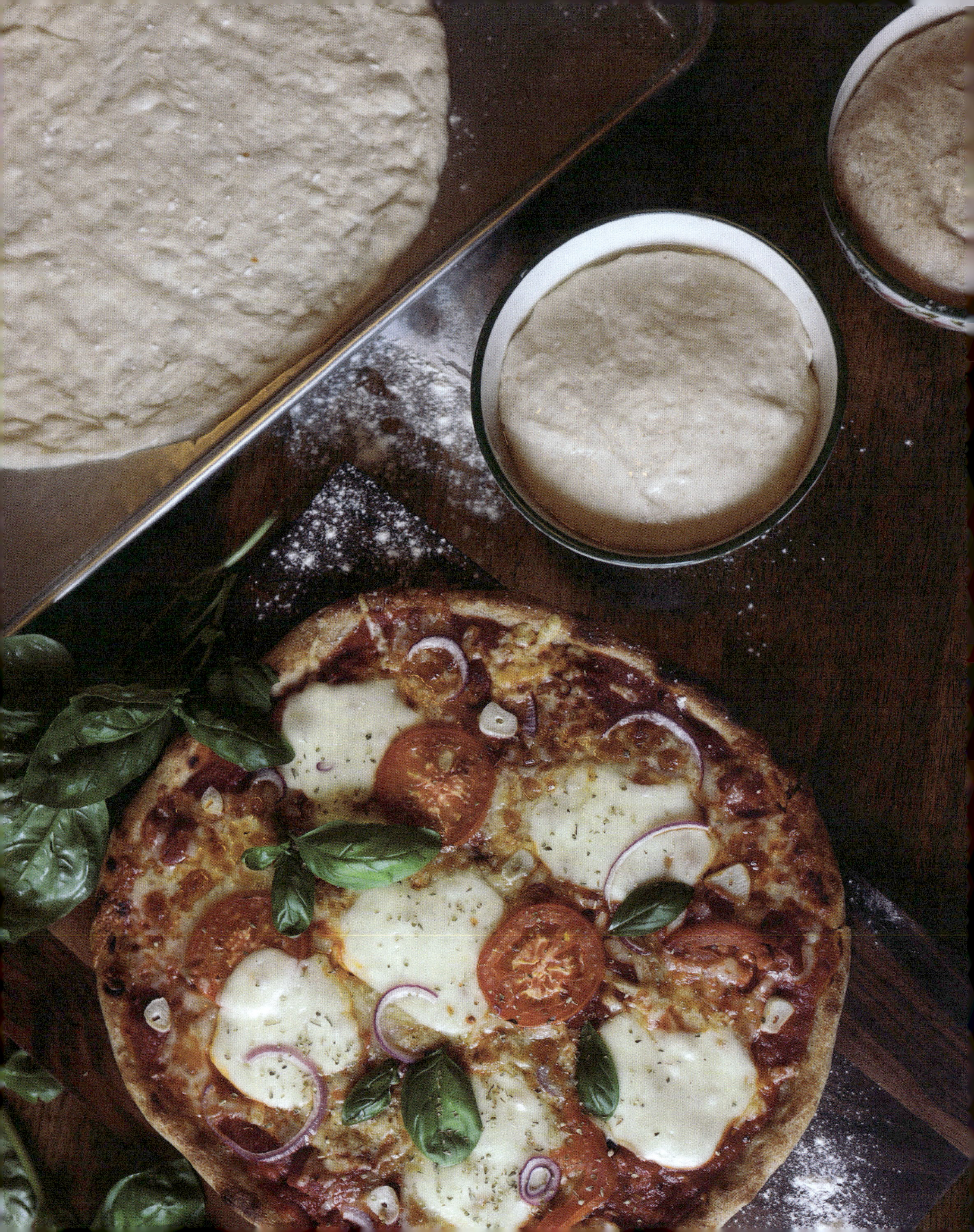

SOURDOUGH PIZZA CRUST

MAKES 4 SMALL PIZZAS

Rest: *9 hours*
Prep: *15 minutes*
Cook: *25 minutes*

Anti-Inflammatory
Dairy Free
Gut Healthy
Low FODMAP

Homemade pizza is one of my most nostalgic meals—I can call to mind right now the smell and taste of Mom's pizza, with a whole wheat crust that somehow tasted even better than the store-bought kind, thick layers of homemade sauce, and *mature cheddar*. It was always a group effort; I couldn't even tell you how many times I helped my mom shape dough and spoon sauce, begging to make my own whole pizza (pepperoni, red onion, sweet corn, and extra cheese, if you must know). It's been one of my favorite traditions to continue with my own family.

360 milliliters (1½ cups) filtered water

100 grams (½ cup) active starter (see page 60), just past peak

2 tablespoons olive oil, plus more for greasing

10 grams (2 teaspoons) sea salt

225 grams (2 cups) whole wheat flour

180 to 240 grams (1½ to 2 cups) unbleached all-purpose flour

Cheese, pizza sauce, and/or other toppings (see Headnote; optional)

1. The evening before pizza night, mix the water, starter, olive oil, and salt in a large bowl. Add the whole wheat flour, mix thoroughly again, and let rest for about 15 minutes so the flour can fully hydrate.
2. Add the all-purpose flour in ½ cup (63 g) increments until the dough comes together into a rough, shaggy ball. (You may not need all the flour.) Cover with a damp tea towel and let sit at room temperature overnight, or until doubled in size.
3. In the morning, if the dough is already doubled, perform a set of stretches and folds. Wet your hands with cold water and grab the dough on one side of the bowl with both hands. Pull upward, gently shaking the dough as it stretches out. Fold it down to meet the opposite side of the bowl and gently press on it. Rotate the bowl a quarter turn and repeat, stretching and folding on all four "sides." Cover with a damp towel and refrigerate until ready to use. If the dough is not quite doubled (which can happen if it's a cold night), perform two or three sets of stretching and folding, at 20-minute intervals, and then let sit until doubled. Cover and refrigerate.
4. When you're ready to bake, remove the dough from the fridge and allow it to warm up for 20 minutes. Then, divide and shape it into four balls. Place each ball in a small, oiled bowl, cover with a damp tea towel, and let rise for another 30 minutes.
5. Preheat the oven to 475°F (245°C). Plop each dough ball onto its own oiled baking sheet and use your fingers to gently press the dough, stretching it out into a circle or the shape of your tray. Lightly prick each crust all over with a fork. (Alternatively, use a well-seasoned and oiled cast-iron pan under the broiler and cook one pizza at a time.)
6. Parbake two pizza crusts at a time for about 5 minutes, or until the dough just loses its shine. Remove from the oven and add your toppings. Then return to the oven, two at a time, for 20 minutes, or until the cheese is melted and browning. Finish off with a quick broil for extra-bubbly cheese!

NOTE

If you don't want to use all the pizza dough at once, you can store it in a sealed container in the fridge for up to 7 days, or shape and parbake the dough and then freeze it for up to 3 months.

SOURDOUGH DISCARD CRACKERS

MAKES 180 CRACKERS

***Rest:* 30 minutes**
***Prep:* 10 minutes**
***Cook:* 30 minutes**

Anti-Inflammatory
Gut Healthy
Low FODMAP

Anytime someone tries to tell me how they feed their starter just enough to make no discard, I say, "Hey! What if I want discard, huh? What if my favorite homemade crackers rely on that yeasty goodness?" But these crackers can also be made without discard: Just sub in a mixture of equal parts flour and water, and you're good to go.

240 grams (1 cup) sourdough discard (unfed sourdough starter)
120 grams (1 cup) unbleached all-purpose flour, plus more for dusting
57 grams (¼ cup) unsalted butter or coconut oil, softened
25 grams (¼ cup) shredded Parmesan or Asiago, plus more for sprinkling
1 tablespoon dried rosemary, thyme or other dried herbs, plus more for sprinkling
¾ teaspoon sea salt, plus more for sprinkling
2 tablespoons unsalted butter or coconut oil, melted, divided

1. Mix the discard, flour, softened butter, Parmesan, herbs, and salt in a medium bowl to form a smooth, somewhat tacky dough. Start mixing with a spoon and then use your hands to gently knead the dough until it comes together nicely.
2. Divide the dough into halves, shape each into a rough rectangle, wrap individually in parchment paper, and refrigerate for at least 30 minutes.
3. When you're ready to bake, preheat the oven to 350°F (180°C).
4. Place half of the dough on a lightly floured piece of parchment paper. Then, lightly flour the dough and cover with a second sheet of parchment paper. Gently roll the dough to ½ to 1 inch (1 to 2.5 cm) thick. Aim to make a rectangle, but don't stress about perfection—the funky edges are always the yummiest!
5. Remove the top piece of parchment paper and lift the bottom piece of parchment paper and dough onto a baking sheet. Prick with a fork in rows (this will keep the crackers from puffing into balls in the oven), and brush with 1 tablespoon melted butter. Sprinkle with extra salt, Parmesan, and herbs.
6. Use a knife or pizza roller to cut the dough into bite-size squares, 1 to 1½ inches (2.5 to 4 cm) each.
7. Repeat steps 4 through 6 with the second half of the dough.
8. Bake for 25 to 30 minutes, until the edges are golden. You may need to rotate the pans in the oven halfway through for even baking.
9. Let cool completely, then store in an airtight jar or other container. The crackers will keep for up to 2 weeks at room temperature.

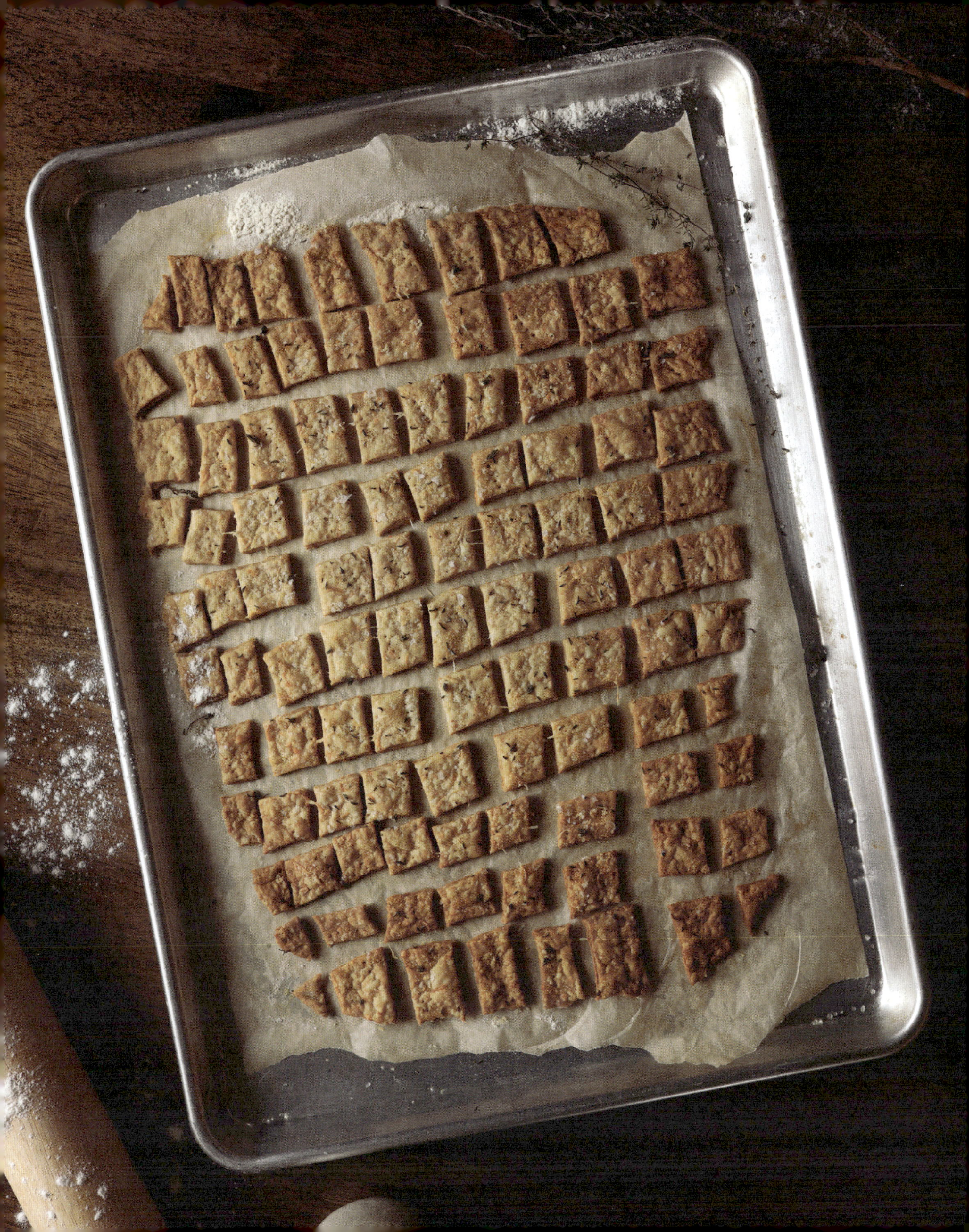

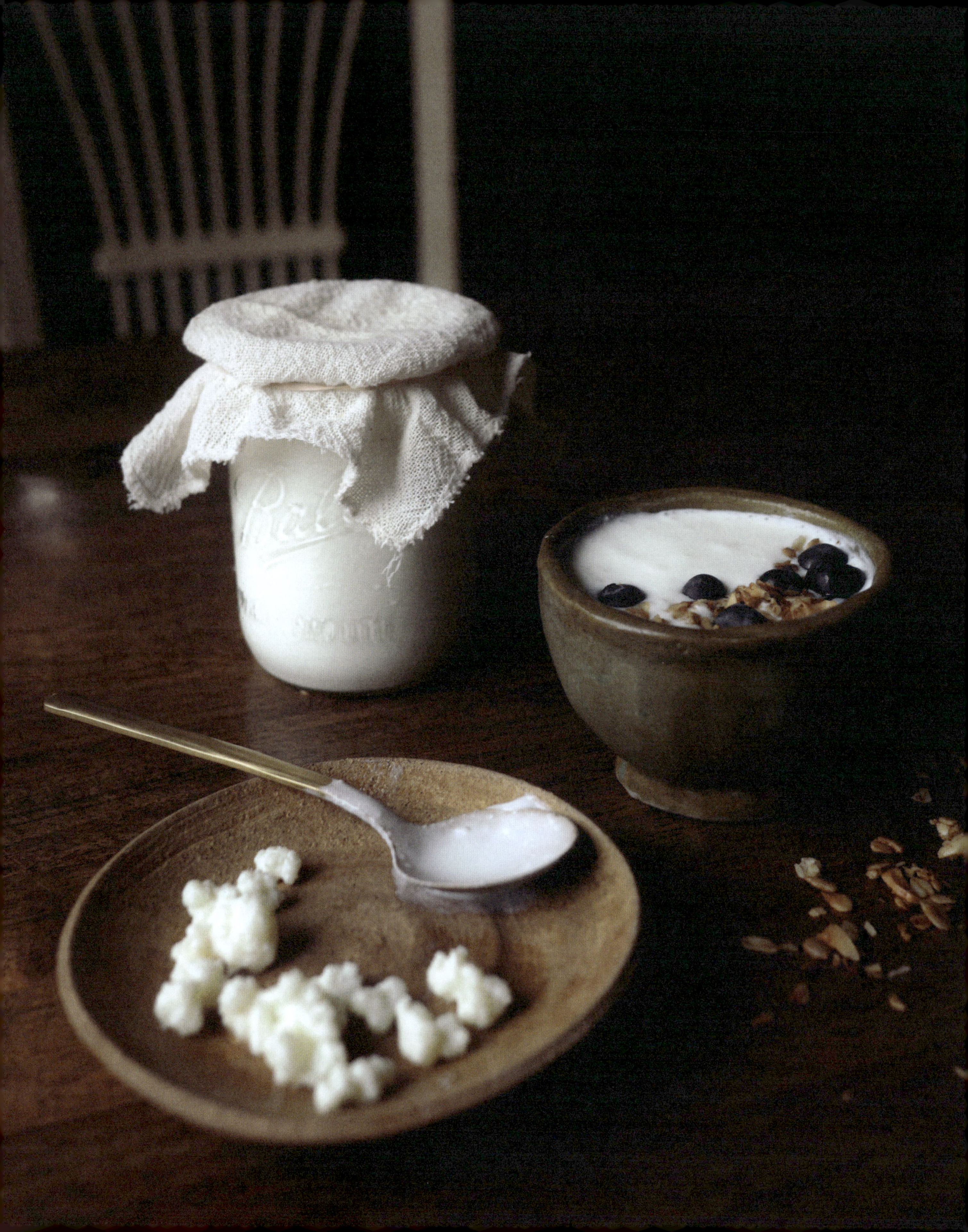

KEFIR

MAKES
1¾ CUPS
(420 ML)

Prep: *5 minutes*
Fermenting: *24 hours*

Anti-Inflammatory
Gluten Free
Gut Healthy

Step aside, yogurt: Kefir has entered the chat. Kefir is yogurt's older, sassier, sourer, and far more powerful sister, and she truly is an enigma. Originating in Eastern Europe, kefir is so easy to make, but it contains up to 60 unique probiotic strains and 15 to 20 billion CFUs (colony-forming units), in comparison to yogurt's 1 to 5 active cultures and 6 billion CFUs. The bacteria in kefir grains also feeds on lactose, making it pretty easy for many to tolerate even if they are lactose intolerant. It is super sour, so my favorite uses for it are in a morning smoothie, pancakes (page pages 81, 82), or my Kefir Ranch (page 211).

At least 2 tablespoons live, active kefir grains (see Notes 1 and 2)
2 cups (480 ml) whole milk

1. Add the kefir grains and milk to a quart-sized (1 L) wide-mouth mason jar. Stir to combine. Cover with a cheesecloth and secure with a mason jar ring to allow airflow.
2. Let sit on the counter for 12 to 24 hours, stirring every 6 to 12 hours, until the milk is thick and sour. The timing will depend on your kitchen's temperature and the health and amount of your kefir grains.
3. Use a plastic strainer (see Note 3) to strain the kefir into another jar, removing and reserving the grains for your next batch.
4. Use immediately in smoothies or sauces, or cover and refrigerate for up to 1 week.
5. If you're using kefir regularly, immediately start a new batch with your grains. No need to rinse them—leave all of that good-bacteria kefir juice on them. If you aren't ready to make another batch, put the grains in a small jar, just barely cover them with milk, and return to the fridge. They will last pretty much indefinitely, until you are ready to make another batch.

NOTES

1. To make kefir, you will need kefir grains, which can be sourced online (Cultures for Health is great).

2. If you are working with new kefir grains, reviving grains that haven't been used in a long time, or only have a few grains, you may need to halve the amount of milk and make a few batches that you toss before you are able to use the kefir. If using dehydrated grains, follow the package instructions for rehydration. The more you feed the grains, the more they'll multiply. Once they are awake and happy, and you have a good ½ cup (100 to 150 g) of grains, you should be able to make a batch of kefir easily in 1 day (or even overnight if your kitchen is warm).

3. It is important to use a plastic strainer for this, as the bacteria in kefir will slowly erode a metal one.

SAUERKRAUT

Sauerkraut is the perfect first foray into ferments! It has an immense and diverse probiotic profile, and cabbage itself is full of prebiotic fiber (the stuff that probiotic bacteria need to thrive). So by including it regularly in your diet, you're both feeding your gut bacteria and continually introducing more! Once you have the recipe down, experiment with different combinations of flavors: For a classic sauerkraut, add caraway seeds or juniper berries. For a bolder flavor, add sliced garlic or grated ginger, or herbs like dill, parsley, and cilantro.

MAKES 1 QUART (900 G)

Prep: *30 minutes*
Fermenting: *1 to 4 weeks*

Anti-Inflammatory
Dairy Free
Gluten Free
Gut Healthy

1 large head green cabbage (around 2½ pounds/1.1 kg)
5 teaspoons sea salt (1½ to 2 teaspoons per pound of cabbage), plus more as needed

1. Remove the outer leaves of the cabbage and any that look damaged or moldy. Keep one good-looking outer leaf whole to use later. Cut the cabbage into quarters, cut out the core, give it a rinse, and drip dry.
2. Slice the cabbage very thinly with a knife, food processor, or mandoline.
3. Throw the cabbage into a large bowl, sprinkle it with the salt, and toss well to distribute. Let sit for about 15 minutes to allow the salt to draw the moisture out of the cabbage.
4. With clean hands, massage the cabbage—use some elbow grease and really rub it between your fingers—for 5 to 10 minutes. The cabbage will become soft, reduce in volume, and produce a lot of brine.
5. Pack a layer of kraut into a 32-ounce (940 ml) jar. Use your hands or a tamper to really squish the cabbage and ensure there are no air bubbles. Repeat until you have used all the cabbage or the jar is mostly full (leave 2 inches/5 cm of headspace at the top).
6. There should be just enough liquid to cover the cabbage. If there is, skip to step 8.
7. *If you need more liquid, make a saltwater brine:* Dissolve 1 teaspoon of salt in 1 cup (240 ml) hot water. Let the brine cool, then add just enough to barely cover the cabbage, maintaining the 2 inches (5 cm) of headspace.
8. To ensure none of the cabbage pops up as it ferments and gets exposed to air, take the reserved cabbage leaf, fold it up, and place it on top, pressing it down to submerge.
9. Place clean fermentation weights on top. You can also use a ziplock bag filled with stones or any other clean, heavy object that can fit inside the jar.
10. If you're using a fermentation lid, place the lid on the jar. If you're using a mason jar lid, screw it on very loosely. The fermentation process will produce gases that need to escape, so it's important not to seal the jar too tightly, or you will have an explosion!
11. Store in a cool, dark place, as lactic acid bacteria grow better in the dark.
12. Ferment for 1 to 4 weeks, depending on the temperature of your house (the warmer the environment, the quicker the kraut will ferment). Check on your kraut every couple of days, looking for bubbles on the sides. If it's really bubbly, you can begin tasting it around day 3: Remove the weights and cabbage leaf and use a clean fork to taste. It should be sour and a little fizzy, with a pleasant smell and taste. You can stop fermenting at the first sign of sourness or let it continue to develop a sharper flavor.
13. Once the kraut is fermented to your liking, remove the weights and the leaf, seal with a lid, and store in the fridge. Ferments will keep almost indefinitely if kept clean!

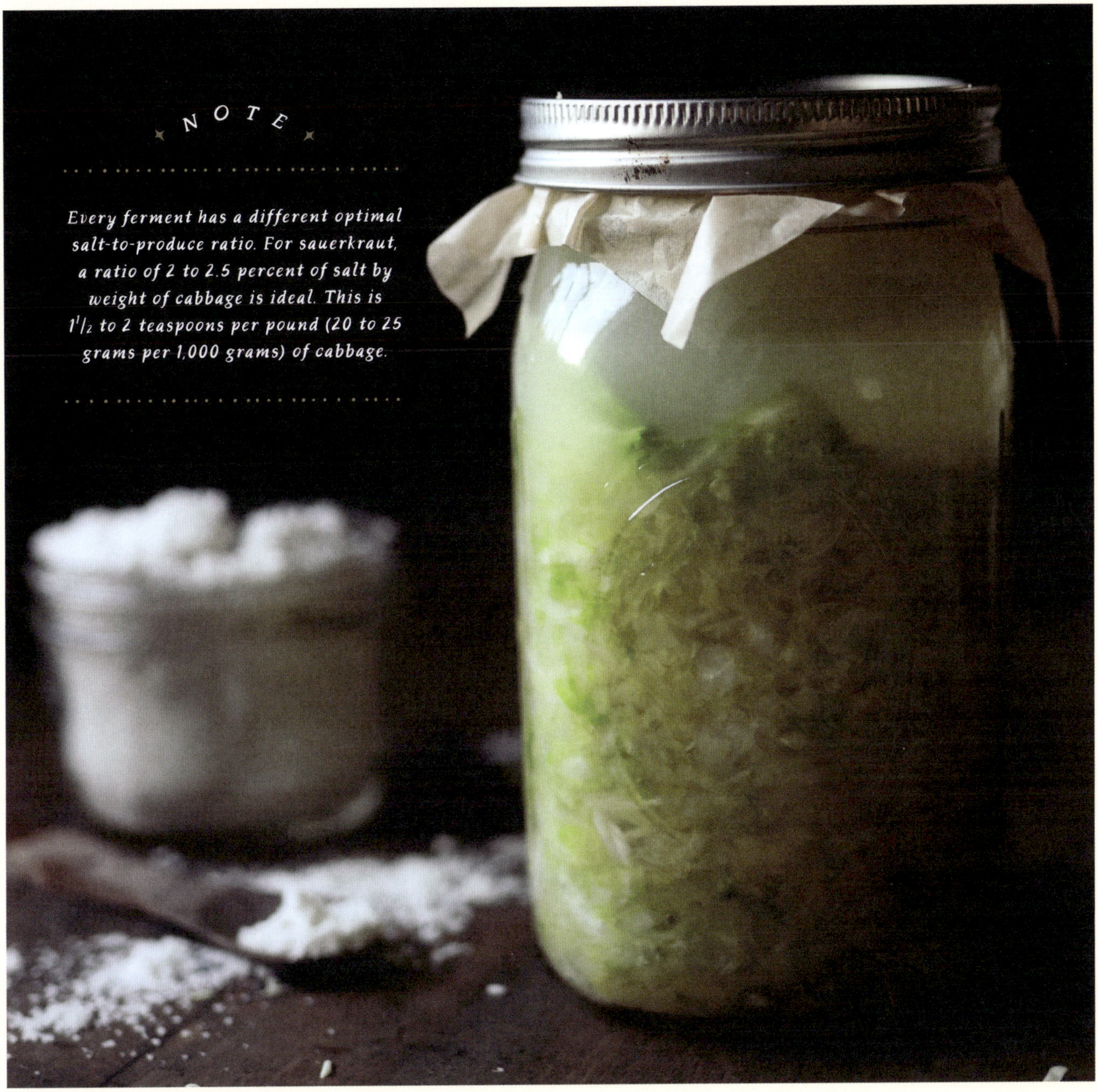

NOTE

Every ferment has a different optimal salt-to-produce ratio. For sauerkraut, a ratio of 2 to 2.5 percent of salt by weight of cabbage is ideal. This is 1½ to 2 teaspoons per pound (20 to 25 grams per 1,000 grams) of cabbage.

Troubleshooting

- *My kraut is not producing enough brine:* Your cabbage is probably not super fresh! The fresher the cabbage, the juicier it will be.
- *My kraut is kind of soft and slimy:* You likely don't have enough salt, as salt prevents slime mold. Discard this batch and try again.
- *My kraut isn't fermenting, it's just . . . existing:* You likely have too much salt, which can impede the fermentation process.
- *My kraut has a layer of white scum on top:* This is just kahm yeast, a harmless byproduct of fermentation. You can skim it off and eat the kraut.
- *My kraut has fuzzy black, pink, green, or red mold on it:* It's best to discard the kraut, as the spores so easily contaminate the whole lot.

LACTO-FERMENTED SALSA

MAKES 1 QUART (1 L)

Prep: 10 minutes
Fermenting: 2 to 3 days

Anti-Inflammatory
Dairy Free
Gluten Free
Gut Healthy
Ovulation Phase

This is one of the recipes that opened my eyes to how simple and widely applicable fermenting can be, and it's one of the quickest ferments you can make. As long as you have the correct salt ratio for the ingredients you're using, the world is your oyster! This simple salsa tastes super good pre-fermentation, but once it's fermented, it has a lovely, complex flavor with a little sourness, and it's incredibly beneficial for the good bacteria in your gut. Stop! I can't make enough.

4 or 5 large Roma tomatoes
½ large bell pepper, any color, finely chopped
1 jalapeño, finely chopped
½ small red onion, finely chopped
3 garlic cloves, minced
Juice of 2 limes
2 teaspoons sea salt
Handful of chopped cilantro

1. Chop half of the tomatoes and place them in a medium bowl with as much of their juice as possible. Cut the remaining tomatoes in half and grate them with a box grater into the bowl, discarding the skins.
2. Add the bell pepper, jalapeño, onion, and garlic and mix.
3. Add the lime juice and salt to the vegetables and mix thoroughly to combine.
4. Scoop everything into a clean quart-sized (1 L) mason jar, working in batches and using the handle of a spoon or a tamper to gently pack the vegetables and remove any air bubbles. Ensure at least 1 inch (2.5 cm) of headspace on top (you may have a little leftover salsa to snack on right away).
5. Place a fermentation weight or clean ziplock bag with small stones or weights in it on top of the ingredients to keep them submerged by at least ½ inch (1 cm) of liquid (see Note).
6. Cover the jar with a square of parchment paper, then place the lid on the jar and loosely screw on the ring. Leave it somewhere visible for 24 hours.
7. After 24 hours, you should start to see some bubbles and hear a small pop or fizz when you open the jar. Burp the jar by unscrewing the ring and removing the lid briefly to allow air to escape.
8. Use a clean spoon to taste the salsa. It should taste fresh and flavorful with a slight sour zing. If you're happy with the flavor, you can stop fermenting.
9. If your salsa isn't sour enough yet, replace the lid and repeat steps 6 through 8 to let it ferment for 1 or 2 more days.
10. Stir in the cilantro and store in the fridge for up to 2 months.

NOTE

If you don't have enough liquid to cover the salsa, you can dissolve ½ teaspoon salt in ½ cup (120 ml) water and add that to the jar.

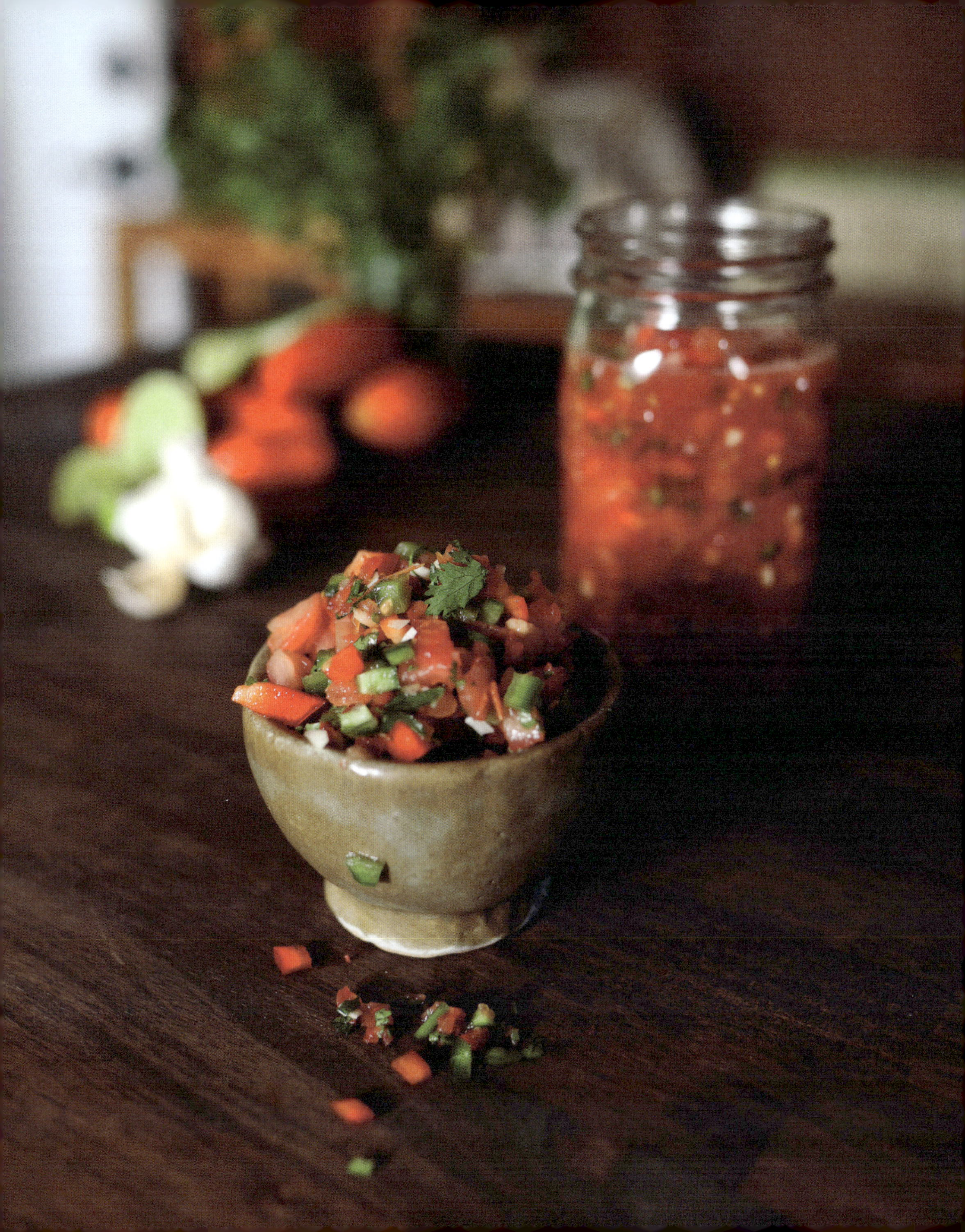

CHAPTER TWO

BREAKFAST

NOT TO SOUND LIKE MY LITERAL MOTHER,

but breakfast might actually be the most important meal of the day. Like many, I used to religiously skip breakfast. "It makes me feel sick," "If I eat breakfast, I get hungry so quickly afterward," or "I just don't have time," I would say. I was partial to the champions' breakfast of a quad shot of espresso and a cigarette, myself, but I was a victim of the early 2000s "heroin chic" Tumblr era and had a raging eating disorder, so let's not take notes from teen Rebekah.

Little did I know that this breakfast habit was having the opposite of the desired effect, wreaking havoc on my metabolic health, cortisol function, and hormone balance. It took a long time to undo and relearn those habits.

These days, I don't skip breakfast. In fact, I don't have coffee until I've eaten breakfast, which I try to do within 30 minutes to an hour of waking up. Here's why: Regular daily breakfast habits are associated with a major decrease in cardiovascular and metabolic disease, type 2 diabetes, obesity, hypertension, and stroke—among other things. Eating breakfast, particularly foods high in fiber and protein, improves insulin sensitivity and helps stabilize blood sugar, preventing sudden blood glucose spikes. This in turn signals the body to reduce the elevated cortisol levels that wake us up in the morning. Eating breakfast also provides the nutrients you need to begin producing essential hormones and other functions for the day.

Consistently skipping breakfast is correlated with higher average daily cortisol levels. Elevated cortisol levels have a domino effect through the endocrine system and can contribute to hormone imbalances as the body tries to make up for the dysregulation.

For women, breakfast is especially important for our monthly hormone cycle. Eating a protein-rich breakfast decreases hunger hormones and signals fullness hormones, which improves satiety and helps regulate appetite throughout the day. So when I said eating breakfast made me hungrier, it was because I wasn't eating a substantial, balanced breakfast (half a grapefruit and half a piece of toast isn't really going to cut it).

So eat breakfast. Eat soon after waking. Try to avoid sugar and simple carbs, and really lean into protein, healthy fats, and lots of fiber. The recipes in this chapter, which range from easy meal-prep brekkies to slow weekend brunches, will inspire your journey!

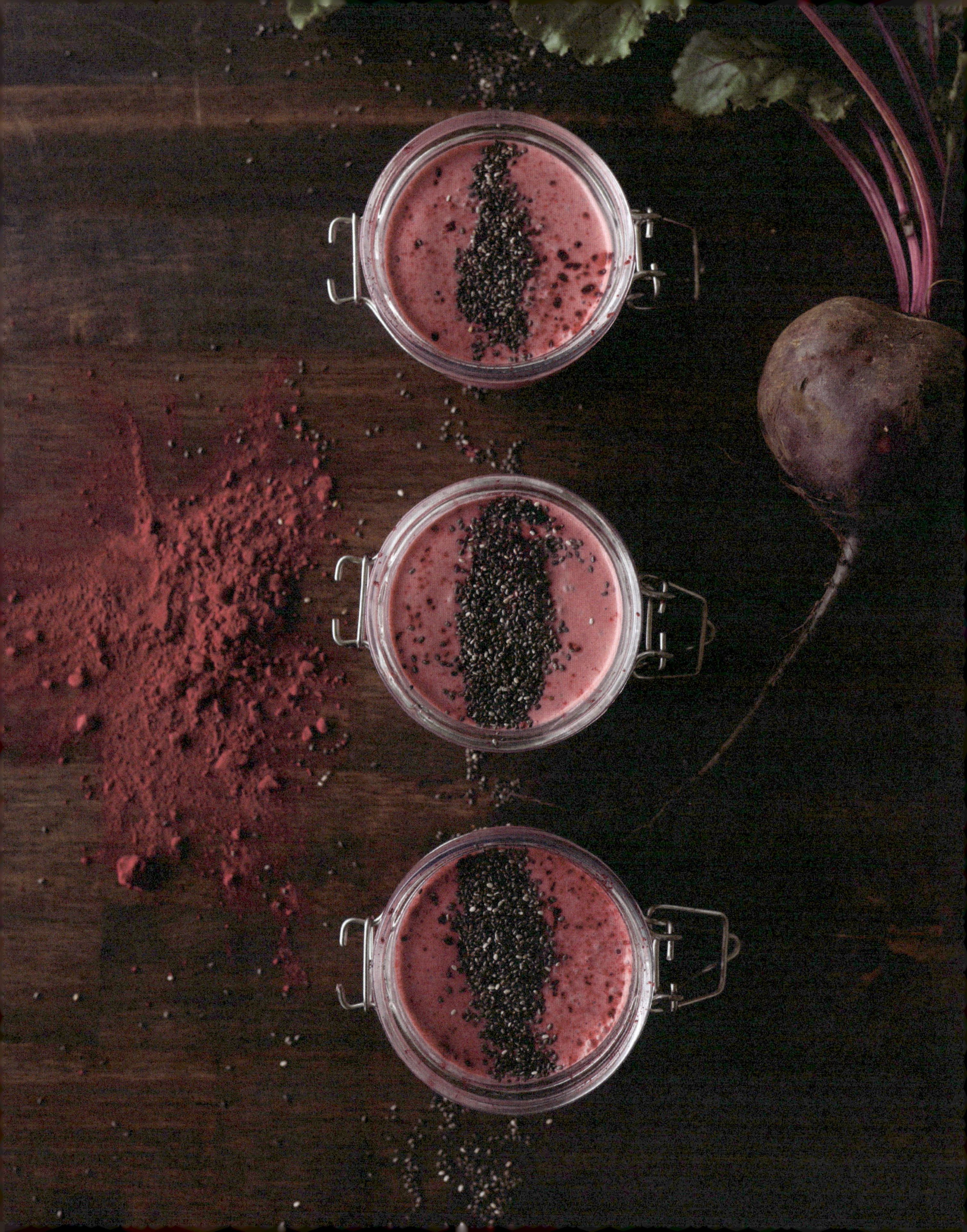

BEET-BERRY CHIA PUDDING

SERVES 8

Rest: 8 hours, 30 minutes
Prep: 10 minutes

Dairy Free
Gluten Free
Menstrual Phase

If you need a make-ahead, fiber-rich, blood sugar-balancing, hormone-healthy breakfast, this is the one. Chia seeds are so powerful for such teeny tiny seeds. They're rich in omega-3s, which are essential for brain function and fighting inflammation, plus they're mineral rich and high in fiber. Don't eat them dry, though; they soak up so much moisture and expand, so they can gum up the works in your gut. The best way to get all their goodness is to soak them in liquid until they have fully expanded, and the yummiest way to do that is with an overnight chia pudding recipe like this one! The beets bring in extra fiber and nutrients like folate. This is so good on its own or topped with whipped coconut cream and berries.

2 small (120 g) beets, cooked (see Note), or 2 tablespoons beet powder
3 cups (720 ml) coconut milk
½ cup (75 g) frozen berries
¾ cup (125 g) chia seeds
¼ cup (60 ml) maple syrup
½ teaspoon vanilla extract
Pinch of sea salt

1. Add the beets, coconut milk, and berries to a blender and blend on high until smooth, about 20 seconds.
2. Add the chia seeds, maple syrup, vanilla extract, and salt, and blend again briefly, about 10 seconds.
3. Pour into one large, lidded container or eight individual jars. Cover and place in the fridge for 30 minutes.
4. Remove from the fridge and stir the mixture once. Return to the fridge and let rest for at least 8 hours or overnight. Store in the fridge for up to 1 week.

NOTE

To cook the beets, you can boil them whole in a small pot of water for 20 to 30 minutes, until fork tender, or cut them into 1-inch (2.5 cm) chunks and roast them in a 400°F (200°C) oven for about 40 minutes, or until tender. You can also buy precooked beets.

OATS

I'm an oat lover. You'll see throughout this book that they pop up in the strangest of places! Sometimes they get a bit of a bad rap, and I think that's unfair. Let me convert you.

Oats are a carb, yes. But carbs are not our enemy! Carbohydrates are essential for so many basic bodily functions (though they can spike blood glucose and cause issues for those with insulin disorders or who are on a weight-loss journey).

But oats, our besties, are low-glycemic, meaning their high fiber content slows our digestion of their carbs and absorption of their sugars. Oats can actually help regulate blood sugar.

When it comes to hormone health, oats reign again. They contain lignans, a type of phytoestrogen. Phytoestrogens mimic estrogen (one of our sex hormones) in the body, and while some people get nervous that this could cause an excess of estrogen, that's actually not the case. Lignans help regulate estrogen in the body, supporting estrogen production if levels are too low or signaling estrogen to decrease if levels are too high. Oats have fewer phytoestrogens than foods like soy or flax, making them gentle for estrogen-dominant individuals, and their other components further support balanced hormone production. Oats are also good for your heart; the phytoestrogens and beta-glucans in oats can help lower cholesterol. They are full of polyphenols and antioxidants that combat inflammation, too. Oats are amazing!

What's Not to Love: Glyphosate

Oats tend to be sprayed more heavily with pesticides and herbicides than other crops, so they usually contain particularly high levels of the herbicide glyphosate. Glyphosate is known to cause gastrointestinal distress and is linked to other significant health risks. If consuming oats regularly, it is ideal, if not essential, that you choose organic oats to avoid this issue altogether.

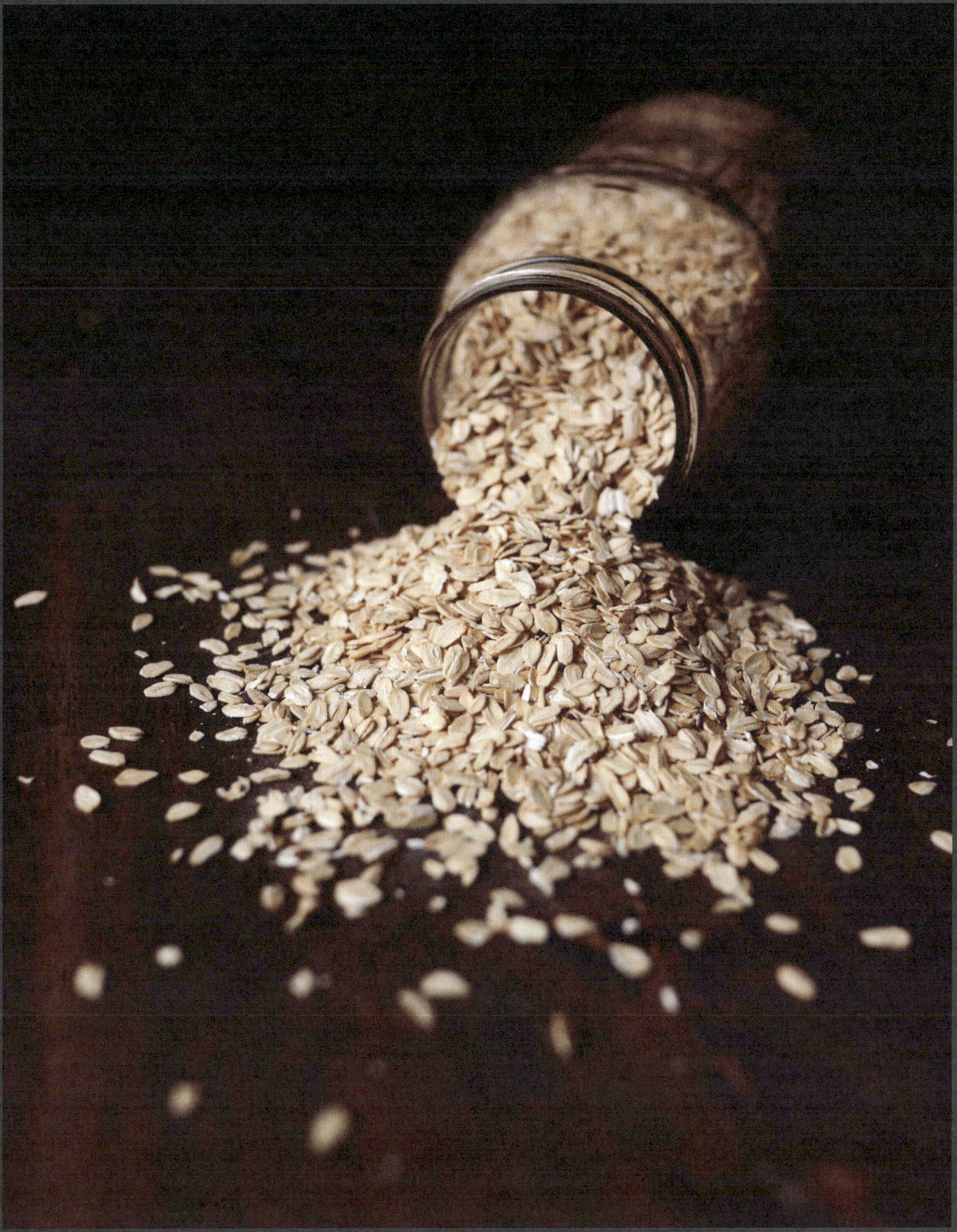

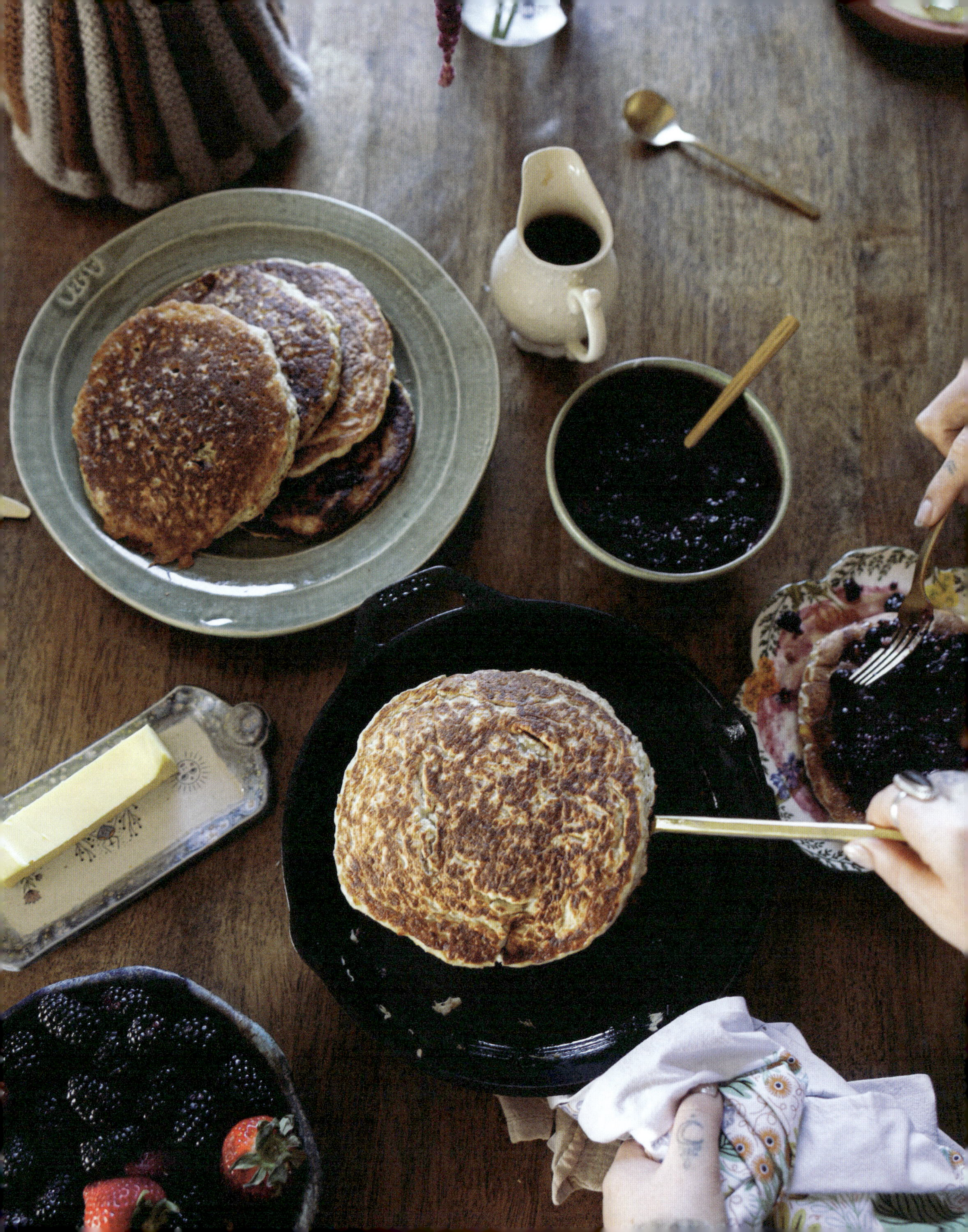

MAMA TESSA'S OVERNIGHT OAT PANCAKES

SERVES 4

Rest: 8 hours
Prep: 10 minutes
Cook: 12 minutes

Follicular Phase

These pancakes will give you a good dose of protein and fiber and keep you full till lunch! The overnight soak at room temperature helps neutralize phytic acid and makes these pancakes super digestible. My mom's simplified recipe is three ingredients at night (buttermilk, quick oats, and flour) and three in the morning (eggs, baking powder, and baking soda). So easy! I've adapted the recipe slightly over the years, but these pancakes are very forgiving and can handle adaptations. If you have seeds on hand, include them; if you don't, leave them out. I love to eat these pancakes with berry compote and a little Greek yogurt to make them extra filling.

1½ cups (360 ml) milk, divided
1 cup (240 ml) plain whole-milk yogurt or Kefir (page 69)
1 cup (80 g) quick oats
1 cup (80 g) rolled oats
½ cup (60 g) whole wheat flour
2 tablespoons chia seeds (optional)
2 tablespoons flaxseeds (optional; see Note 1)
3 large eggs
1 teaspoon baking powder
1 teaspoon baking soda
1 tablespoon coconut oil

BERRY COMPOTE

2 cups (300 g) frozen berries
1 tablespoon coconut oil
1 tablespoon maple syrup or honey

1. *Make the batter:* The night before you want to cook the pancakes, combine 1 cup (240 ml) of the milk, the yogurt, quick oats, rolled oats, flour, and chia seeds and flaxseeds (if using) in a large bowl. Cover with a plate and let rest at room temperature for 8 hours or overnight.
2. In the morning, add the remaining ½ cup (120 ml) of milk and the eggs, baking powder, and baking soda. Stir to combine.
3. *Make the berry compote:* Heat the berries, coconut oil, and maple syrup in a small saucepan over medium heat. Let cook while you make the pancakes, until the berries have broken down, about 10 minutes.
4. *Cook the pancakes:* Heat a 10-inch (25 cm) pan or skillet over medium heat until a sprinkle of water from your fingers dances when it hits the pan. Add the coconut oil to the pan and let it melt.
5. Use a ¼ cup or ⅓ cup (60 to 80 ml) measure to scoop the batter onto the hot pan—it should sizzle but not smoke. Cook until the top has a few bubbles and the edges puff and Begin to look cooked, 2 to 3 minutes. Flip to cook the other side, 2 to 3 more minutes. Repeat with the remaining batter (see Note 2).
6. Serve with the berry compote on top.

NOTES

1. If you use the flaxseeds, add ¼ cup (60 ml) milk in step 2, as the seeds will soak up a little more liquid.

2. As you continue cooking pancakes, you may need to turn down the heat a little, especially if you're using a cast-iron pan. The toughest part of cooking pancakes is finding the correct temperature so that they cook through without burning!

GLUTEN-FREE BANANA PANCAKES

SERVES 4

Prep: 5 minutes
Cook: 15 minutes

Dairy Free

Gluten Free

Hormone Supportive

Ovulation Phase

This is one of my go-to recipes—quick, easy, forgiving, and simple to adapt. I started making a version of these without the oats when I was eating a Paleo diet, and later, I added the oats to make the pancakes a bit more substantial and easier to flip. They're filling and easy on the tummy, with a good amount of protein to kickstart the day. These pancakes already have some sweetness, so I love to eat them with just a bit of butter or coconut oil, yogurt, berries, or even completely plain! The leftovers also make a really great running-out-the-door snack.

1 tablespoon coconut oil
2 bananas
3 egg whites
½ cup (40 g) quick oats
⅓ cup (85 g) peanut butter or other nut butter
2 tablespoons plus 2 teaspoons maple syrup
½ teaspoon baking soda
½ teaspoon ground cinnamon

1. Heat a medium pan over medium heat. When the pan is warm, add the coconut oil. It should quickly melt and cover the bottom but not smoke.
2. Place the bananas, egg whites, oats, peanut butter, maple syrup, baking soda, and cinnamon in a blender and blend until almost smooth.
3. Add a drop of the batter to the pan and see if it quickly sizzles but doesn't smoke. If so, you are good to go! Add the batter to the pan about ¼ cup (60 ml) at a time. Cook until the edges are slightly cooked and the pancake releases when you slide a spatula underneath, about 2 minutes. I find they are best flipped a little earlier than you'd think—when the batter on top is still quite wet.
4. Cook on the other side until the sides are dry, 1 or 2 more minutes. Repeat with the remaining pancake batter and then serve.

VARIATIONS

- These pancakes are incredibly customizable. You can replace the oats with ¼ cup (30 g) of flour or leave them out altogether. You can also add a scoop of your favorite protein powder. These variations will all change the texture slightly—thinner, thicker, fluffier, eggier—but I promise you that the pancakes will still be so good!

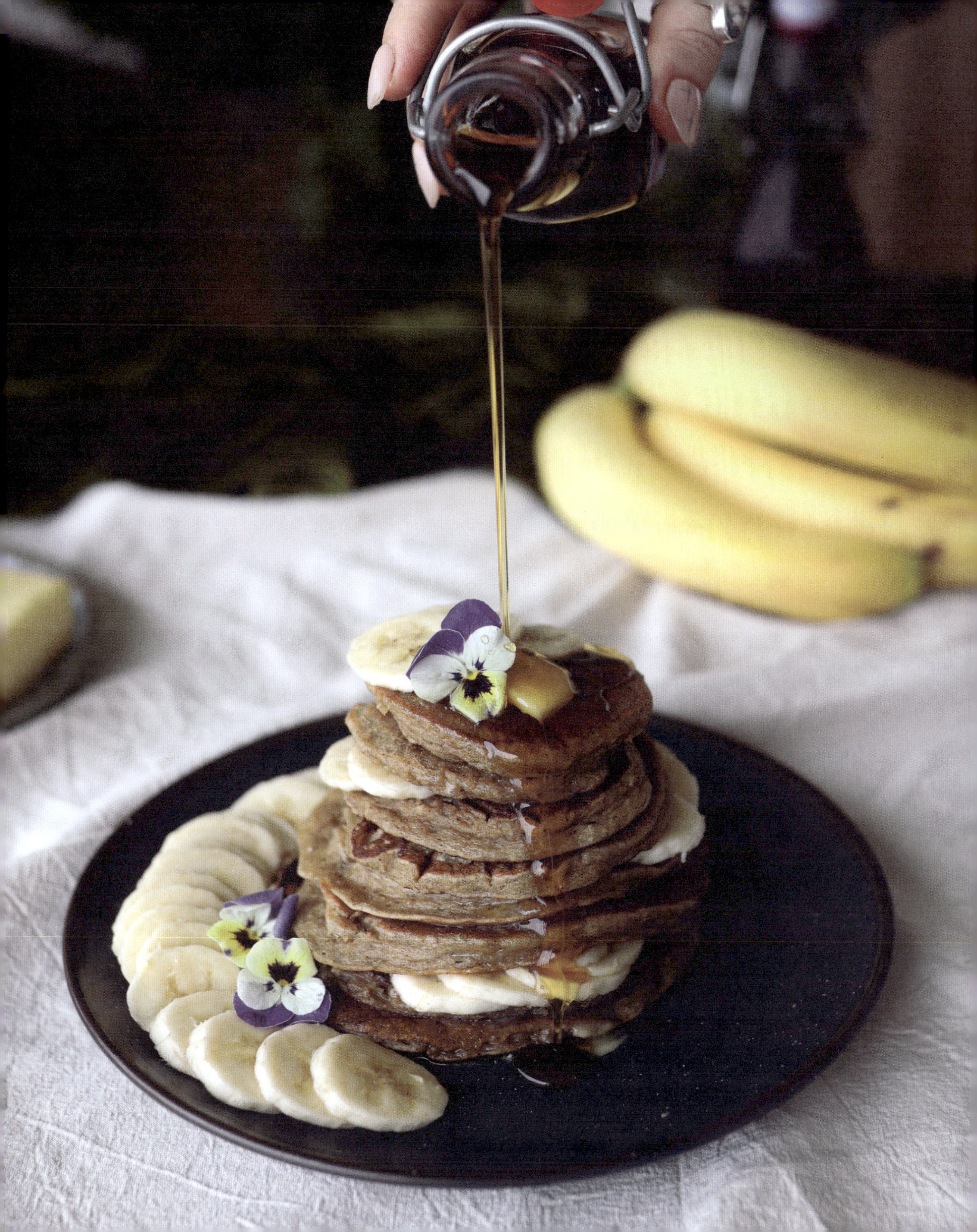

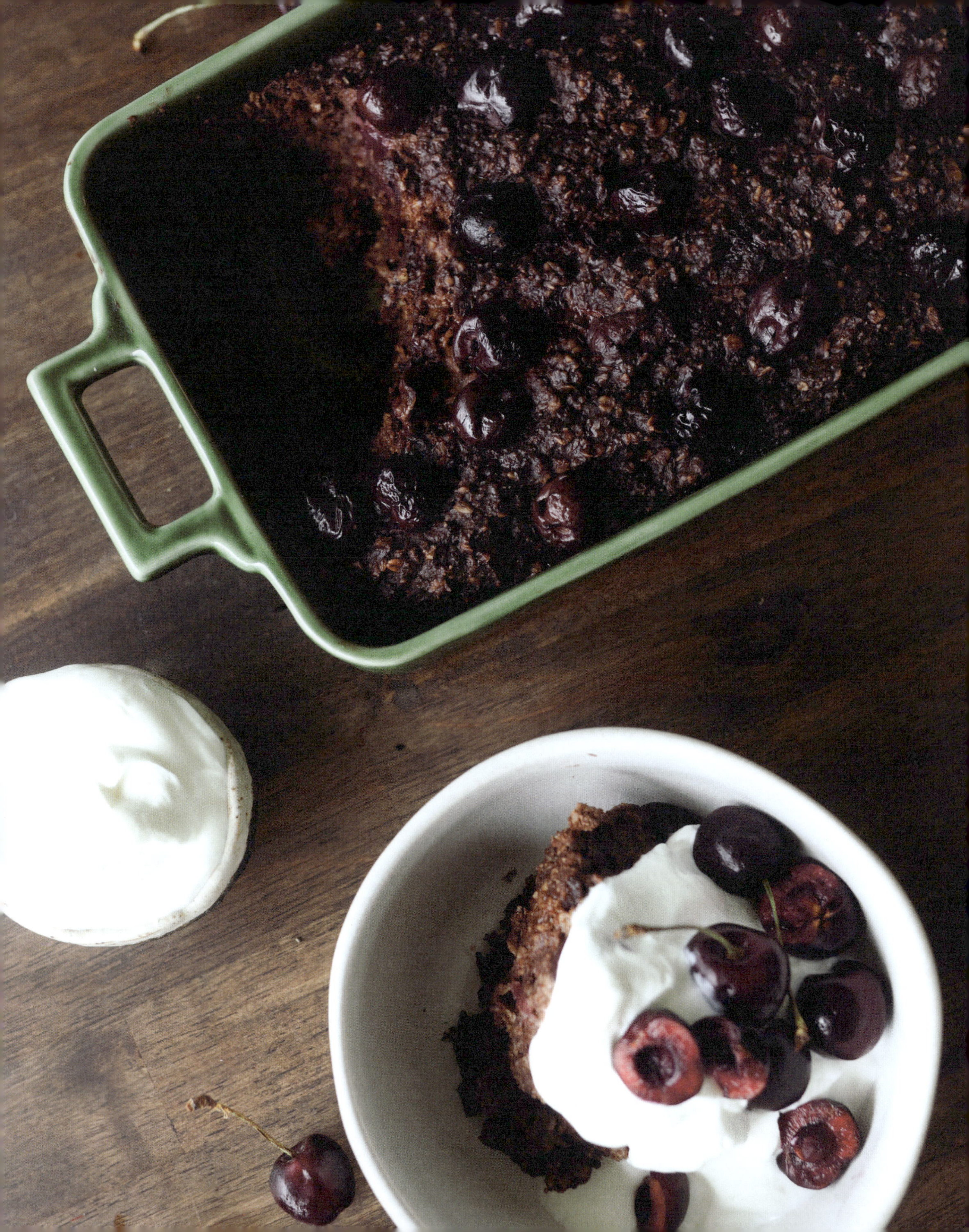

CHOCOLATE-CHERRY OVERNIGHT BAKED OATMEAL

SERVES 8

Rest: 8 hours
Prep: 10 minutes
Cook: 35 minutes

Anti-Inflammatory
Blood Sugar Balancing
Gluten Free
Hormone Supportive
Menstrual Phase

The fact that I can mix this up *right in the baking dish* and just shove it in the oven the next morning is magical. Soaking the oats overnight breaks down the starches and phytic acid, making them easier to digest and giving them a fluffier texture. This recipe tastes like dessert but will keep the crew full till lunch. It's mildly sweet, so you can drizzle on honey or maple syrup to taste, and it's best served with a dollop of Greek yogurt, which provides healthy fats to help metabolize the nutrients in the oatmeal and keep you satiated. I love this for a nourishing menstrual phase meal or a meal train delivery, as it's so full of good minerals and fiber while still feeling like a treat. Cue the music.

Butter, for greasing
2 cups (160 g) quick oats
⅓ cup (40 g) cacao powder
¼ cup (28 g) flax meal
½ teaspoon baking soda
½ teaspoon ground cinnamon
1 cup (240 ml) full-fat Greek yogurt, plus more for serving
½ cup (120 ml) smooth peanut butter
1 cup (240 ml) water or milk
3 eggs
½ cup (120 ml) maple syrup
1½ cups (200 g) frozen cherries
Honey, for serving

1. Grease a 9-inch (23 cm) square glass baking dish with butter.
2. Add the oats, cacao, flax meal, baking soda, and cinnamon, and stir.
3. Add the yogurt, peanut butter, water, eggs, and maple syrup. Beat the eggs into the mixture and stir thoroughly until no globs of egg or yogurt remain.
4. Brazenly scatter the cherries over the top. Cover and place in the fridge for at least 8 hours or overnight.
5. Remove the baking dish from the fridge and place it straight into a cold oven (the glass dish may crack if you transfer it directly from a cold fridge to a hot oven).
6. Heat the oven to 350°F (175°C). Bake the oatmeal for 35 to 40 minutes, until the edges are browned and the center is cooked but still soft.
7. Serve with generous dollops of Greek yogurt and drizzles of honey.

SHAKSHUKA

This is the perfect weekend breakfast or lazy lunch for an ovulation phase meal. Light, flavorful, full of vitamin C, and with plenty of protein to start the day, shakshuka will give you energy without weighing you down. The feta and herbs add dimensions of flavor that you don't want to miss! Serve it up in a skillet with generous hunks of warm sourdough or pita bread and grass-fed butter and dive in with some friends, because you are going to want to share this one.

SERVES 5

***Prep:* 15 minutes**
***Cook:* 55 minutes**

Anti-Inflammatory
Blood Sugar Balancing
Gluten Free
Hormone Supportive
Ovulation Phase

2 tablespoons olive oil
1 medium yellow onion, finely chopped
½ medium red bell pepper, chopped
Sea salt
4 garlic cloves, grated or crushed
2 teaspoons smoked paprika
1 teaspoon ground coriander
1 teaspoon ground cumin
½ to 1 teaspoon chili powder, to taste
Black pepper, to taste
2 tablespoons tomato paste
One 28-ounce (794 g) can crushed fire-roasted tomatoes
One 28-ounce (794 g) can diced tomatoes
5 large eggs
½ cup (75 g) crumbled feta

HERB DRIZZLE

⅓ cup (80 ml) olive oil
4 garlic cloves
1 small bunch fresh parsley, roughly chopped
Juice of 1 lemon, or more to taste
½ teaspoon sea salt, or more to taste

1. Heat a large heavy-bottomed skillet or cast-iron pan over medium heat. Add the olive oil, followed by the onion, bell pepper, and ½ teaspoon salt. Stir and sauté until the onions are translucent and the peppers begin to brown, about 5 minutes.
2. Add the garlic and cook until fragrant, 3 to 4 minutes, stirring to prevent it from burning.
3. Add the paprika, coriander, cumin, chili powder, pepper, and a good pinch of salt. Stir continuously for 1 or 2 minutes to bloom the spices. Add the tomato paste, stirring until it's softened and evenly distributed.
4. Pour in the crushed tomatoes and diced tomatoes and stir. Reduce the heat to low and let simmer slowly for 20 to 30 minutes, stirring occasionally, until the sauce is thickened and deeper in color. Taste and add salt and pepper if needed.
5. Use the back of a serving spoon to make five little divots in the sauce, one in the center and the rest around the outside.
6. Crack an egg into each divot, season with salt and pepper, and scatter the feta around the pan. Cover and cook until the whites are set and the yolks are cooked to your liking, 8 to 10 minutes. For sunny-side up eggs, use a fork to break up the whites a little and jiggle them down into the sauce, and cook uncovered.
7. *Meanwhile, make the herb drizzle:* Add the olive oil, garlic, parsley, lemon juice, and salt to a blender and blend on high until combined but not completely smooth, about 10 seconds. You can also use a jar and an immersion blender.
8. Once the eggs are cooked, remove from the heat, drizzle generously with the herb sauce, and serve.

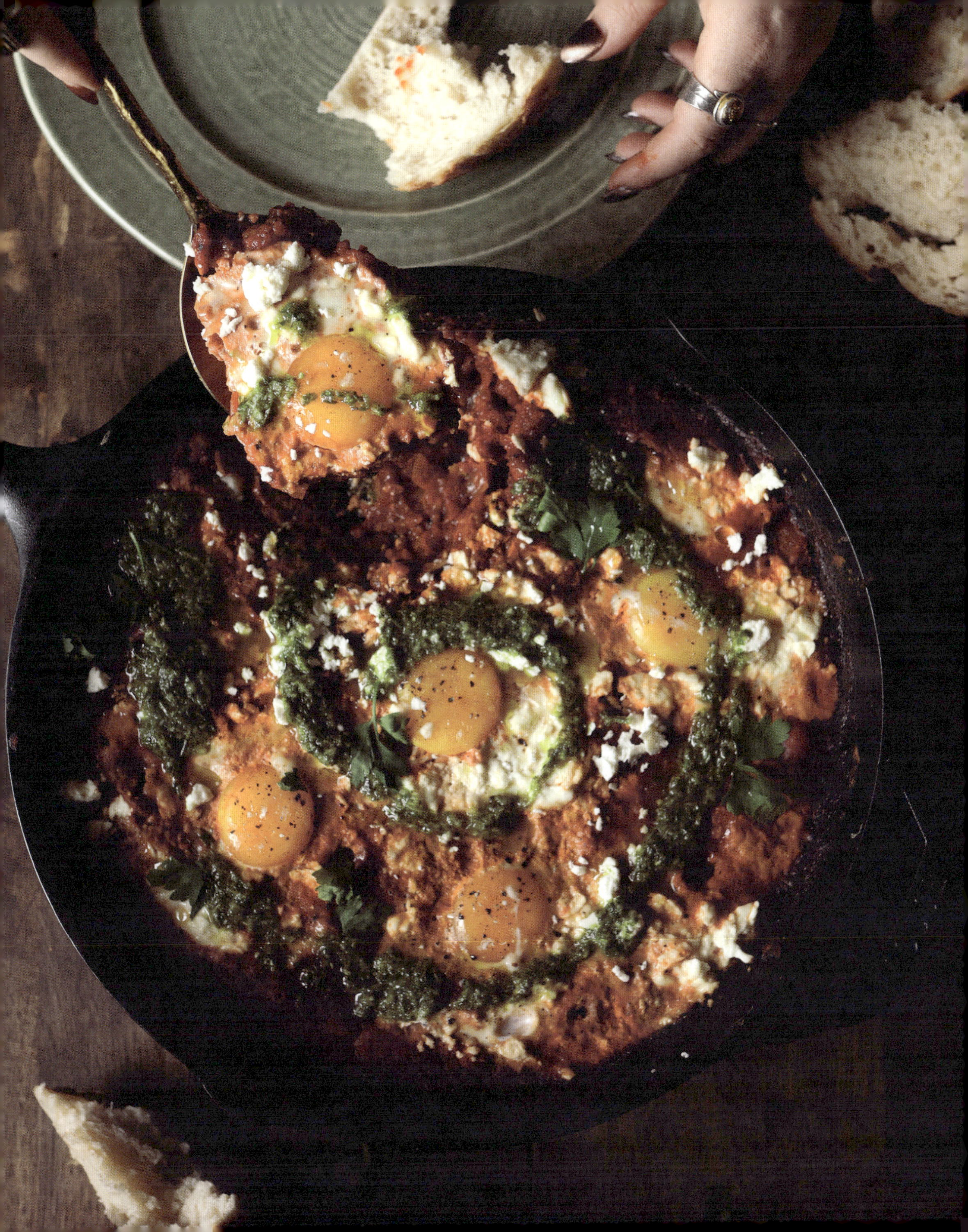

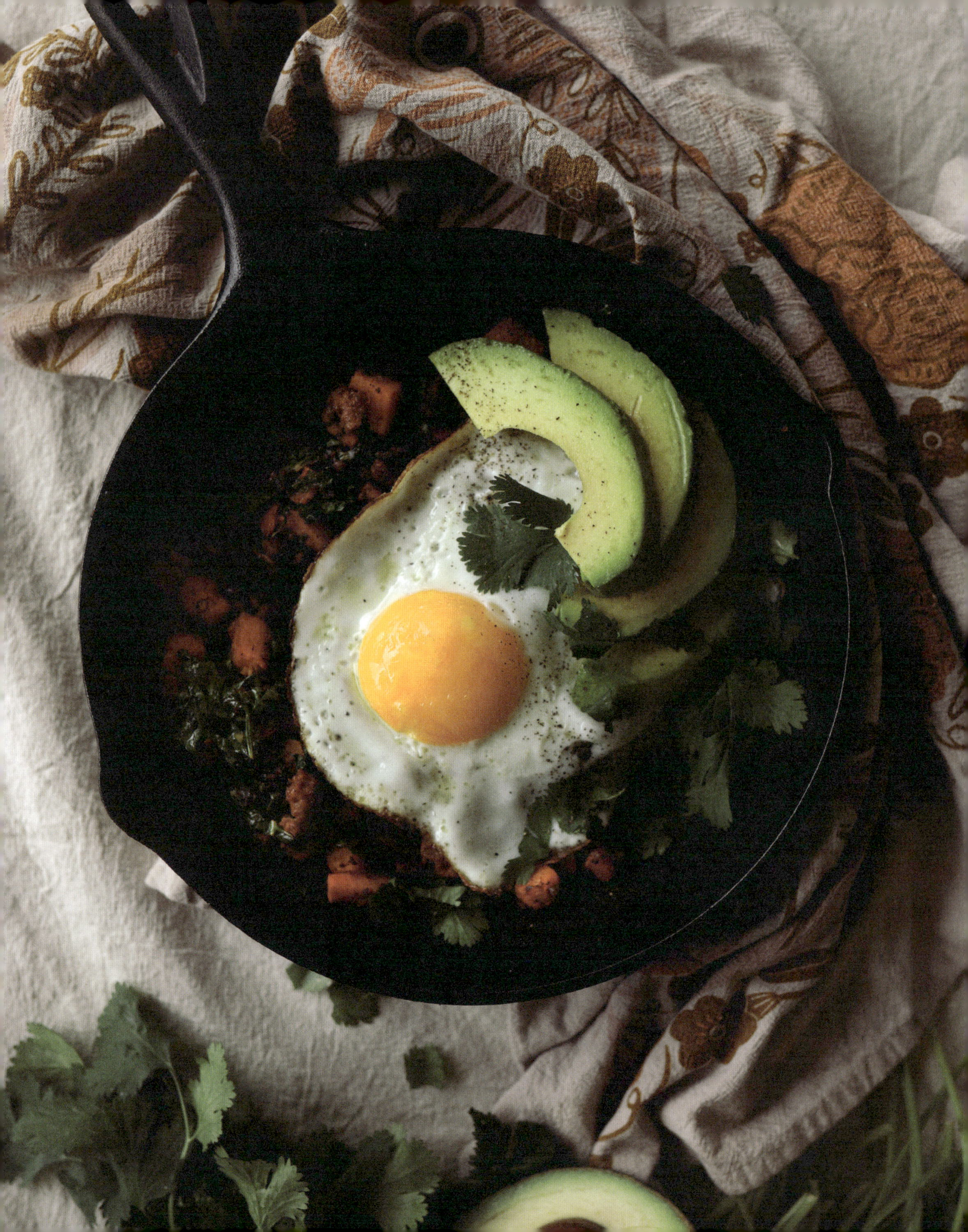

CHORIZO SWEET POTATO HASH

SERVES 4 TO 6

Prep: 10 minutes
Cook: 30 minutes

Gluten Free
Luteal Phase
Menstrual Phase

I go weak at the knees for a breakfast hash, and this one is elite. It's a fuel-your-whole-day type of breakfast. It's quick and easy if you've prepped the Smoked Paprika Sweet Potatoes (page 134) ahead of time, but even if you haven't, you can just throw them in the oven before prepping the rest of the ingredients, and they will be done in time! If you aren't a pork fan, I highly recommend Foodies Pumfu Chorizo Crumble, a meat substitute made of pumpkin seeds that makes this a killer combo for the menstrual phase. Choose your own adventure with the eggs: Scramble them in or add them on top at the end, and don't forget some extra yummy garnishes.

2 tablespoons avocado oil
½ medium red onion, chopped
½ large red bell pepper, chopped
Sea salt
1 pound (454 g) ground chorizo or Foodies Pumfu Chorizo Crumble
2 garlic cloves, crushed or grated
2 cups (400 g) Smoked Paprika Sweet Potatoes (page 134)
1 bunch kale (6 to 8 stems), julienned
4 to 6 large eggs
¼ cup (60 ml) milk (if scrambling eggs)
Black pepper, to taste

FOR SERVING

Cotija or feta crumbles
Sliced avocado
Harissa dollops

1. Heat a large skillet over medium heat. Add the avocado oil and swirl to coat the pan.
2. Add the onion, bell pepper, and ½ teaspoon salt, and sauté, stirring often, until the veggies begin to soften, 3 to 4 minutes.
3. Add the chorizo and cook until mostly browned, breaking it up with a spatula to form small crumbles, about 7 minutes.
4. Make a little space in the center of the pan and add the garlic (see Tip 1), stirring while it browns to keep it from burning, about 1 minute, then stir it into the chorizo mixture.
5. Reduce the heat to medium-low and add the sweet potato and kale, stirring to combine. Sauté until the sweet potato is heated and browning on the edges and the kale has softened, 5 to 10 minutes (see Tip 2). Stir occasionally to keep everything from sticking.
6. *To make a scramble*, whisk the eggs with the milk, ¼ teaspoon salt, and ⅛ teaspoon pepper in a small bowl. Pour them over the mixture in the pan and cook, scraping the bottom often, 2 to 3 minutes. To fry the eggs, create little wells in the chorizo and vegetable mixture and crack an egg into each. Sprinkle with salt and pepper and cook for 3 to 5 minutes, until cooked to your preference. You can place a lid on the pan to help the eggs cook through if you like. Remove from the heat.
7. Sprinkle with cotija and top with avocado and a dollop of harissa for extra heat and flavor!

TIPS

1. If the pan looks dry, you can add a little oil before cooking the garlic.

2. You can continue to sauté until the ingredients reach your preferred level of crispness. I like my chorizo extra browned and my veggies a little caramelized on the edges.

EGG BITES

MAKES 24

Prep: 15 minutes
Cook: 50 minutes

Blood Sugar Balancing

Gluten Free

Hormone Supportive

If you prep one thing ahead, make it breakfast! And if you're gonna prep breakfast, it should be these fluffy, perfect egg bites. They're simple, versatile, and easy to store and reheat. Protein, fats, and some good veggies—choose your own add-ins, catering to exactly to exactly what you need to start your day well. I've made four variations, one for each phase of the hormone cycle, so you can just pick your ingredients and slot them into the recipe!

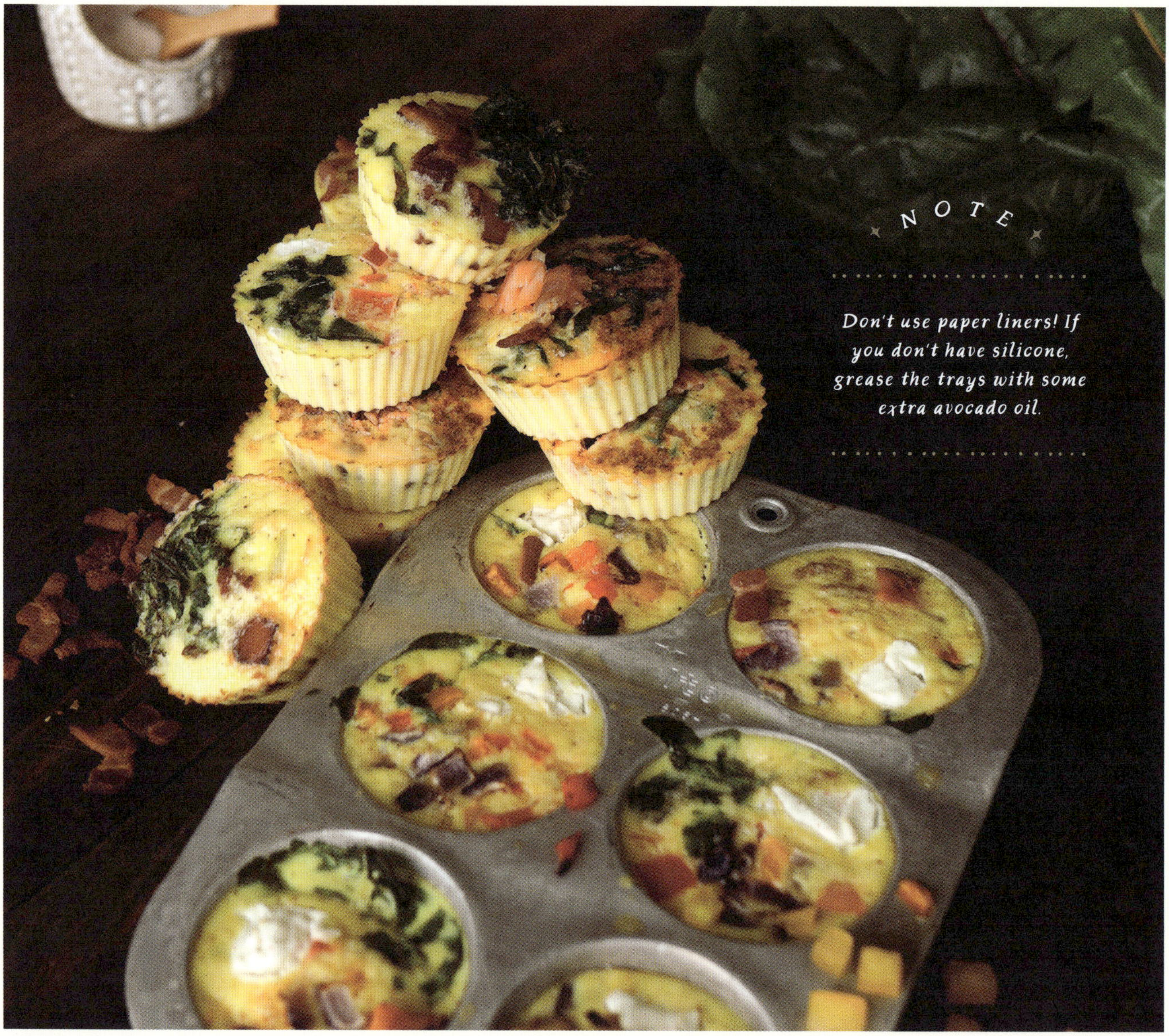

NOTE

Don't use paper liners! If you don't have silicone, grease the trays with some extra avocado oil.

1. Choose and make the filling.

MENSTRUAL PHASE

1 cup (225 g) raw chopped bacon

1 cup (150 g) finely chopped potato

Sea salt, to taste

2 cups (50 g) chopped kale

- Toss the bacon in a large, cold skillet and cook over medium heat until crispy, about 10 minutes. Transfer to a plate, reserving about 2 tablespoons of bacon fat in the pan.
- Add the potato to the pan, sprinkle with salt, cover with a lid, and cook until soft, stirring occasionally, about 10 minutes.
- Return the bacon to the pan and add the kale. Cook until the kale softens, 1 to 2 minutes, then remove from the heat.

FOLLICULAR PHASE

2 tablespoons avocado oil, divided

1 cup (130 g) Foodies Pumfu Chorizo Crumble or other plant-based chorizo

¾ cup (100 g) diced zucchini

¼ cup (35 g) diced bell pepper

¼ cup (40 g) diced onion

Sea salt, to taste

2 cups (70 g) chopped Swiss chard

- Warm a large skillet over medium heat, add 1 tablespoon of avocado oil and the Pumfu, and cook until heated through and beginning to crisp, breaking it apart with a spatula as it cooks, about 5 minutes. Transfer to a plate and set aside.
- Add the remaining avocado oil to the pan, then add the zucchini, bell pepper, and onion, sprinkle with salt, and cook until tender, 5 to 7 minutes.
- Return the Pumfu to the pan and add the chard. Cook until the chard softens, 1 to 2 minutes, then remove from the heat.

OVULATION PHASE

1 tablespoon avocado oil

1 cup (180 g) diced tomato

Sea salt, to taste

2 packed cups (70 g) chopped spinach

1 cup (150 g) finely chopped smoked salmon

- Warm a large skillet over medium heat and add the avocado oil.
- Add the tomato, sprinkle with salt, and cook until the juices have released and evaporated, 3 to 5 minutes.
- Add the spinach and salmon to the pan. Cook until the spinach softens, 1 to 2 minutes, then remove from the heat.

LUTEAL PHASE

1 cup (130 g) minced turkey sausage

1 tablespoon avocado oil

1 cup (150 g) finely chopped sweet potato

½ cup (80 g) diced onion

Sea salt, to taste

1 cup (70 g) chopped arugula

- Heat a large skillet over medium heat. Add the sausage and cook, breaking it apart with a spatula until browned, about 5 minutes. Transfer to a plate and set aside.
- Add the avocado oil to the pan, then add the sweet potato and onion, sprinkle with salt, cover with a lid, and cook, stirring occasionally, until softened, about 10 minutes.
- Return the sausage to the pan and add the arugula. Cook until the arugula softens, 1 to 2 minutes, then remove from the heat.

2. Make the egg base.

14 large eggs

1 cup (210 g) full-fat cottage cheese

½ cup (60 g) grated cheddar

1 teaspoon sea salt

½ teaspoon black pepper

- Preheat the oven to 350°F (175°C). Line two muffin pans with silicone liners (see Note).
- Place the eggs, cottage cheese, cheddar, salt, and pepper in a blender. Blend on high until just combined, 5 to 10 seconds.
- Fill each muffin liner about three-fourths of the way with the egg mixture. Add about 1 tablespoon of filling to each (if you have leftover filling, save it to make with scrambled eggs within a week).

3. Add the toppings.

- *Menstrual Phase:* Top the egg bites with **½ cup (60 g) grated cheddar.**
- *Follicular Phase:* Top the egg bites with **½ cup (120 ml) harissa.**
- *Ovulation Phase:* Top the egg bites with **½ cup (120 g) cream cheese.**
- *Luteal Phase:* Top the egg bites with **½ cup (90 g) goat cheese.**

4. Bake the egg bites.

- Place each muffin pan in a slightly larger baking dish and fill the larger pans with hot water halfway up the sides of the muffin pans. This will ensure fluffy egg bites!
- Carefully transfer the pans to the oven and bake for 30 to 35 minutes, until firm.
- Remove from the oven and let cool completely. Remove the egg bites from the muffin pans. Store in an airtight container in the fridge for up to 1 week or in a ziplock bag in the freezer for up to 1 month.

BREAKFAST BOWLS

EACH RECIPE SERVES 2

Menstrual Phase

Buckwheat Breakfast Bowl

Prep: 5 minutes • Cook: 20 minutes

Buckwheat is restorative, easy to digest, and rich in the iron and minerals you need during the menstrual phase. Beets and kale support circulation and blood flow, and pumpkin seeds provide micronutrient goodies that support your hormone balance and help you feel your best.

2 cups (480 ml) Bone Broth (page 159) or water
1 cup (160 g) buckwheat, soaked overnight and rinsed
2 tablespoons salted butter
Pinch of sea salt
⅓ cup (45 g) roasted beets (see Note)
1 packed cup (40 g) rubbed kale from Rubbed Kale and Acorn Squash Salad (page 108)
¼ cup (35 g) pumpkin seeds
¼ cup (30 g) crumbled goat cheese
Honey, to taste
Soy sauce or liquid aminos, to taste

1. Bring the broth to a boil in a medium saucepan and stir in the buckwheat, butter, and a pinch of salt. Return to a boil and then reduce to a simmer, cover, and cook for 15 minutes, or until the liquid has absorbed.
2. Scatter the pumpkin seeds onto a parchment paper–lined baking sheet and place on the center rack of the oven. Broil on high on the center rack for about 5 minutes, until they begin to brown and smell nutty. Remove from the oven and set aside.
3. Divide the buckwheat between two bowls. Top with the beets, rubbed kale, toasted pumpkin seeds, goat cheese, a generous drizzle of honey, and a dash of soy sauce.

NOTE

To roast the beets, cut them into 1-inch (2.5 cm) chunks and roast them in a 400°F (200°C) oven for about 40 minutes, until tender.

Follicular Phase, Gluten Free

Savory Oats Breakfast Bowl

Prep: 5 minutes • Cook: 30 minutes

Phytoestrogens in oats balance rising estrogen, support blood sugar regulation, and reduce inflammation to support follicle development. The avocado provides healthy fats to protect cells from oxidative stress, and cashews, which are rich in zinc, help to prepare for healthy ovulation.

1 tablespoon olive oil, plus more for drizzling
¼ small white onion, diced
1 garlic clove, chopped
1 cup (80 g) steel-cut oats
2 cups (480 ml) Bone Broth (page 159) or water
1 to 2 cups (240 to 480 ml) water (see Note)
Sea salt
Black pepper
1 avocado, pitted, peeled, and sliced
½ cup (75 g) crumbled feta
2 tablespoons cashew butter
Lemon zest, to taste
Honey, to taste

1. Warm the olive oil in a medium pot over medium-low heat. Add the onion and sauté until softened, 2 to 3 minutes. Add the garlic and stir until fragrant, 1 minute.
2. Add the oats and stir to coat them in the oil, onion, and garlic mixture. Let cook gently until fragrant, 2 to 3 minutes.
3. Pour in the broth and water and bring to a boil. Reduce the heat to a simmer, cover, and cook, stirring occasionally, until the oats are tender, 15 to 30 minutes (see Note). Add salt and pepper to taste.
4. Divide the oats between two bowls and top each with avocado, feta, cashew butter, lemon zest, honey, and an extra drizzle of olive oil.

NOTE

For a chewier texture, use 1 cup (240 ml) water and cook for 15 to 20 minutes. For a creamier texture, add 2 cups (480 ml) water and cook for 20 to 30 minutes.

Ovulation Phase, Dairy Free, Gluten Free

Quinoa Breakfast Bowl

Prep: 5 minutes • Cook: 25 minutes

Quinoa provides fiber to detox extra estrogen and protein to support high-energy days during the ovulation phase. Almonds provide vitamin E, fats, and and magnesium, protecting egg health and combating egg health and combat oxidative stress caused by ovulation, and the veggies boost the vitamins and iron that help support the transition into the luteal phase.

1 cup (185 g) quinoa, thoroughly rinsed
1¾ cups (420 ml) Bone Broth (page 159) or water
½ cup (45 g) sliced almonds
1 tablespoon white or apple cider vinegar
2 eggs
2 cups (60 g) chopped baby spinach
Handful of parsley, chopped
2 tablespoons harissa, or to taste
Roasted peppers from Mediterranean Summer Veg (page 135; optional)

1. Place the quinoa and broth in a medium saucepan and bring to a boil, then reduce the heat to low, cover tightly with a lid, and simmer for 15 minutes. Remove from the heat and let sit for 10 minutes, then remove the lid and fluff with a fork.
2. Meanwhile, spread the almonds on a parchment paper–lined baking sheet and place on the center rack of the oven. Broil on medium for 5 minutes, or until the almonds are starting to brown and smell nutty. Remove and set aside.
3. Bring 3 inches (7.5 cm) of water to a boil in a medium saucepan, then reduce the heat to barely a simmer. Add the vinegar and then gently crack the eggs into the pan one at a time. Cook for exactly 4 minutes, then lift the eggs out with a slotted spoon. If you prefer firmer eggs, keep the water at a simmer and cook for 30 more seconds at a time, lifting out in between to check for doneness.
4. Divide the quinoa between two bowls and top each with a poached egg.
5. Drop the spinach into the simmering water for 30 seconds to blanch. Remove with a slotted spoon and drain for a few seconds. Divide the spinach between the bowls.
6. Top with the toasted almonds, parsley, harissa, and roasted peppers (if using).

Luteal Phase

Farro Breakfast Bowl

Prep: 5 minutes • Cook: 20 minutes

Farro helps increase insulin sensitivity, which decreases with the rise in progesterone during the luteal phase. Farro and beef are full of B vitamins that fight PMS and iron to prep for menstruation. Sweet potatoes help satisfy sweet cravings, and sunflower seeds contain targeted minerals for this phase!

½ cup (75 g) farro, soaked overnight and rinsed
1½ cups (360 ml) Bone Broth (page 159) or water
Sea salt
1 tablespoon avocado oil
¼ medium yellow or white onion, finely chopped
½ pound (227 g) minced beef chorizo
2 cups (70 g) thinly sliced Swiss chard
2 eggs
1 cup (150 g) Smoked Paprika Sweet Potatoes (page 134)
¼ cup (35 g) raw sunflower seeds
2 tablespoons salted butter, divided

1. Place the farro and broth in a medium pot with a generous pinch of salt. Bring to a boil and cook for 20 minutes, or until the farro is soft with a little chew. Drain.
2. Meanwhile, heat a medium pan over medium heat. Add the oil and onion and cook until the onion is translucent, 4 to 5 minutes.
3. Add the chorizo and break it up, stirring regularly, until browned, 4 to 5 minutes.
4. Add the chard and stir until wilted and incorporated, then remove the mixture from the pan and set aside in a warm spot. Leave some of the oil in the pan.
5. Crack the eggs into the pan and cook to your liking. For sunny-side up, cook for 3 to 4 minutes without flipping. For over easy, cook for 2½ to 3 minutes, then flip and cook for for 20 to 30 seconds. For over medium, flip and cook for 45 to 70 seconds. For over hard, flip and cook for 2 to 3 minutes.
6. Divide the farro between two bowls. Top with the chorizo mixture, eggs, sweet potato, sunflower seeds, and butter.

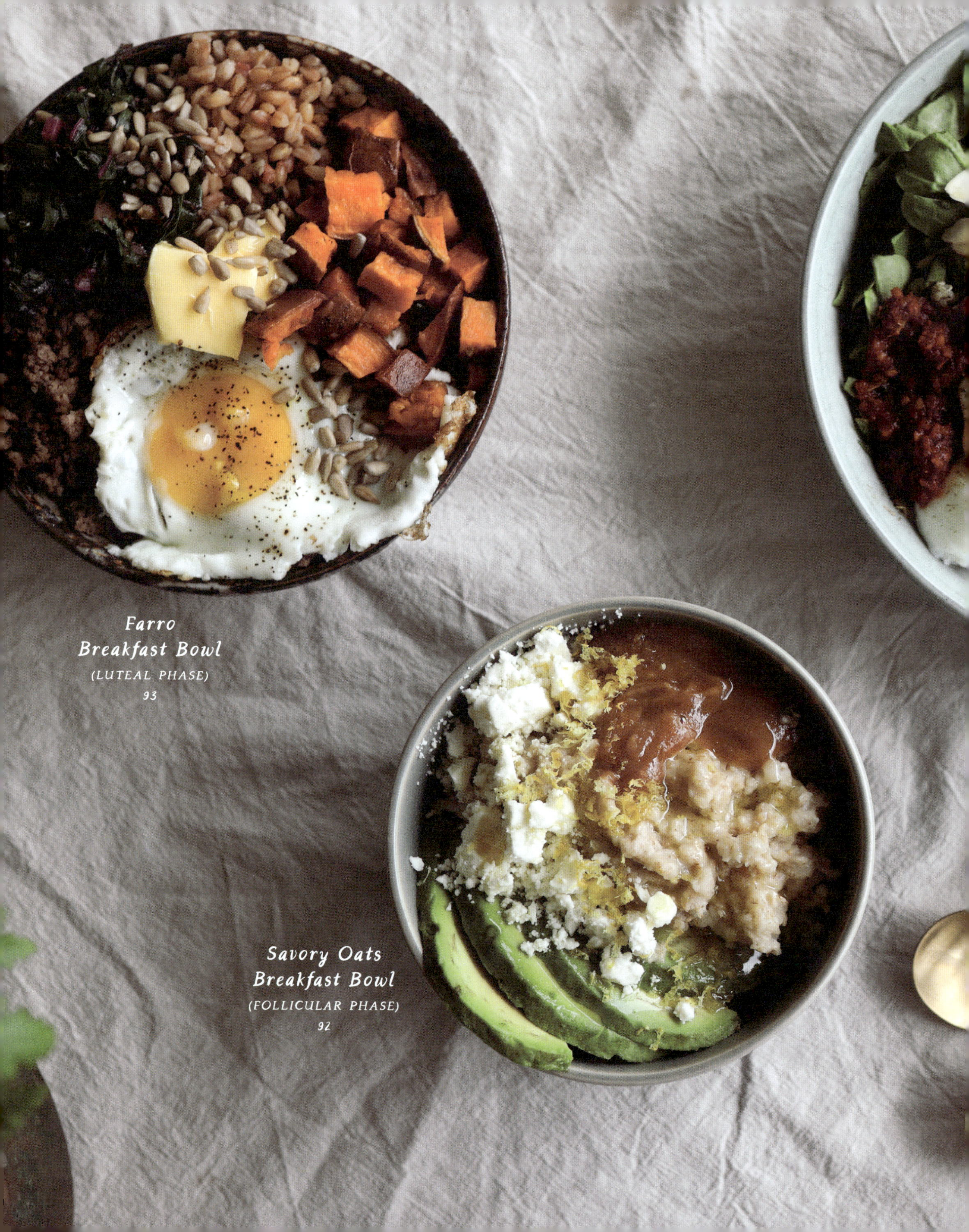
Farro
Breakfast Bowl
(LUTEAL PHASE)
93
Savory Oats
Breakfast Bowl
(FOLLICULAR PHASE)
92

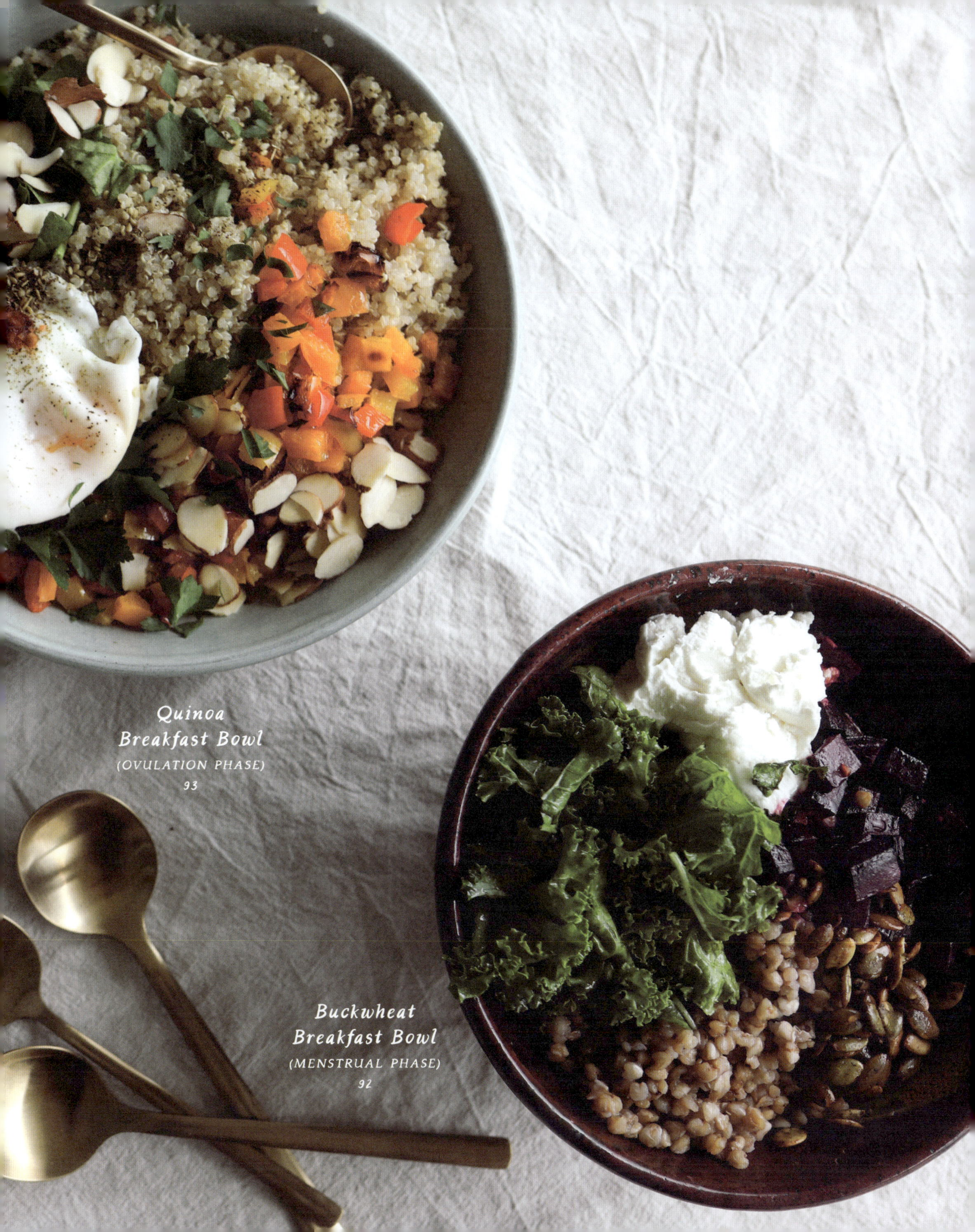
Quinoa
Breakfast Bowl
(OVULATION PHASE)
93
Buckwheat
Breakfast Bowl
(MENSTRUAL PHASE)
92

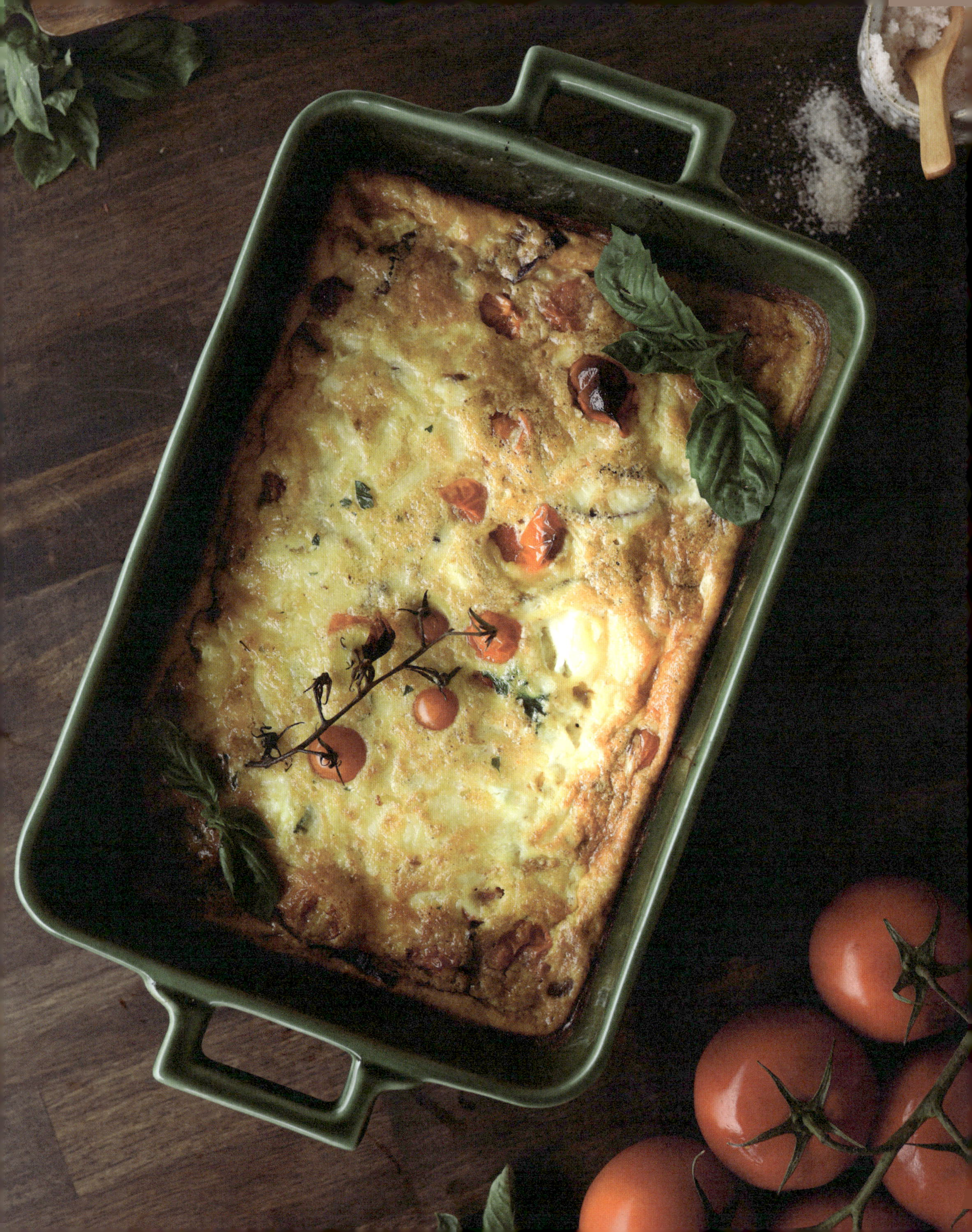

ROAST TOMATO AND GOAT CHEESE FRITTATA

SERVES 8

Prep: 10 minutes
Cook: 1 hour, 10 minutes
Rest: 15 minutes

Anti-Inflammatory
Blood Sugar Balancing
Follicular Phase
Gluten Free
Hormone Supportive

Super easy breakfast prep : check. Impressing everyone at the brunch potluck : check. Simple ingredients with major flavors : check, check, check! I will eat this *daily* on top of some steamed kale with a li'l sliced avocado layered on top and never tire of it.

3 tablespoons olive oil
16 ounces (454 g) cherry tomatoes, plus a small bunch on the vine (optional)
2 tablespoons balsamic vinegar
1 tablespoon sugar
½ teaspoon sea salt, plus more to taste
½ teaspoon black pepper, plus more to taste
½ large red onion, thinly sliced
3 large garlic cloves, unpeeled
12 large eggs
¾ cup (180 ml) whole milk or heavy cream
One 4-ounce (113 g) log goat cheese
½ cup (56 g) finely shredded cheddar
Handful of fresh basil, ribboned

1. Preheat the oven to 350°F (175°C).
2. Add the olive oil to a 10-inch (25 cm) skillet or casserole dish, followed by the tomatoes (including the tomatoes on the vine, if using).
3. Drizzle with the balsamic vinegar and sprinkle with the sugar and a liberal pinch of salt and pepper to taste. Toss in the onion and garlic and shake the pan to coat everything evenly.
4. Roast in the oven for 25 to 30 minutes, until the tomatoes are soft, bursting, and beginning to caramelize.
5. Meanwhile, crack the eggs into a large bowl and add the milk, ½ teaspoon salt, and ½ teaspoon pepper. Whisk to combine.
6. Remove the skillet from the oven, then remove the tomatoes on the vine and set aside. Remove the garlic, smush the cloves out of their peels, and mash them with a fork, then return them to the pan and stir them through the oil.
7. Pour in the egg mixture and stir briefly to evenly distribute the tomatoes and onions.
8. Plop little dollops of goat cheese around the pan and sprinkle with the cheddar and basil. Gently add the tomatoes on the vine, allowing them to peek out of the top of the eggs.
9. Return to the oven and bake for 35 to 40 minutes, until the eggs are just cooked through. Let rest for 10 to 15 minutes before serving.

CHAPTER THREE

GLORY SALADS

OKAY, WE NEED TO CHAT ABOUT SALADS.

Many of us are traumatized by salads—by their role in diet culture as the "healthy option" or by forcing down bowls of leaves coated in lame dressings when we would rather be eating *literally* anything else, all in the name of health. Not here! No, here we uplift salads and also don't pretend they are the only path to health. We're going for nutrient density, not fewer calories. My family makes what we call "glory salads," a term coined by my dad, after my big sis Beth started creating salads that were the star of the show, not a begrudging nod to health. Now, glory salads—giant bowls of lovingly prepared greens, roasted veggies, cheese, nuts, fruit, and delectable dressings, all combined with the intention of mega flavor—are a part of our family culture, and often the best part of the meal.

Of course, I would be remiss not to note that the benefit of a good salad is a huge hit of fiber (which I'll expand on in a minute, but the gist of it is that it's very important and most of us don't get nearly enough) in one fell swoop. And the beauty of making a flavorful, craveable *glory* salad is that it makes fiber easy to get while completely sidestepping the toxic diet culture moment of forcing yourself to eat something just to avoid calories. Some of these salads have a lower caloric load, sure. But some of them don't, and they are substantial enough to be a meal or a hearty snack in their own right.

When crafting a good, nutrient-dense salad, choose mostly dark leafy greens (like spinach, arugula, kale, or mesclun mix) over watery, crunchy lettuce like iceberg or even romaine. Crunchy lettuces are super refreshing, and there's nothing wrong with them, but they don't offer anywhere near the nutrients and minerals that dark greens do. When adding veggies, consider incorporating them roasted or cooked, particularly cruciferous ones like broccoli if your tummy is a little sensitive. Be sure to add a healthy fat source; most often this comes in the form of dressing, but it can also be avocado, nuts, or cheese—those fats are essential for your body to properly metabolize the nutrients in the greens!

Without further ado, this chapter offers up some of my favorite salads in a range of types, from warm and earthy to super light and refreshing. I've kept them fairly simple in the hopes that they will be easy to recreate but offer inspiration for you to go forth and create your own glory salads!

FIBER

Okay, I know we *"KNOW"* that fiber is good for us (especially if you want to stay, ya know . . . *regular*), but most of us vastly underestimate its importance and significantly don't eat enough of it. Lack of fiber is associated with higher risks of GI disorders, obesity, type 2 diabetes, heart disease, stroke, hypertension, and even certain cancers. Most of us (at least in the US) think we are eating enough fiber, but only 5 percent of us are! It doesn't help that there are a lot of misconceptions about fiber, including what foods are actually high in it, that fiber-rich foods taste bad or are expensive, and that fiber should be supplemented.

How Much Is Enough Fiber?

According to the National Academy of Medicine, women and children should eat at least 25 grams of fiber per day, and men should eat at least 38 grams. What does this look like in a day?

- ½ cup (40 g) oats = 8.2 grams fiber
- ⅓ cup (35 g) blueberries = 1.2 grams fiber
- 2 tablespoons nuts and/or seeds = 5 grams fiber
- ½ avocado = 5 grams fiber
- 1 cup (20 g) kale = 1.3 grams fiber
- ½ cup (75 g) broccoli = 1.2 grams fiber
- 1 cup (185 g) quinoa = 5 grams fiber
- 1 ounce (28 g) dark chocolate = 3.5 grams fiber
- Total fiber: around 30 grams

Fiber promotes a happy, healthy gut microbiome and regular bowel movements, and it keeps you feeling satisfied after a meal. It can help lower blood pressure and balance cholesterol and blood sugar, and because it aids the body's natural elimination processes, it helps reduce the risk of so many diseases. Notably, fiber is crucial for hormone health, as excess hormones bind to fiber to be removed from the body. Think of it as the Scrubbing Bubbles of the metabolic system, taking with it everything your body doesn't need and leaving you balanced at the end of the day.

Note that it is possible to get too much fiber! If so, you'll have digestive discomfort. Be wary of processed foods with added fiber, like protein bars, which can have as much as 10 grams of added fiber. Low-carb tortillas, baked goods, cereals, and even yogurt or ice cream can have additional fiber. Fiber supplements aren't ideal either; it's always best to get your fiber from whole food sources (this way it's very hard to get too much in one day).

HIGH-FIBER FOODS

If in doubt, your best bets for fiber are always legumes, whole unprocessed grains, nuts, seeds, fruits, and vegetables that require lots of chewing (although there are some fun exceptions to that rule like dark chocolate and raspberries). Refined grains (like white bread, pasta, and cereals) are going to be low in fiber, so even switching out white bread for seeded whole grain bread will make a difference!

FOOD	SERVING SIZE	FIBER CONTENT
LEGUMES		
Navy Beans	1 cup (180 g)	19 grams
Split Peas	1 cup (200 g)	16 grams
Lentils	1 cup (200 g)	15.5 grams
Black Beans	1 cup (170 g)	15 grams
Cannellini and Great Northern Beans	1 cup (180 g)	13 grams
NUTS & SEEDS		
Chia Seeds	1 ounce (28 g)	10 grams
Almonds	1 ounce (28 g)	3.5 grams
Pistachios	1 ounce (28 g)	3 grams
Sunflower Seeds	¼ cup (32 g)	3 grams
GRAINS		
Whole Wheat Pasta	1 cup (140 g)	6 grams
Barley	1 cup (200 g)	6 grams
Quinoa	1 cup (185 g)	5 grams
Oatmeal	1 cup (235 g)	4 grams
Popcorn	3 cups (24 g)	3.5 grams
Brown Rice	1 cup (195 g)	3.5 grams
Whole Wheat Bread	1 slice	2 grams
VEGETABLES		
Green Peas	1 cup (160 g)	9 grams
Artichoke Hearts	1 cup (160 g)	7.2 grams
Broccoli (Cooked)	1 cup (90 g)	5 grams
Turnip Greens	1 cup (144 g)	5 grams
Brussels Sprouts	1 cup (90 g)	4.5 grams
Potato, with Skin	1 medium	4 grams
Corn	1 cup (160 g)	4 grams
Cauliflower	1 cup (100 g)	2 grams
Carrots, Raw	1 medium	1.5 grams
FRUITS		
Raspberries	1 cup (125 g)	8 grams
Pear	1 medium	5.5 grams
Apple, with Skin	1 medium	4.5 grams
Banana	1 medium	3 grams
Orange	1 medium	3 grams
Strawberries	1 cup (150 g)	3 grams

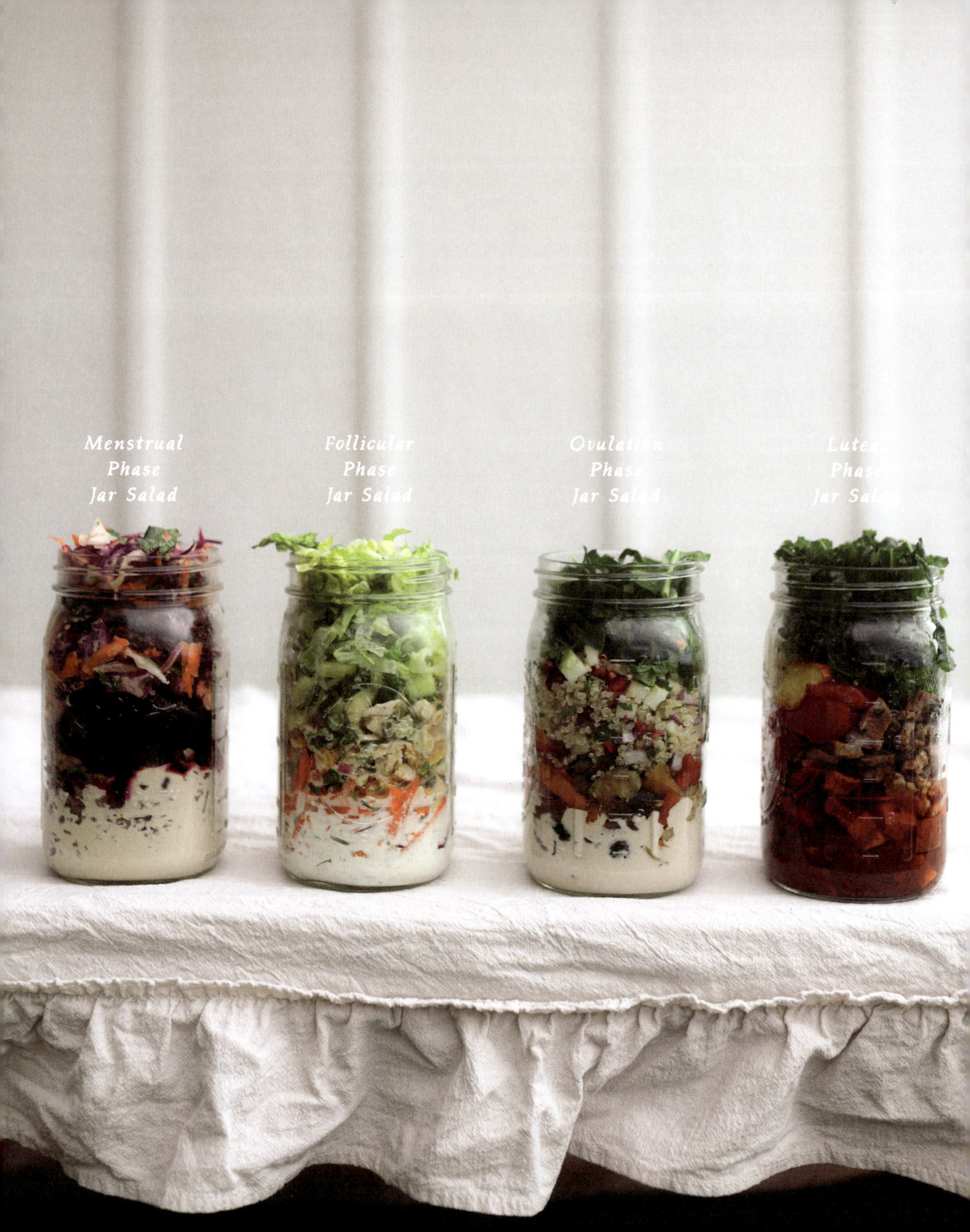
Menstrual Phase Jar Salad
Follicular Phase Jar Salad

JAR SALADS

EACH RECIPE SERVES 1

There is an art to building a good food-prep jar salad! You can utilize leftovers, roasted veggies, beans, grains—whatever you like. Measure with your heart, but I do about a handful of each topping, followed by a generous amount of greens. The key is in the layering. If you want your jars to last a few days, you need to build them in reverse: Put the dressing on the bottom, followed by meat, beans, and/or grains, and finish with fresh greens on top. This will keep the greens from getting soggy and make sure your proteins and grains get plenty of flavor from the dressing!

Menstrual Phase Jar Salad

Miso mayonnaise (from Korean-Style BBQ Beef Bowls; page 196)

+

kidney beans

+

cooked wild rice

+

roasted beets (from Honey Roast Beets with Labneh; page 141)

+

Good Gut Coleslaw (page 111)

Follicular Phase Jar Salad

Kefir Ranch (page 211)

+

Honey Mustard Chicken Salad (page 104)

+

The Carrot Salad (page 120)

+

chopped cucumber

+

butter lettuce leaves

Ovulation Phase Jar Salad

Tahini Dressing (page 208)

+

Quinoa Salad (page 107)

+

Mediterranean Summer Veg (page 135)

+

chopped tomatoes

+

baby arugula

Luteal Phase Jar Salad

Holy Chipotle Dressing (page 210)

+

chopped steak (from Chipotle Steak Bowls; page 205)

+

chopped roasted sweet potato

+

red bell pepper (fresh or roasted)

+

Rubbed Kale and Acorn Squash Salad (page 108)

HONEY MUSTARD CHICKEN SALAD

SERVES 6

Prep: 20 minutes
Cook: 10 minutes

Dairy Free
Follicular Phase
Gluten Free
Ovulation Phase

Chicken salad is so underrated, and I promise you this version is a well-deserved upgrade to the classic. The honey mustard chicken tenders are divine in and of themselves, but paired with the little bursts of apricot, the sweet and savory vibe is top-notch. It's such a good make-ahead recipe to prep for the week!

DRESSING

⅓ cup (80 ml) mayonnaise
2 tablespoons honey
2 tablespoons stone-ground mustard
2 tablespoons olive oil
1 tablespoon apple cider vinegar
Juice of ½ lemon
Sea salt and black pepper, to taste

SALAD

¼ cup (60 ml) stone-ground mustard
3 tablespoons honey
Juice of 1 lemon
1 teaspoon sea salt
½ teaspoon black pepper
1 pound (454 g) chicken tenderloins
1 tablespoon avocado oil
2 celery sticks, chopped (about 1 cup/100 g)
¼ cup (40 g) chopped red onion
5 or 6 apricots, chopped (about 1 cup/150 g) or ½ cup (65 g) chopped dried apricots
½ cup (75 g) pumpkin seeds
1 small bunch parsley, chopped

1. *Make the dressing:* Mix the mayonnaise, honey, mustard, olive oil, vinegar, lemon juice, salt, and pepper in a large bowl. Set aside in the fridge.
2. *Make the salad:* Combine the mustard, honey, lemon juice, salt, and pepper in a large bowl. Add the chicken, stir to coat, cover, and let marinate for 10 to 15 minutes.
3. Heat a large skillet over medium-high heat. Coat the pan with the avocado oil and then add the chicken, making sure the pieces do not touch. They should sizzle loudly as soon as they hit the pan.
4. Cook until browned on the bottom, 3 to 4 minutes, then flip and cook until browned on the other side, 3 to 4 more minutes. Test for doneness by using tongs to bend a piece of chicken in half; it should easily break.
5. Let the chicken cool, then roughly chop or shred it and add it to the bowl with the dressing. Add the celery, onion, and apricots, and mix to combine.
6. Sprinkle in the pumpkin seeds and parsley; you can mix them in or leave them on top as a garnish.
7. Store in an airtight container in the fridge for up to a week!

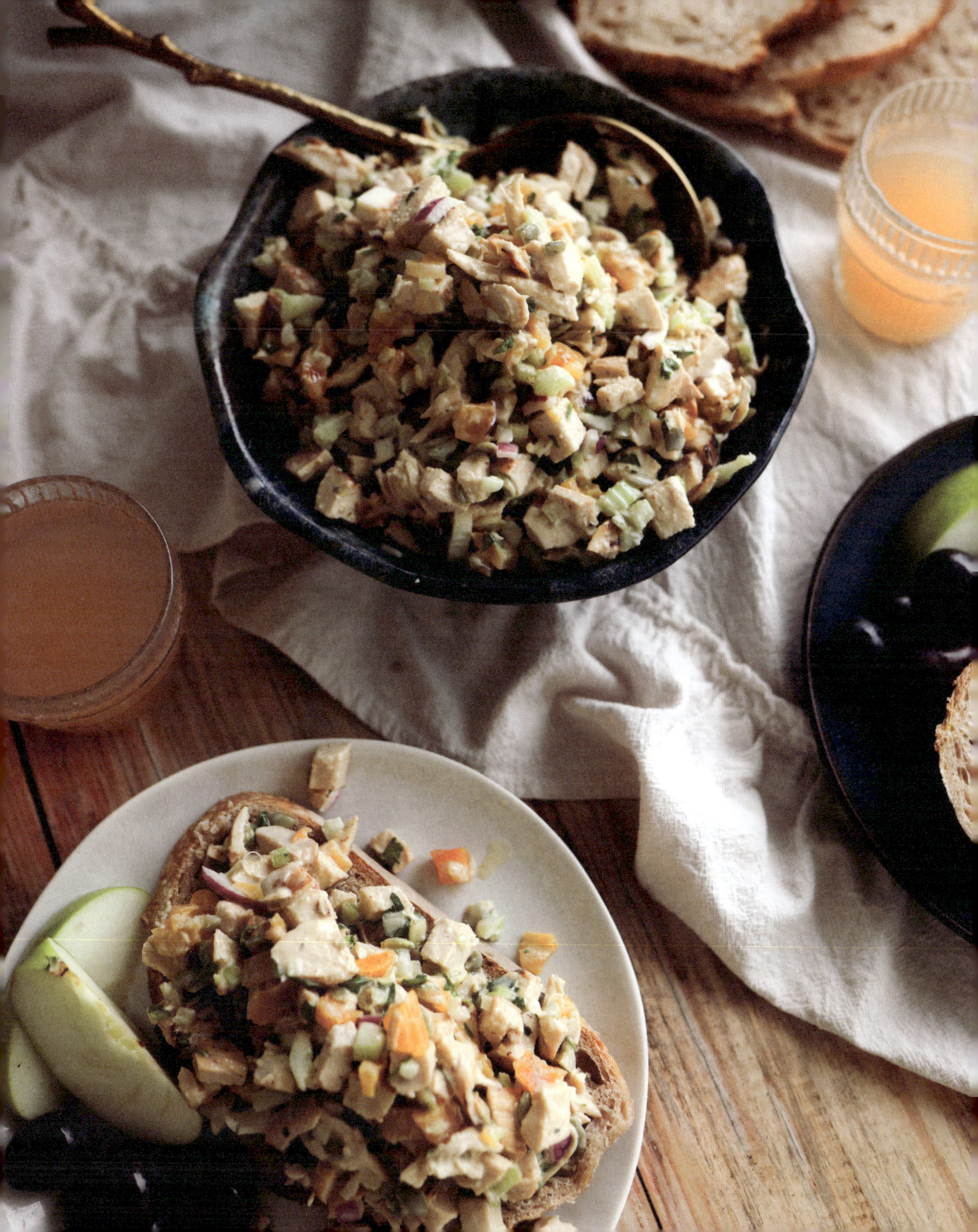

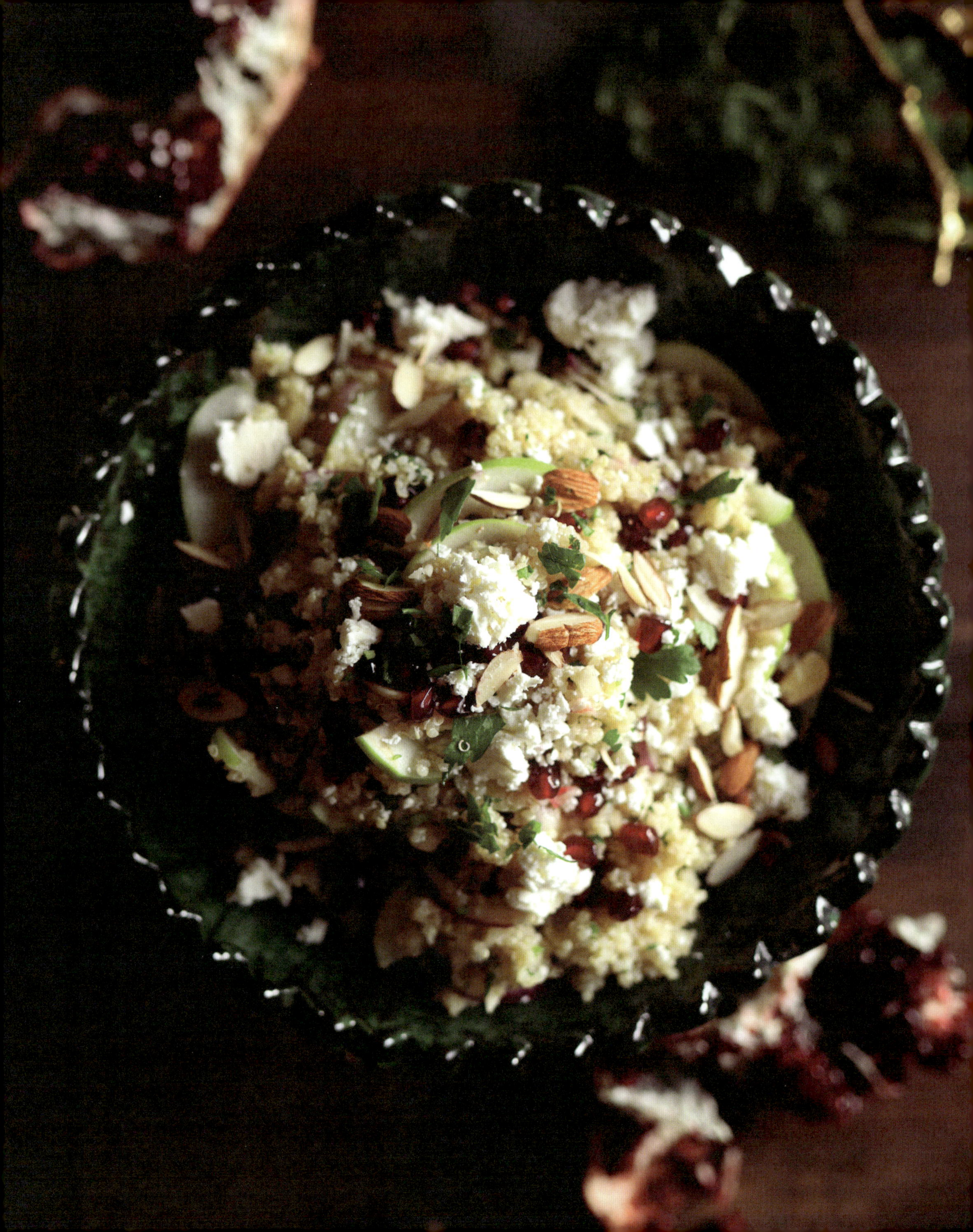

QUINOA SALAD

SERVES 8

***Prep:* 10 minutes**
***Cook:* 20 minutes**

Gluten Free
Ovulation Phase

I didn't used to like quinoa, but I forced myself to eat it because of the nutritional benefits. It contains all nine amino acids, making it one of the few complete plant proteins, plus it offers tons of minerals and fiber. Then I discovered how to make it taste good. First, you absolutely *must* rinse it—super well—and when you think it's rinsed enough, rinse it more. This will remove the bitter saponins that coat the grains and can leave a weird soapy flavor after the quinoa is cooked. Be liberal with salt and seasonings during and after the cooking process, as quinoa is so plain but can really soak up flavor! This salad is one of my favorite ways to eat it. The balanced sweet and sour flavors, crunch from the apples and almonds, and saltiness of the feta make it simple but satisfying.

1 cup (185 g) quinoa
1 cup (240 ml) chicken Bone Broth (page 159)
¾ cup (180 ml) water
Juice of 1½ lemons, divided
1 teaspoon sea salt, divided
6 tablespoons extra virgin olive oil
¼ cup (60 ml) honey
3 tablespoons apple cider vinegar or champagne vinegar
½ green apple, very thinly sliced
¼ medium red onion, very thinly sliced
Small bunch of parsley, cilantro, dill, or basil, finely chopped
½ cup (87 g) pomegranate arils
½ cup (75 g) crumbled feta
⅓ cup (30 g) sliced almonds

1. Place the quinoa in a strainer and rinse thoroughly, until the water runs completely clear. This is important if you don't want bitter quinoa!
2. Transfer the quinoa to a medium saucepan and add the Bone Broth and water. Bring to a boil, then cover the pan and reduce the heat to low. Gently simmer for about 10 minutes.
3. Stir in the juice of ½ lemon and ½ teaspoon salt, then cover and simmer for 5 more minutes, until all of the liquid has been absorbed. Remove from the heat and let sit, covered, for about 10 minutes, then uncover and let cool completely (see Tip).
4. Whisk together the olive oil, honey, vinegar, juice of 1 lemon, and ½ teaspoon salt (or more to taste) in a large bowl. Mix in the quinoa.
5. Add the apple, onion, and parsley to the bowl and stir to combine.
6. Add the pomegranate, feta, and almonds, saving a little of each to sprinkle on top for garnish if you like.

TIP

You can speed up this process by spreading the quinoa thinly on a baking sheet and throwing it in the freezer for a few minutes.

RUBBED KALE AND ACORN SQUASH SALAD

SERVES
6 TO 8

Prep: 10 minutes
Cook: 40 minutes

Gluten Free
Luteal Phase
Menstrual Phase

Fun fact: Kale is super good for you but hard for most people to digest raw. It's a brassica, so it contains tons of insoluble fiber as well as raffinose, a complex sugar that easily ferments during digestion, causing gas and bloating. This can be sidestepped simply by rubbing your kale. Yes, massaging it, particularly with oil, an acid like lemon juice, and an abrasive like salt, helps to begin the process of breaking down the kale before it reaches your stomach. This process eases digestion and makes all that luscious folate, vitamin K, vitamin A, and other goodies more readily available to you. But if you have had gut health issues, it's best to avoid eating any brassicas (like kale, broccoli, cauliflower, and brussels sprouts) raw.

½ medium acorn squash (see Note), halved and deseeded
4 garlic cloves
2 fresh rosemary sprigs or 1 teaspoon dried rosemary
2 tablespoons avocado oil
1 teaspoon sea salt, plus more for sprinkling
Pinch of black pepper
1 bunch kale (6 to 8 stems)
Juice of ½ lemon (about 1 tablespoon)
2 tablespoons olive oil
1 teaspoon honey
¼ medium red onion, thinly sliced
¼ cup (35 g) raw sunflower seeds
¼ cup (37 g) crumbled feta

1. Preheat the oven to 375°F (190°C). Line a baking sheet with parchment paper.
2. Place the squash on the baking sheet with the garlic and rosemary. Drizzle with the avocado oil and sprinkle with salt and pepper.
3. Roast in the oven for 35 minutes, or until the squash is soft throughout. Remove from the oven and let cool slightly, and either slice and leave the skin on or peel and cut into cubes.
4. Meanwhile, rip the kale leaves from the stems, stack them tightly together, and slice into thin ribbons.
5. Place the kale in a large bowl with the lemon juice, olive oil, honey, and 1 teaspoon salt. Massage the kale for a few minutes until it darkens in color, reduces in volume by almost half, and becomes very soft.
6. Add the onion to the bowl.
7. Toast the sunflower seeds in a small dry pan over medium-low heat, constantly keeping an eye on them and stirring often, until they begin to brown, about 5 minutes.
8. Transfer the salad to a platter and add the squash on top.
9. Thinly slice the roasted garlic cloves and sprinkle them onto the salad along with the toasted sunflower seeds. Top with the feta, and serve.

NOTE

Measure this recipe with your heart. Use the whole squash if you like! If not, maybe use any squash left over from the Easy Peasy Roasty Squash Soup (page 163).

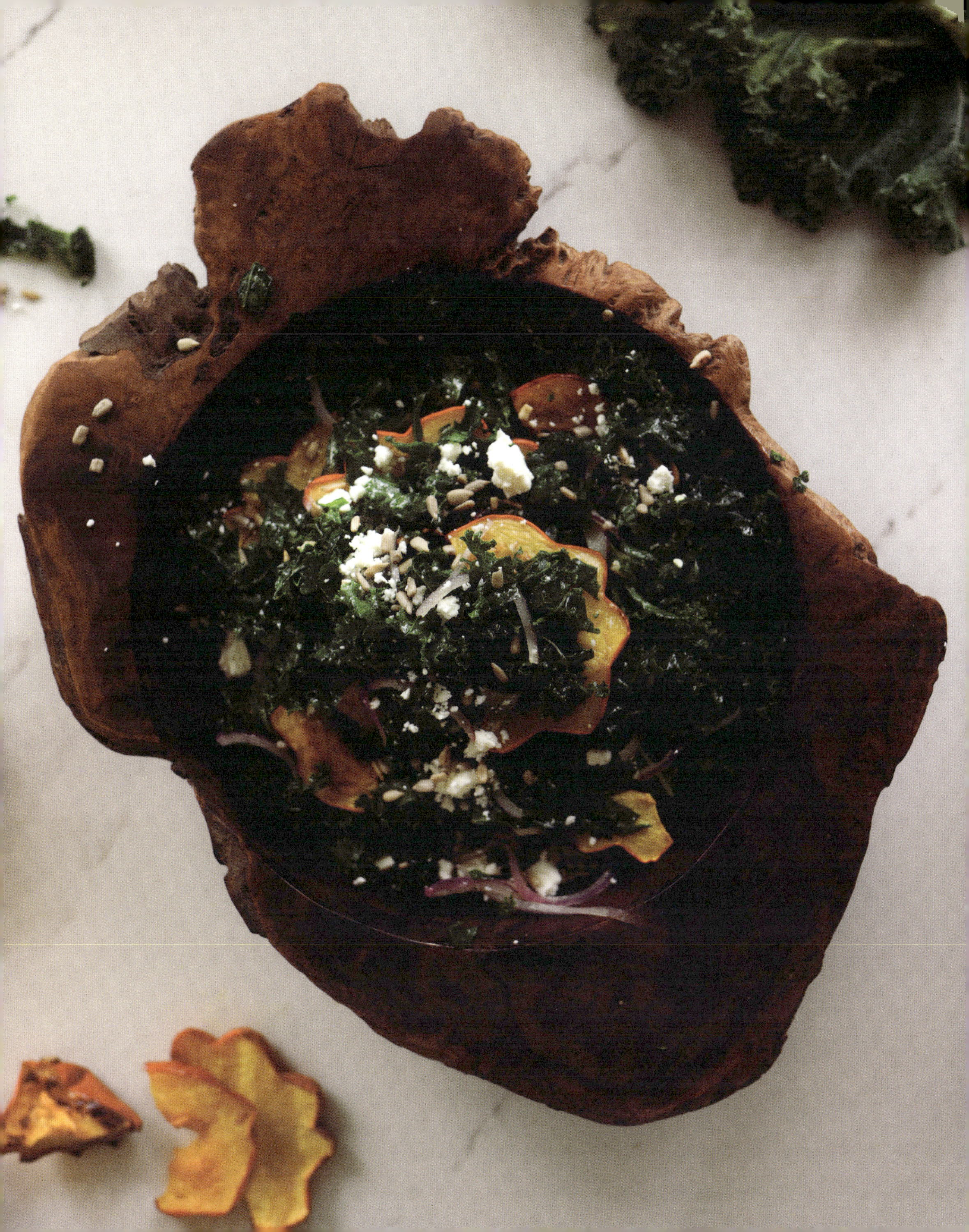

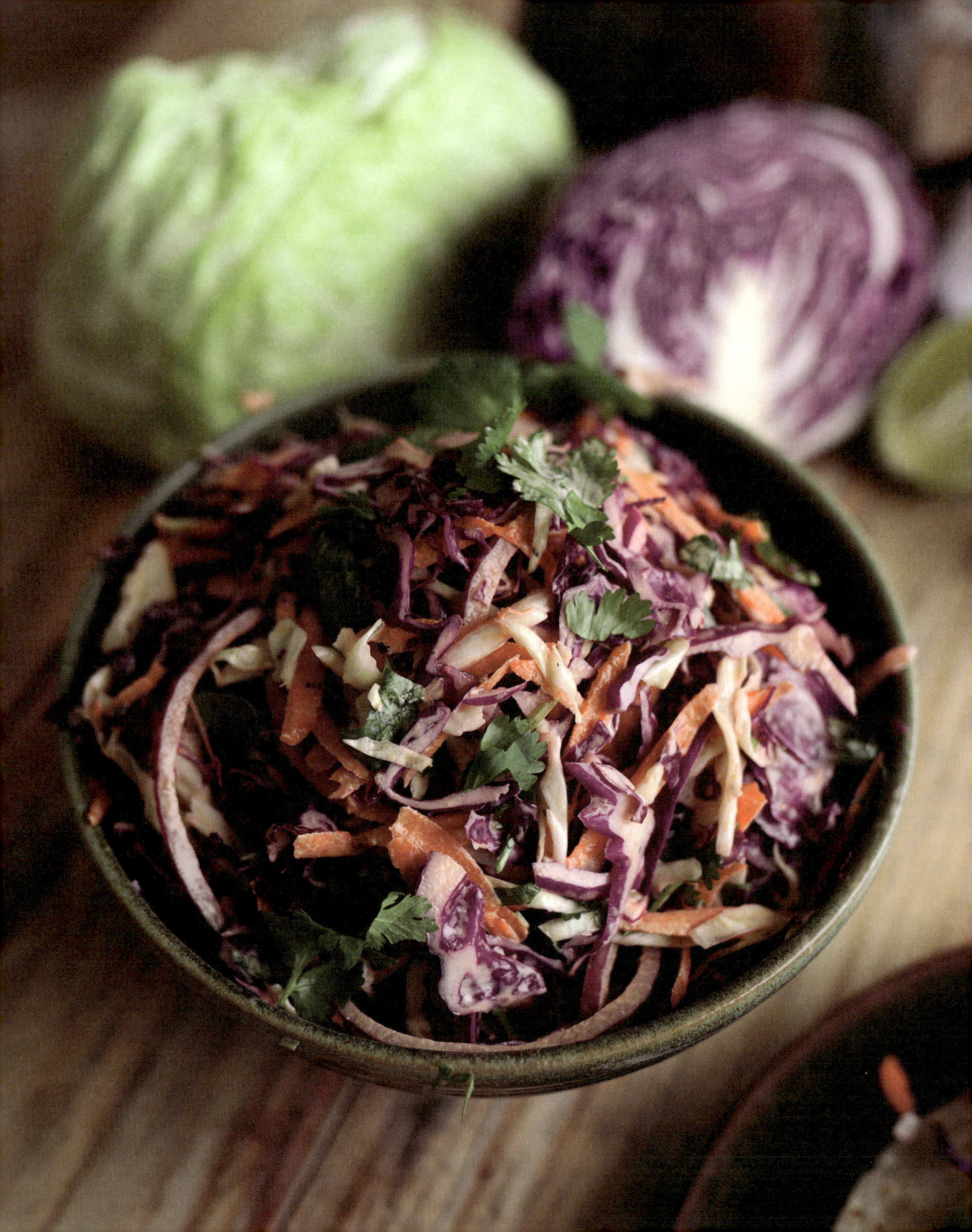

GOOD GUT COLESLAW

SERVES 8 TO 10

***Prep:* 15 minutes**

Dairy Free
Gluten Free
Luteal Phase
Ovulation Phase

Forget the sweet-mayo-and-onion slaw of neighborhood BBQs of yore—this coleslaw is fresh, tangy, and complex, and it genuinely makes people say, "I never liked coleslaw until now." The raw cabbage and carrots provide both prebiotic and insoluble fiber to feed your healthy gut bacteria and help bind to and eliminate excess hormones and waste. This keeps well in the fridge, making it a great prep-ahead item to keep on hand and add to any meal for digestive support.

½ medium head red cabbage, cored and thinly sliced
½ medium head green cabbage, cored and thinly sliced
3 tablespoons extra virgin olive oil
2 tablespoons apple cider vinegar
2 teaspoons lemon juice
½ teaspoon sea salt
3 medium carrots, grated
½ small red onion, finely sliced
1 small bunch fresh cilantro, chopped
¼ cup (60 ml) Avocado Oil Mayo (page 212)
Zest of ½ lemon (about 1½ teaspoons)
2 teaspoons honey
2 teaspoons red miso
Black pepper, to taste

1. Place the red and green cabbage in a large bowl. Drizzle with the olive oil, vinegar, and lemon juice, and sprinkle with the salt.
2. Mix and massage the cabbage with your hands until it softens, 1 or 2 minutes. (This will begin to break down the fibers, making the cabbage easier to digest.)
3. Add the carrots, onion, and cilantro to the bowl.
4. Mix the mayonnaise, lemon zest, honey, miso, and pepper in a small bowl or jar until smooth.
5. Pour the dressing into the large bowland stir thoroughly to combine. This will keep in the fridge for up to 1 week.

ARUGULA CITRUS SALAD

The combination of arugula and citrus in this salad feels intuitively light and refreshing because it actually is anti-inflammatory and cleansing. Fun fact: Arugula is not a lettuce; it's a cruciferous vegetable. It provides many of the same benefits as vegetables like kale or broccoli—lots of fiber, cancer-fighting glucosinolates, tons of micronutrients, and vitamin C—while being much easier to digest! It can support the body's toxin elimination processes and protect the liver, among other things.

SERVES 4

Prep:* *10 minutes

Dairy Free
Follicular Phase
Gluten Free
Ovulation Phase

3 tablespoons olive oil
2 tablespoons honey
Zest of ½ lemon
Juice of 1 lemon
1 teaspoon sea salt
5 ounces (142 g) baby arugula
1 large ruby red grapefruit, peeled and sliced into ¼- to ½-inch-thick (6 to 13 mm) rounds and half moons
1 large orange, peeled and sliced into ¼ to ½-inch-thick (6 to 13 mm) rounds
1 large avocado, pitted, peeled, and thinly sliced
¼ cup (30 g) hemp seeds
¼ teaspoon red pepper flakes, or more to taste

1. Whisk the olive oil, honey, lemon juice, and salt in a jar or small bowl.
2. Place the arugula in a large bowl and drizzle it with half the dressing mixture. Toss to coat, then pile onto a serving plate.
3. Scatter the citrus across the arugula and tuck some of it under the edges. Make it cute!
4. Add the avocado slices and sprinkle the hemp seeds on top.
5. Drizzle the remaining dressing over the top of the salad as generously as you'd like, followed by a dusting of red pepper flakes and freshly grated lemon zest.

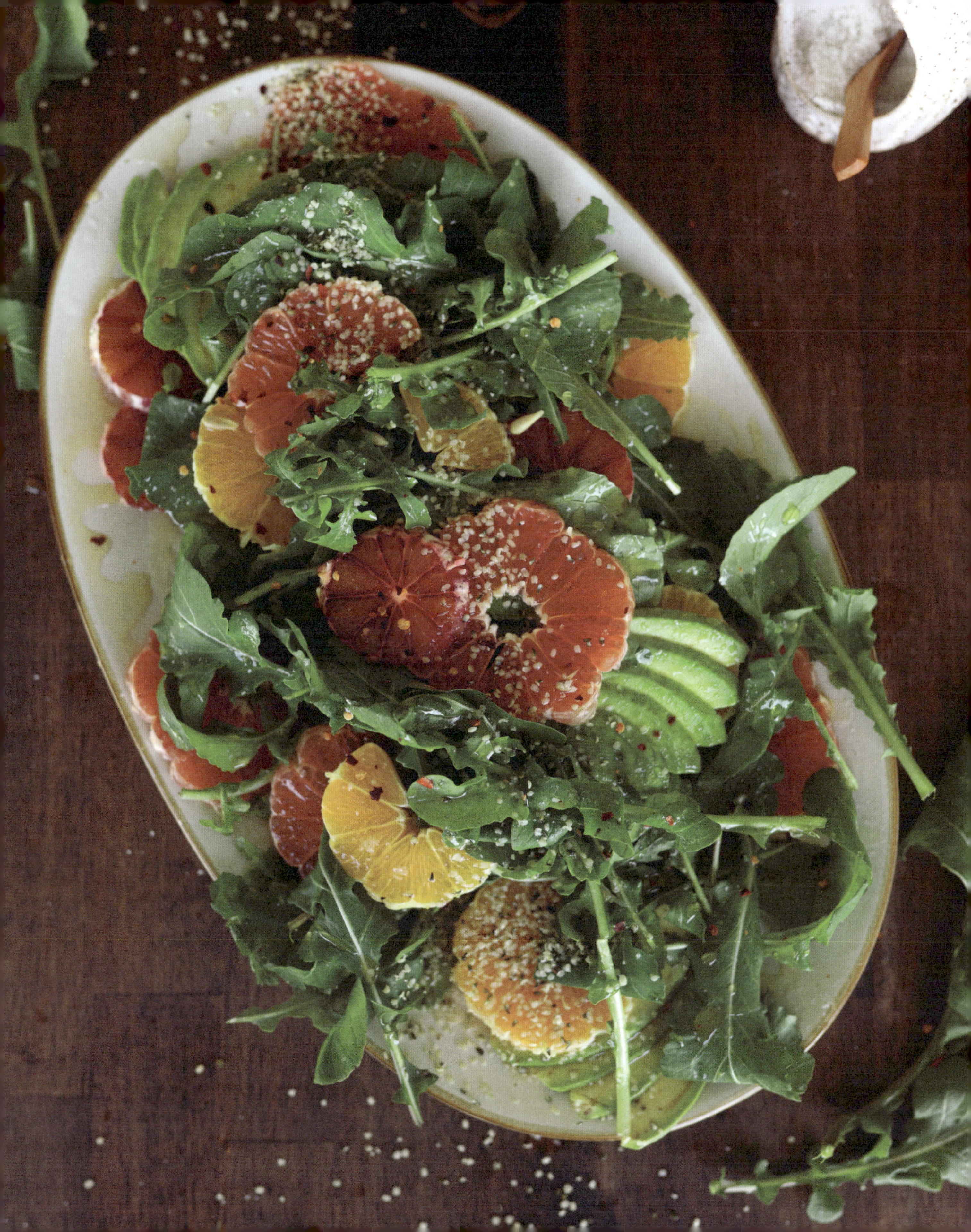

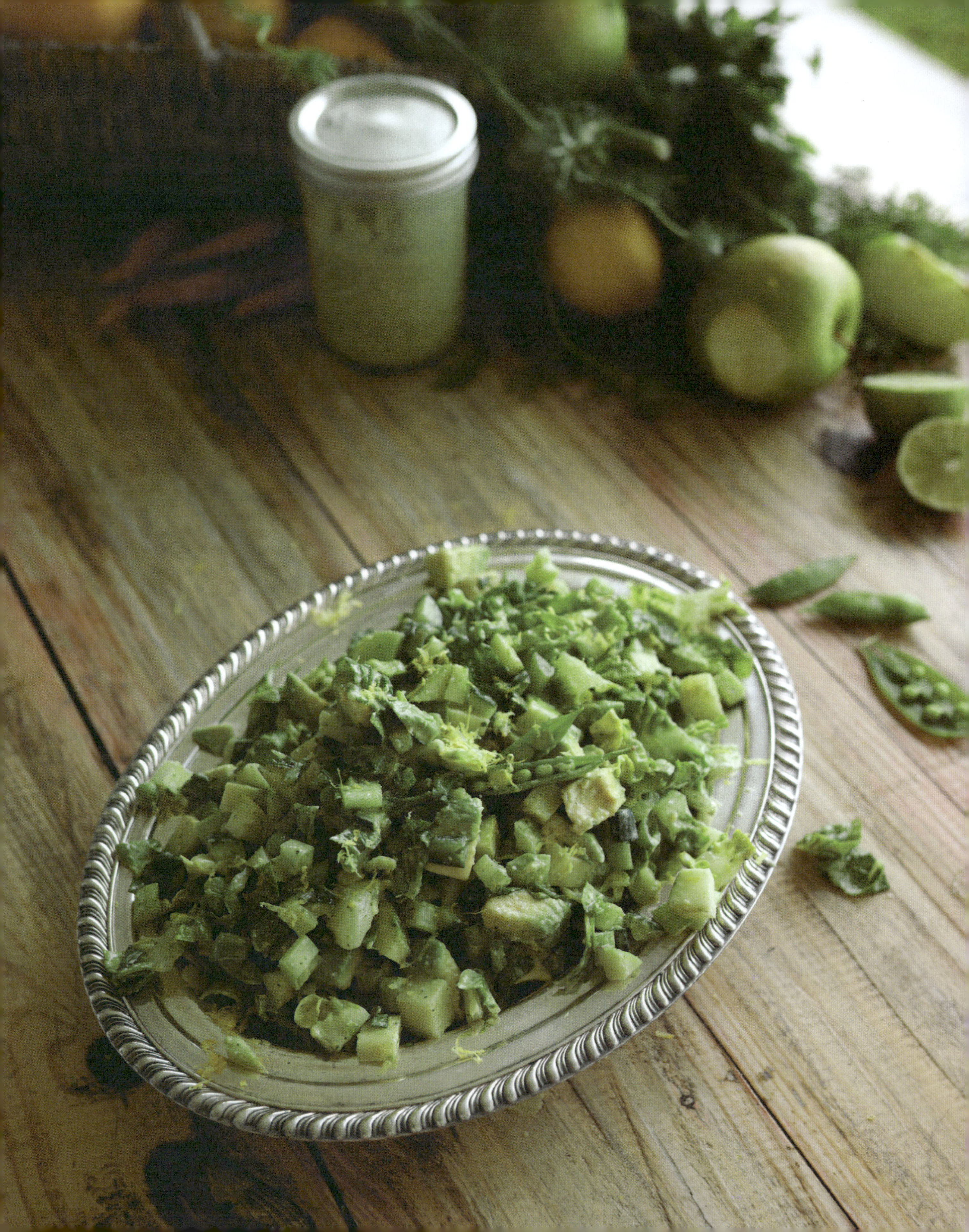

EXCESSIVELY GREEN SALAD

SERVES 10

Prep: 25 minutes

Dairy Free
Follicular Phase
Gluten Free
Ovulation Phase

Here's what to eat when you feel heavy, bloated, and stuck. This salad is incredibly fiber-rich, which will help your body eliminate all kinds of waste. Fiber picks up and carries out excess hormones (like estrogen and cortisol), cholesterol, and environmental toxins. All the greens are full of chlorophyll, which fights inflammation and free radicals. Arugula, fennel, parsley, and mint are also known to stimulate digestive enzymes and support the liver. What makes this salad especially delicious is chopping everything tiny, the creaminess of the avocado, and a really good dressing. To prep this salad ahead, leave it undressed and add the avocado fresh when serving!

5 ounces (142 g) baby arugula
1 large or 2 small green apples
1 medium English cucumber
2 to 3 celery stalks
1 medium fennel bulb
1½ cups (200 g) sugar snap or snow peas
Handful of mint leaves
Handful of parsley leaves
Zest and juice of 1 lemon
Generous pinch of sea salt
1 to 2 ripe avocados, peeled, pitted, and cut into bite-size chunks
Herbaceous Green Dressing (page 210), Tahini Dressing (page 208), or Mama's Vinaigrette (page 211)

1. Find the biggest bowl you can and throw your arugula into it.
2. Chop the apple, cucumber, celery, fennel, and peas into ½-inch (1 cm) pieces and finely chop the herbs. Transfer to the bowl with the arugula and add the lemon zest, lemon juice, and salt. Toss to mix.
3. Right before serving, add the avocado, drizzle with dressing, and toss again to coat.

ADZUKI BEAN SALAD

SERVES
8 TO 10

Prep: 15 minutes

Dairy Free
Gluten Free
Menstrual Phase

Beans can be scary if you've had gut health issues—at least they were for me for a long time! But they are so rich in fiber and prebiotics that they can also be incredibly good for your gut health. What's a girl to do? The answer: 1. Slowly introduce beans to your diet. 2. Get dry beans and soak them to release phytic acid and make them easier to digest. 3. Eat them with herbs and aromatics that improve digestion—like the ginger, turmeric, and cilantro in this salad! The addition of fermented veggies gives you a boost of good bacteria to further help things along. Prep this salad and eat a little every day to train your tum!

1 tablespoon extra virgin olive oil
1 egg yolk (ideally pasture-raised)
Juice of 1 lemon or lime
1 teaspoon ground cumin
1 teaspoon grated fresh ginger
1 teaspoon sea salt
½ teaspoon ground black pepper
¼ teaspoon ground turmeric
Pinch of cayenne pepper (optional)
2 cups (360 g) soaked, sprouted, and cooked adzuki beans (see page 116)
1 cup (96 g) finely chopped cucumber
1 cup (150 g) chopped cherry tomatoes
½ cup (70 g) Sauerkraut (page 70)
¼ cup (40 g) finely chopped red onion
Small handful of chopped fresh cilantro or parsley

1. Whisk the olive oil, egg yolk, lemon juice, cumin, ginger, salt, pepper, turmeric, and cayenne (if using) in a large bowl until creamy.
2. Add the beans, cucumber, tomatoes, Sauerkraut, onion, and cilantro, and toss to combine.
3. Let rest for at least 30 minutes before serving to let the flavors develop.

NOTE

Adzuki beans are higher in minerals, fiber, and antioxidants than many other kinds of beans and are one of the easiest varieties to digest.

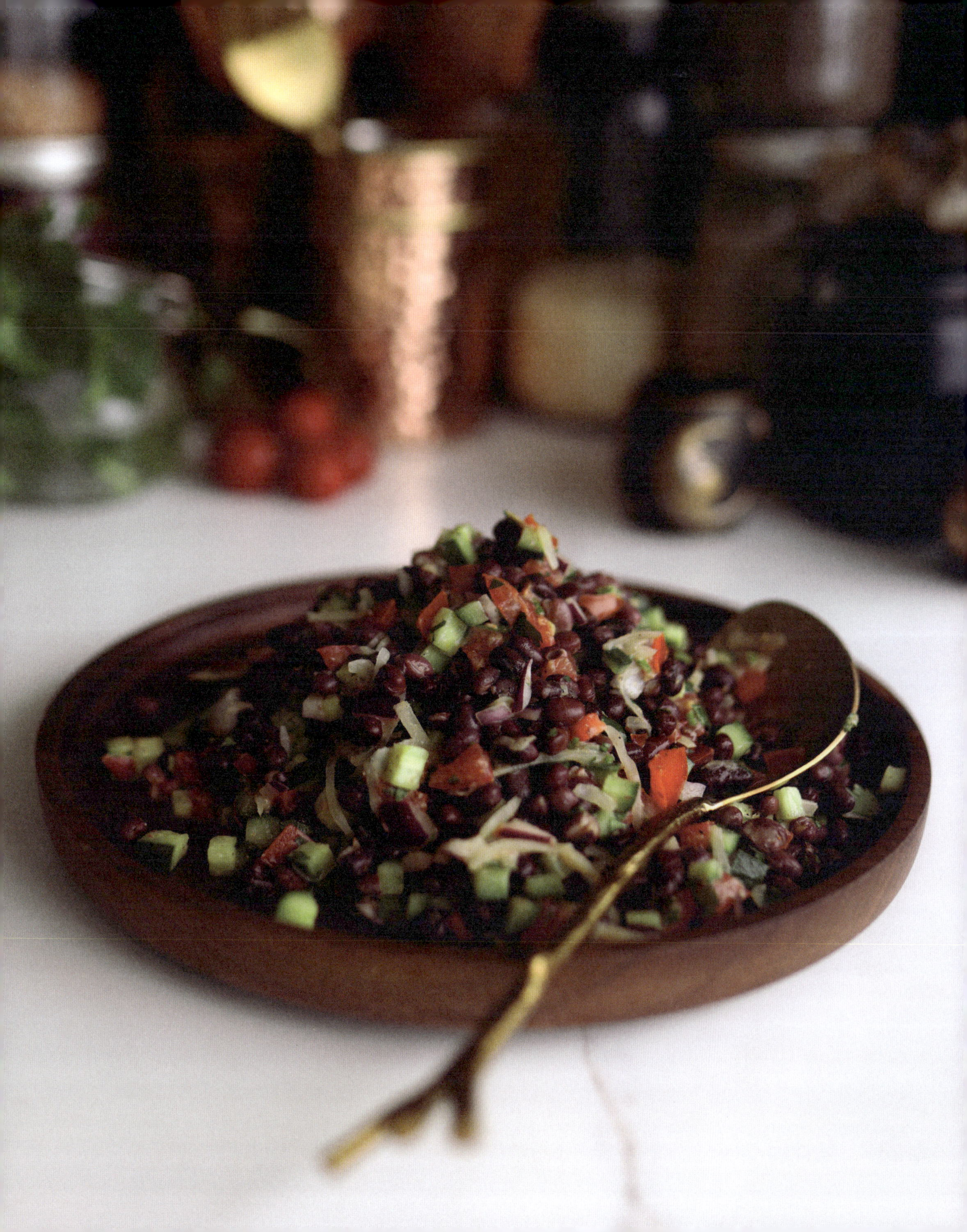

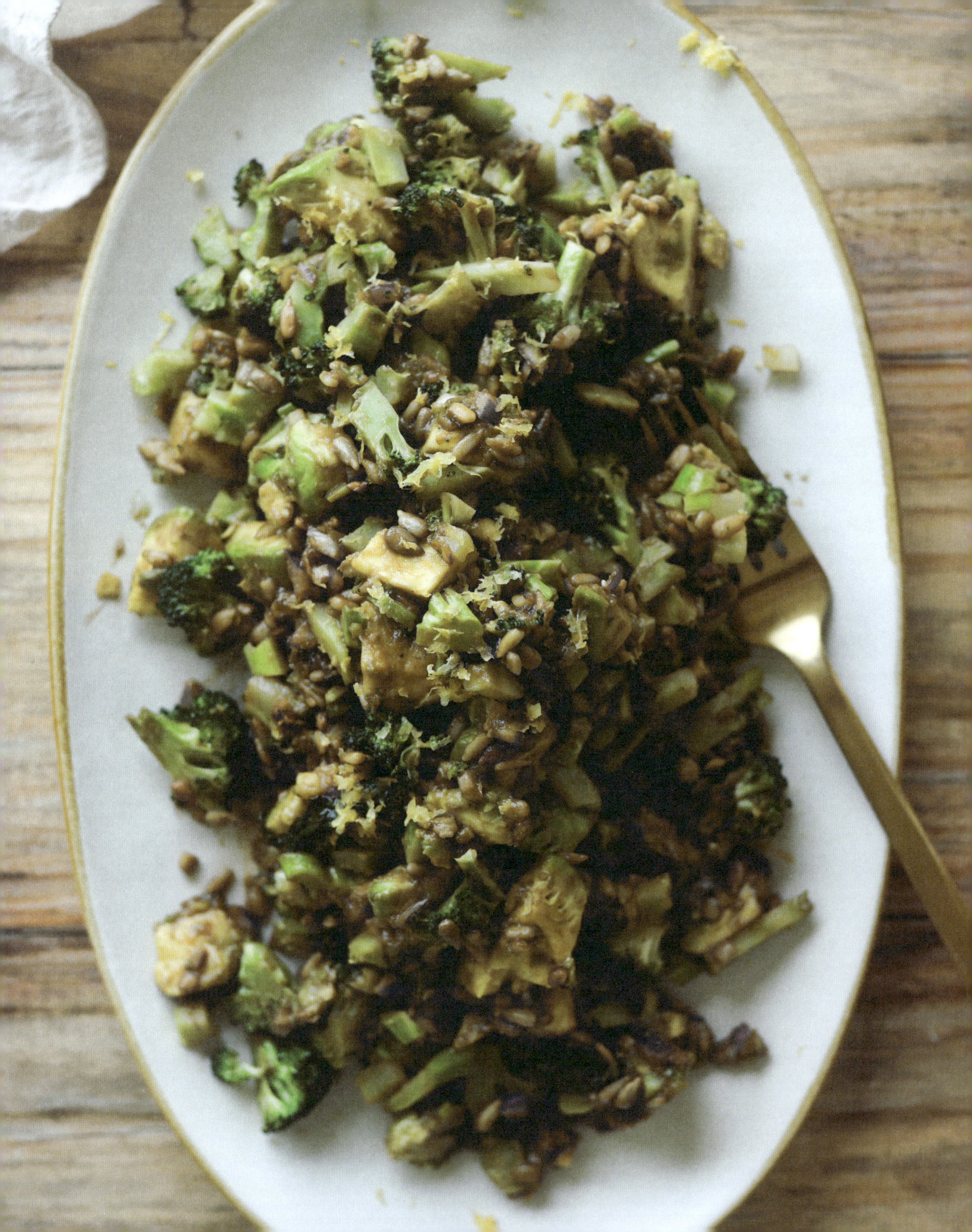

BROCCOLI AVO SALAD

SERVES 6

***Prep:* 10 minutes**
***Cook:* 15 minutes**

Dairy Free
Follicular Phase
Gluten Free

One day, I realized that my vegetable waste was out of control—as in, I kept stocking up on vegetables that went bad before I could use them. This is a common problem for a lot of us, if the lack of fiber epidemic in the West is to be believed. My solution was to just start sautéing vegetables at any opportunity. Thus, the crunchy, creamy, green dream that is this salad was born. It's follicular phase perfection—eat the leftovers through ovulation and you'll thank me! (I highly recommend drizzling it with the Herbaceous Green Dressing on page 210.)

2 tablespoons avocado oil, plus more as needed
1 large head broccoli, chopped into ½- to 1-inch (1 cm to 2.5 cm) pieces
½ teaspoon sea salt
¼ cup (60 ml) water
Zest of ½ lemon, plus more to taste
Juice of 1 lemon
⅓ cup (40 g) raw sunflower seeds
2 or 3 medium avocados
¼ medium red onion, finely chopped
Small handful of fresh basil, finely ribboned
2 tablespoons balsamic vinegar
1 tablespoon honey

1. Heat a large skillet over medium heat. Add the oil to coat the pan, then throw in the broccoli.
2. Add the salt, pour in the water, and quickly cover with a lid. Cook for about 5 minutes, or until the water has evaporated. Uncover, stir the broccoli, and cook until browned on a few sides, another 5 minutes, adding 1 more tablespoon of avocado oil if needed.
3. Add the lemon juice, quickly deglazing by scraping the pan as you mix the broccoli.
4. Add the sunflower seeds and stir occasionally, until they begin to brown, 2 or 3 minutes. Remove the pan from the heat and tip the mixture into a medium bowl.
5. Halve the avocados and remove the pits. Reserve 1 avocado half. Cut the flesh of the other halves into small squares, then scoop them into the bowl. Mash the reserved avocado in its skin and then add the mashed flesh to the bowl. Add the onion and basil and toss to combine.
6. Combine the balsamic vinegar, honey, and lemon zest in a small jar. Pour over the salad, toss, and serve!

THE CARROT SALAD

SERVES 6

Prep: 10 minutes

All Phases
Dairy Free

Will eating carrot salad every day heal your hormones? I'm not promising it will. But I'm also not promising it won't... The claims made about this dish seem pretty wild, but carrots do have a unique blend of insoluble fiber and prebiotic fiber that helps the gut break down and eliminate excess estrogen, as well as tons of beta-carotene, which converts to vitamin A, an essential nutrient for hormone metabolism. Can you just Bugs Bunny a raw carrot? Totally. (All of that chewing is great for your jaw, but that's a whole other tangent.) But adding healthy fats and fermented vinegar will help your body get the most out of it. And it's yummy, so...

3 cups (330 g) shredded carrots, skin on
¼ small red onion, very thinly sliced
½ packed cup (10 g) fresh cilantro, chopped
3 teaspoons apple cider vinegar
1 medium garlic clove, minced
2 teaspoons olive oil
2 teaspoons sesame oil (see Note)
2 teaspoons lime juice
2 teaspoons soy sauce or liquid aminos
½ teaspoon red pepper flakes, or more to taste
¼ teaspoon sea salt, or more to taste
Sesame seeds, for garnish

1. Place the carrots, onion, and cilantro in a medium bowl.
2. Combine the vinegar, garlic, olive oil, sesame oil, lime juice, soy sauce, red pepper flakes, and salt in a small cup or jar.
3. Pour the dressing over the salad and mix thoroughly to combine. Sprinkle with the sesame seeds.
4. Store in an airtight container in the fridge for up to 1 week and eat a handful-sized portion every day.

NOTE

The sesame oil and seeds make this an extra hormone-healthy powerhouse. Switch to pumpkin seed oil or flaxseed oil during your menstrual or follicular phase if you're seed cycling.

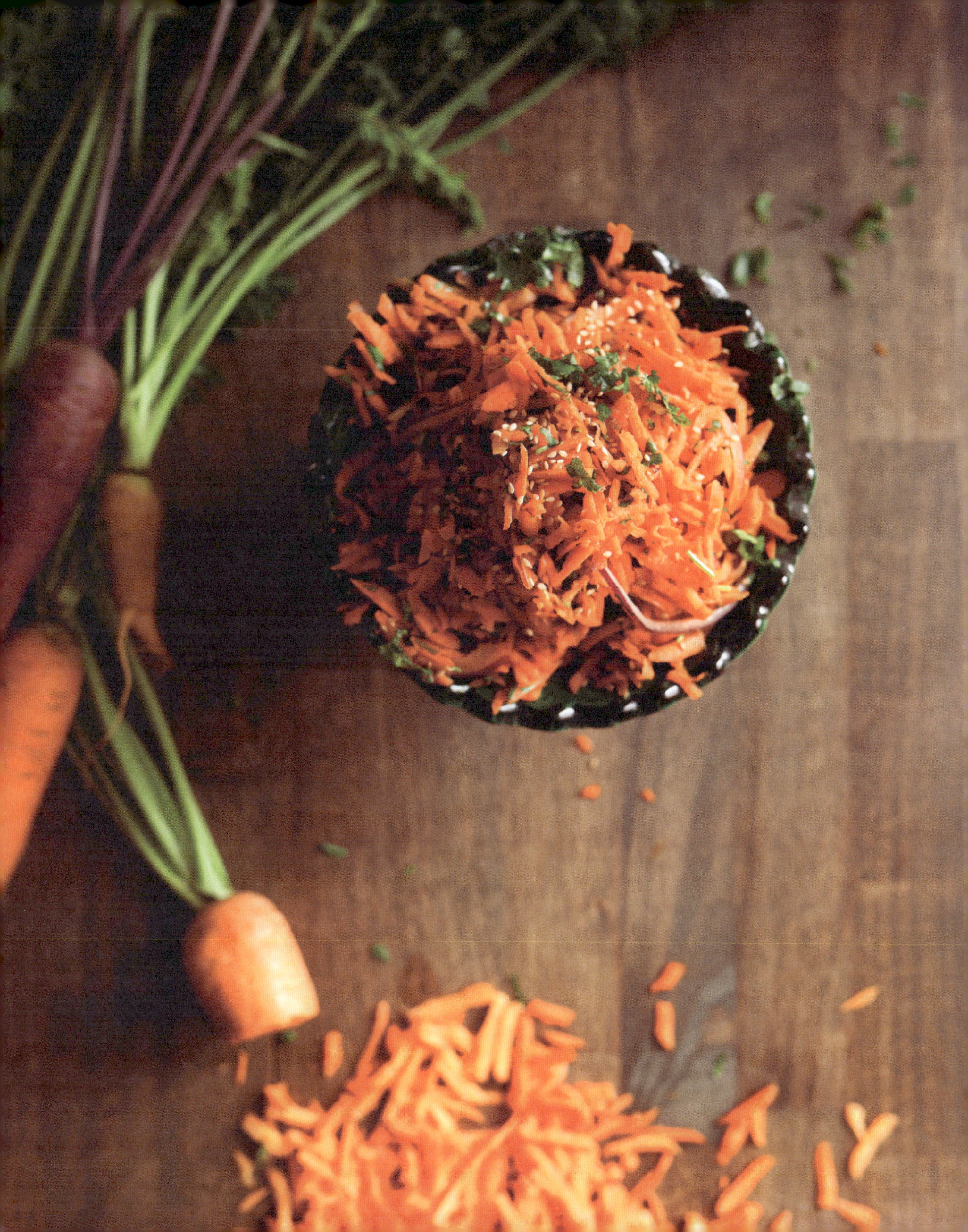

CHAPTER FOUR

VEG SIDES

CAST YOUR MIND BACK TO THE VERY START OF THIS BOOK,

where we talked about the discovery of cooking and what a transformational moment that was for human development. That was largely because chomping on raw vegetables all day is a really inefficient way to get nutrients and calories. Not only does it take ages, but the raw fibers are also much more challenging to digest. And for many vegetables, you can actually get *more* nutrients out of them when they're cooked properly. By "properly," I basically mean not boiling them; you will not find a single basic boiled brussel in this book. Not to be a hater, but boiling veggies is a great way to pull all their nutrients out of them and into the water—and also a great way to make them have the least flavor and worst texture.

You can get so creative with vegetables. They have such diverse uses and flavor profiles, but since we are focusing on *simple* kitchen magic, I've mostly included simple vegetable sides with intentional elevations. It's so easy to draw rich, complex flavor out of veggies, so sometimes the simplest preparations are the best! You'll find a lot of roasting because it is A. really easy and B. a great way to preserve nutrients. Most of these recipes let the vegetable shine but incorporate ingredients that elevate the vegetable's particular flavor profile—like the gorgeous, smoky Harissa Baked Eggplant (page 146), one of the easiest things I've ever made, or Miso Braised Cabbage (page 150), humble in appearance but rich and comforting in flavor. The addition of fats, salt, and spices does so much more than just make these recipes mouthwatering; it increases the bioavailability of the minerals and vitamins in the vegetables, which I think is pure magic.

POTATOES

(AND WHY WE LOVE THEM)

Poor potatoes. They are such a humble and friendly vegetable and yet they seem to have been ostracized by the health community. I don't know why, but I'm here to tell you that potatoes are vastly misrepresented and to present my argument as to why they deserve a place on your table.

Potatoes are a carb, yes. But they are a whole-food, complex carb full of vitamins and minerals like vitamin C, vitamin B6, and potassium. They are low in calories and sodium-free, while being a pretty solid source of fiber.

It's worth noting that potatoes will affect your blood sugar more than some other complex carbs because they are high in starch. Some varieties are more forgiving than others. Here's how they stack up on the glycemic index (GI) scale.

LOWER GI

- Sweet potatoes (not technically potatoes, but we'll include them): Due to their fiber content, they have a lower glycemic index than potatoes.
- Yellow or gold waxy potatoes
- Red and purple potatoes

MID GI

- Yukon Gold potatoes (boiled)
- White potatoes (boiled)
- Fingerling potatoes

HIGHEST GI

- Russet potatoes
- Instant mashed potatoes
- Yukon gold (baked)
- White potatoes (baked)

Eating potatoes as part of a balanced meal shouldn't be a problem, unless you have health-related reasons to be particularly strict about blood sugar.

RESISTANT STARCHES

Here's a little bit of culinary alchemy: creating resistant starch. Resistant starch is a type of carbohydrate that digests slowly, making its way to the bowel before digesting. This keeps you fuller for longer, slows the release of sugars into your bloodstream, and acts as a prebiotic, feeding your gut microbiome. Certain foods are naturally high in resistant starch: beans, legumes, some whole grains, and green bananas, for example.

But you can also create resistant starch. By cooking high-carbohydrate foods, such as potatoes, sweet potatoes, pasta, white rice, or oats, and then letting them cool completely (refrigerating or freezing) before reheating, some of the digestible starch converts into resistant starch. This is super helpful for low-fiber, high-carb foods, particularly if you are being extra careful about your blood sugar.

It's also a great food prep hack: By roasting up some potatoes and putting them in the fridge, you are creating a blood-sugar-friendly and gut-healthy resistant starch to eat later in the week.

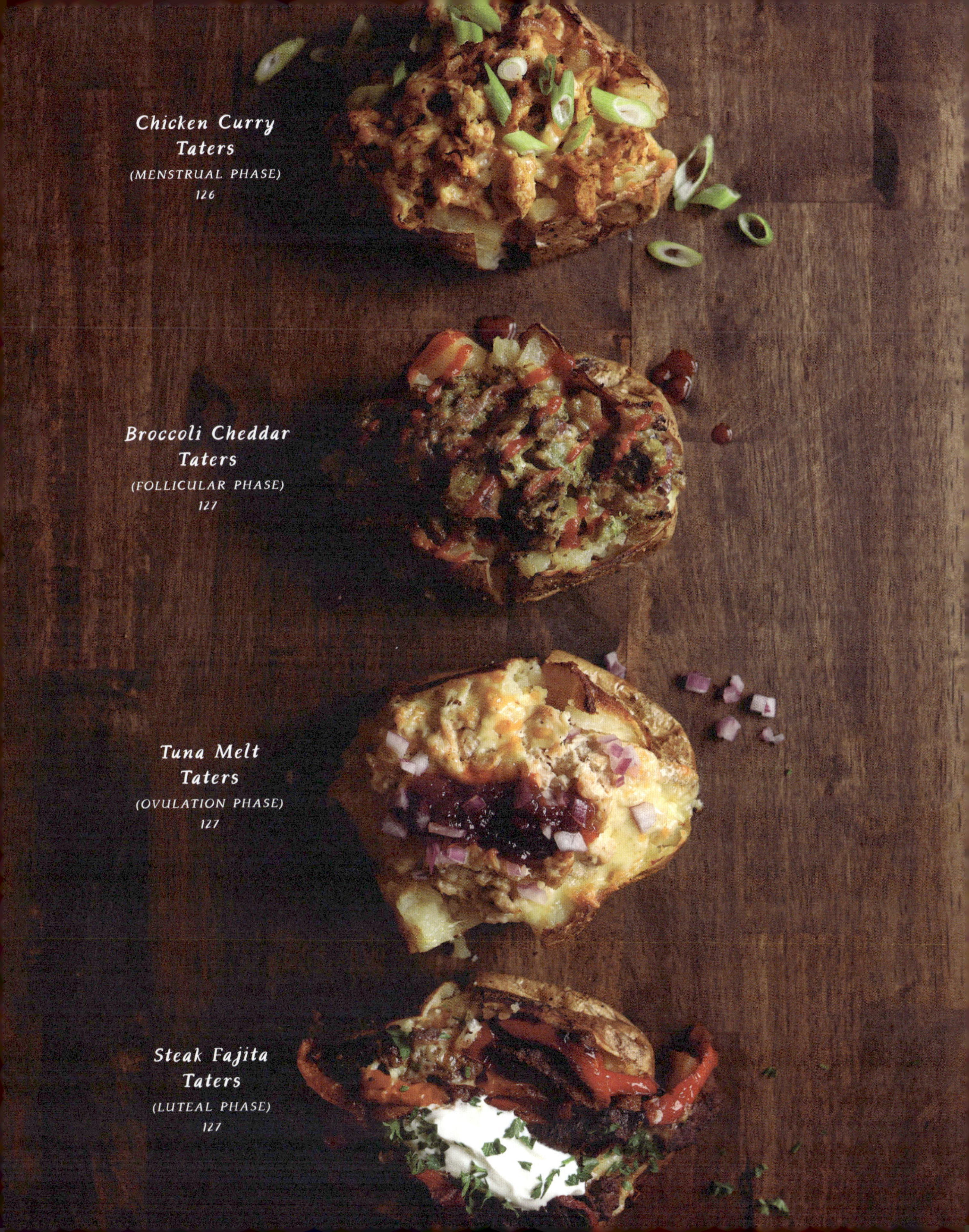

Chicken Curry Taters
(MENSTRUAL PHASE)
126

Broccoli Cheddar Taters
(FOLLICULAR PHASE)
127

Tuna Melt Taters
(OVULATION PHASE)
127

Steak Fajita Taters
(LUTEAL PHASE)
127

BAKED POTATOES

MAKES 4 POTATOES

Prep: *10 minutes*
Cook: *60 minutes*

All Phases

Gluten Free

Baked potatoes are the OG easy-peasy midweek budget meal, and there are so many ways to eat them. They're also so good for you. We need carbs. Say it with me: *We need carbs!* Carbs are an essential energy source and super important for brain function and for thyroid, cortisol, and sex hormone regulation. The type of carb does matter, though: Complex, fiber-rich carbs with lots of minerals and vitamins are what we want, and that's exactly what potatoes are! The beauty of a potato is that you can put literally anything on it (trust me, I've tried), but I've included some of my favorite topping combinations in the recipes that follow.

4 large russet potatoes
4 tablespoons avocado oil
1 teaspoon sea salt
Black pepper, to taste
Butter, to taste

1. Preheat the oven to 425°F (220°C).
2. Thoroughly wash and dry the potatoes, then use a sharp knife to carefully prick each potato a few times on each side.
3. Place the potatoes in a large cast-iron skillet or on a baking sheet.
4. Drizzle each with 1 tablespoon of avocado oil and sprinkle with salt and pepper. Rub the oil, salt, and pepper all over each potato.
5. Bake for 45 to 60 minutes, flipping halfway through, until fork-tender and soft all the way through.
6. Split open and top with lots of butter and one of the following combinations of toppings, with whatever your heart desires!

Chicken Curry Taters

Prep: *10 minutes*
Cook: *10 minutes*

Menstrual Phase

2 tablespoons avocado oil
½ medium yellow onion, thinly sliced
2 garlic cloves, grated or crushed
4 cups (600 g) shredded rotisserie chicken
1 cup (240 ml) Greek yogurt
3 tablespoons mild Indian curry paste
Sea salt, to taste
4 Baked Potatoes, split in half and buttered to taste
1 cup (120 g) grated mature cheddar (optional)

1. Heat the oil in a large pan over medium heat. Add the onion and garlic and cook until softened and browning, about 5 minutes.
2. Add the chicken, yogurt, curry paste, and salt. Give it a good mix and cook until until juicy and delicious, 5 to 10 minutes.
3. Top the potatoes with the chicken mixture and cheddar, if you like.

Broccoli Cheddar Taters

Prep: 10 minutes
Cook: 12 minutes

Follicular Phase

1 tablespoon avocado oil
1 medium red onion, chopped
¼ teaspoon sea salt, or more to taste
¼ teaspoon black pepper, or more to taste
4 cups (360 g) Teriyaki Roast Broccoli (page 134), chopped
1 cup (120 g) grated mature cheddar, plus more for topping
½ cup (120 g) softened cream cheese, cubed
4 Baked Potatoes, split in half and buttered to taste
Drizzle of sriracha

1. Heat the oil in a small pan over medium-low heat. Add the onion, salt, and pepper, and sauté until soft and golden brown, 5 to 7 minutes.
2. When the onions are almost done, preheat the broiler on high.
3. Add the broccoli, cheddar, and cream cheese to the pan, and stir, cooking until combined and melty. Top the potatoes with the mixture and sprinkle with a little more cheddar.
4. Place on a baking sheet and broil in the oven for 3 to 4 minutes, until the cheese is bubbly and browned. Garnish with sriracha.

Tuna Melt Taters

Prep: 5 minutes
Cook: 5 minutes

Ovulation Phase

Three 5-ounce (142 g) cans tuna in water, drained
½ cup (120 ml) mayonnaise
½ cup (120 ml) plain yogurt
½ teaspoon sea salt
¼ teaspoon black pepper
Juice of ½ lemon
4 Baked Potatoes, split in half and buttered to taste
1 cup (120 g) grated mature cheddar
4 tablespoons caramelized onion chutney or chili jam
¼ medium red onion, finely chopped

1. Mix the tuna, mayonnaise, yogurt, salt, pepper, and lemon juice in a medium bowl.
2. Preheat the broiler on high. Top the potatoes with the tuna salad, then add the cheese.
3. Place on a baking sheet and broil in the oven for 5 minutes, or until bubbly and browned. Top with a dollop of chutney and the red onion.

Steak Fajita Taters

Prep: 5 minutes
Cook: 15 minutes

Luteal Phase

2 tablespoons avocado oil
1 red or orange bell pepper, sliced
1 small yellow onion, sliced
¼ cup (32 g) fajita seasoning
2 pounds (907 g) raw marinated steak from Chipotle Steak Bowls (page 205), sliced
4 Baked Potatoes, split in half and buttered to taste
1 cup (120 g) grated mature cheddar
½ cup (120 ml) sour cream
Handful of chopped cilantro

1. Heat the oil in a medium pan over medium-high heat.
2. Add the pepper, onion, and fajita seasoning and cook until the vegetables are softened and browning, about 10 minutes. Add the steak and cook to your desired temperature.
3. Top the potatoes like you're building a taco, with steak, peppers, onion, cheddar, sour cream, and cilantro.

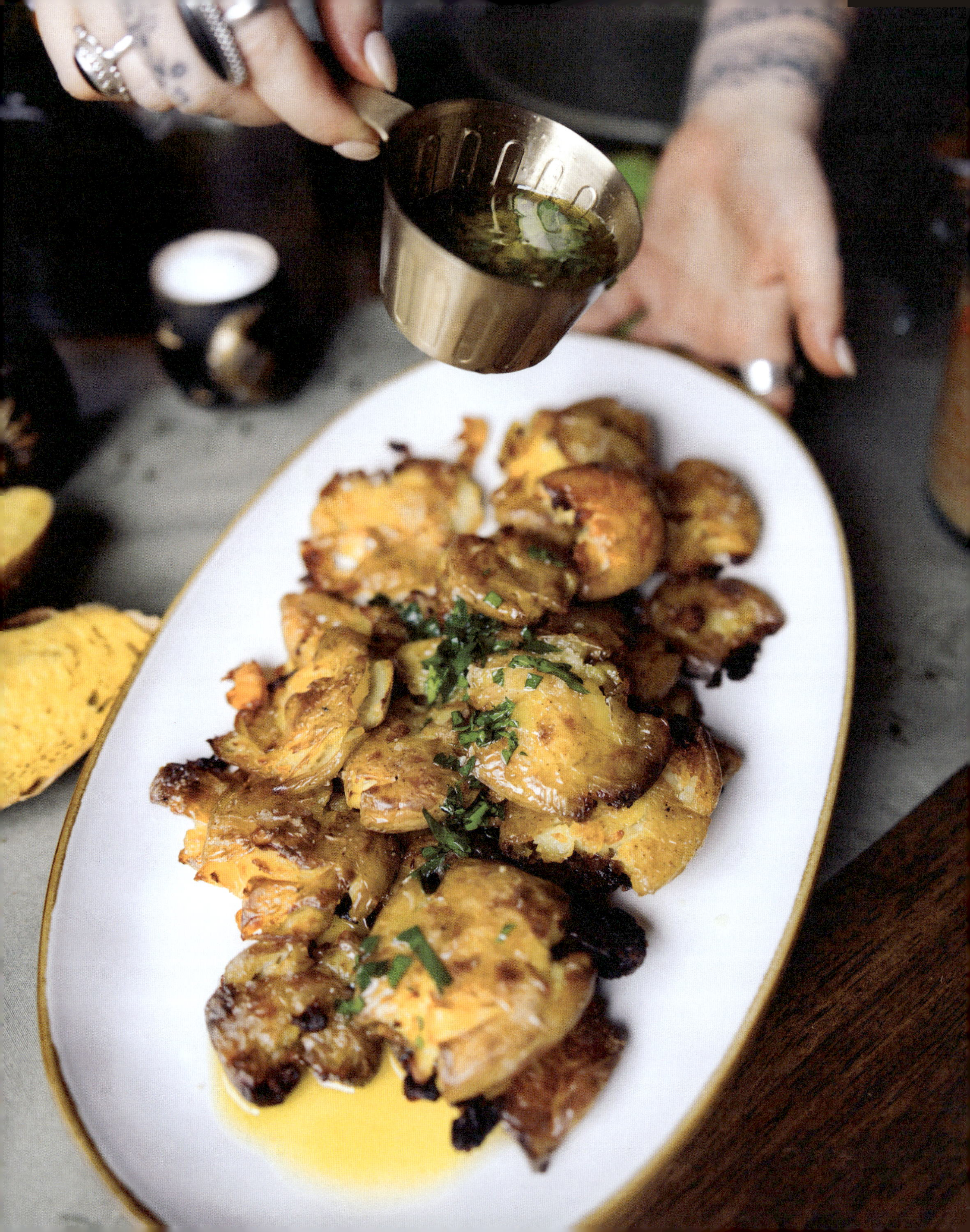

CRISPY SMASHED TATERS

SERVES 6

Prep: 10 minutes
Cook: 75 minutes

Gluten Free
Luteal Phase
Menstrual Phase

It's impossible not to adore these potatoes. They're soft and fluffy inside, super crispy outside, decadent but simple, and always impressive. The ultimate fat for cooking these is goose fat—it makes an incredibly crispy tater, but it can be a bit harder to find, so I often use ghee, tallow, or in a pinch avocado oil, which still does well with high heat, though it doesn't have the crisping power of the solid fats. The garlic butter is an incredible topping, but you can mix it up and try Parmesan cheese, hot honey butter, or Tahini Dressing (page 208). These are an absolute must alongside a Sunday Roast Chicken (page 200).

1 tablespoon sea salt, plus more to taste
2 pounds (907 g) baby potatoes, washed but not peeled (see Note)
4 tablespoons goose fat, ghee, beef tallow, or avocado oil
Black pepper, to taste
1 or 2 fresh rosemary sprigs

GARLIC BUTTER

½ cup (113 g) salted butter
3 garlic cloves, crushed or grated
1 small bunch fresh parsley, finely chopped

1. Sprinkle 1 tablespoon of salt into a large pot of water and bring it to a boil. Carefully drop in the potatoes.
2. Boil for 20 to 25 minutes, until the potatoes are fork-tender but not mushy. Drain the potatoes and let them steam-dry or tip them onto a towel to air-dry for 1 or 2 minutes.
3. Preheat the oven to 400°F (200°C). Dollop the goose fat into a roasting pan or a large cast-iron skillet and place the pan in the oven for about 10 minutes, until the fat is melted and piping hot.
4. Place the potatoes in the oiled pan and carefully toss the potatoes to cover them with the fat.
5. Use a large jar to gently smush each potato. The potatoes should be about ½ inch (1 cm) thick and not totally breaking apart.
6. Generously sprinkle salt and pepper over the potatoes, then add the rosemary to the pan, coating it in fat.
7. Place the pan in the oven and roast for 45 minutes to 1 hour, flipping the potatoes about halfway through, until they are crisped to your liking.
8. *Meanwhile, make the garlic butter:* Melt the butter in a small pan over medium heat, add the garlic, and cook, stirring frequently, until the garlic begins to brown, 2 to 3 minutes. Remove from the heat and mix in the parsley.
9. Remove the potatoes from the oven, generously drizzle them with the garlic butter, and serve.

NOTE

Choose mini red or yellow potatoes for this recipe. You may want to use two pans to ensure each potato has space to crisp around the edges.

ROAST CAULIFLOWER AND FENNEL

SERVES 8

***Prep:** 10 minutes*
***Cook:** 20 minutes*

Gluten Free
Luteal Phase
Ovulation Phase

The beauty of this recipe is in its simplicity: Each ingredient shines, and roasting brings out a glorious depth of flavor! The other beauty is the pairing of cauliflower and fennel. Cauliflower, like other cruciferous vegetables, is an incredible low-carb, high-fiber food. It helps with the body's elimination processes, it's great for hormone health, and it has tons of cancer-combating compounds, but it can be hard to digest. Unless your gut health is really tip-top, I recommend cooking or fermenting it to get the benefits without irritating your belly. Fennel, however, is particularly good for digestion. It soothes the digestive tract and stimulates digestive enzymes, making it the perfect ingredient if you find your gut is a little sensitive.

1 medium head cauliflower, outer leaves removed
1 fennel bulb
2 tablespoons avocado oil
2 teaspoons sea salt
1 teaspoon black pepper

FOR SERVING

3 or 4 tablespoons shaved Parmesan (optional)
Avocado oil or olive oil, for drizzling
Roasted Beet Dip (page 142; optional)

1. Preheat the oven to 400°F (200°C). Line a baking sheet with parchment paper.
2. Quarter the cauliflower and then cut into ½-inch-thick (1 cm) wedges.
3. Strip off and reserve the fennel fronds for later. Cut off the thin green stalks right at the base where they meet the bulb (these can be saved for stock but are too tough to eat). Cut the bulb in half and then into slender wedges.
4. Arrange the cauliflower and fennel flat on the baking sheet. Drizzle with the avocado oil and sprinkle with the salt and pepper. Flip each piece to cover it in oil.
5. Bake for 15 to 20 minutes, without flipping, until soft and browned on one side.
6. Remove from the oven and serve immediately, sprinkling generously with Parmesan, the reserved fennel fronds, and an extra drizzle of oil. I highly recommend serving this on a bed of Roasted Beet Dip (page 142)!

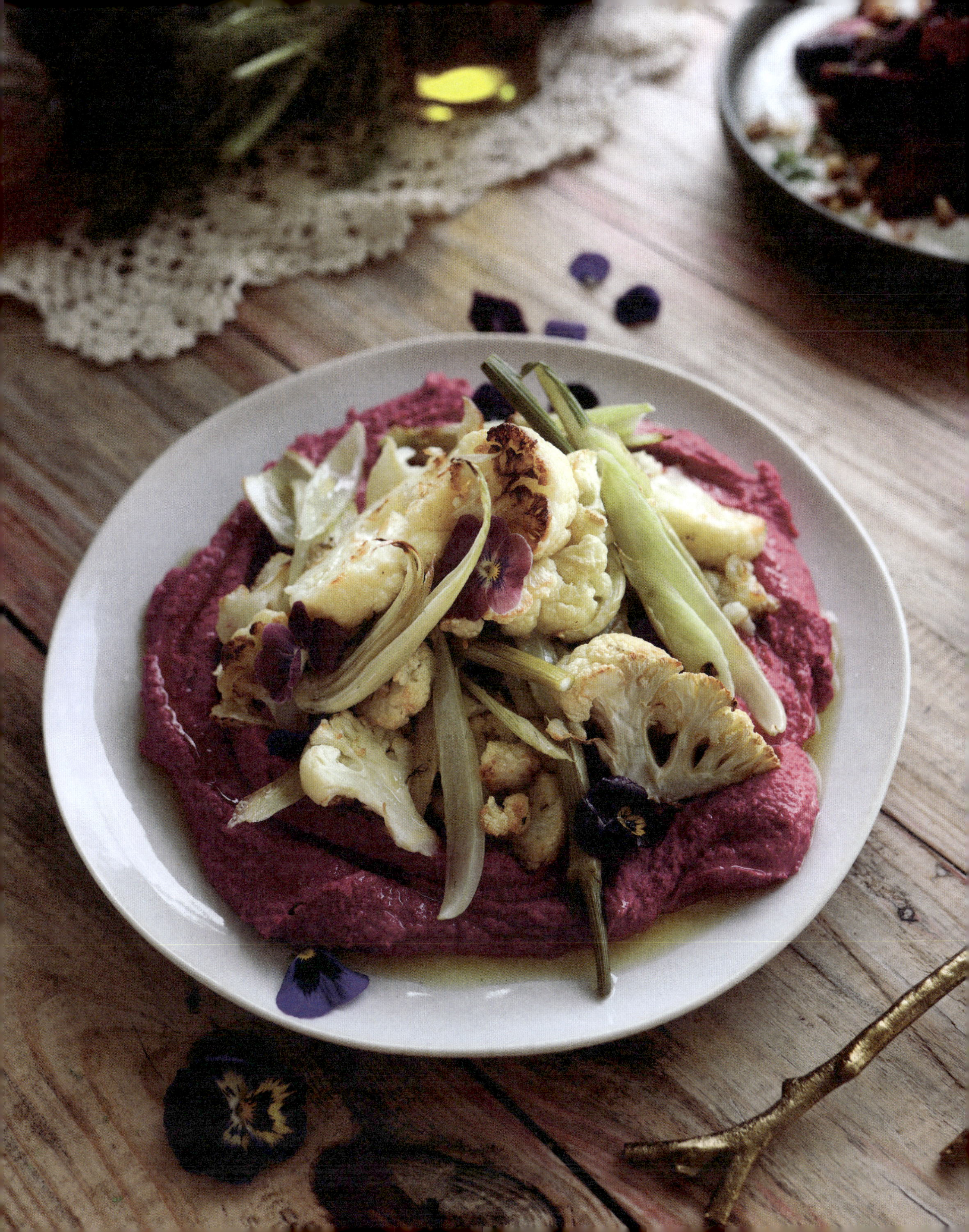

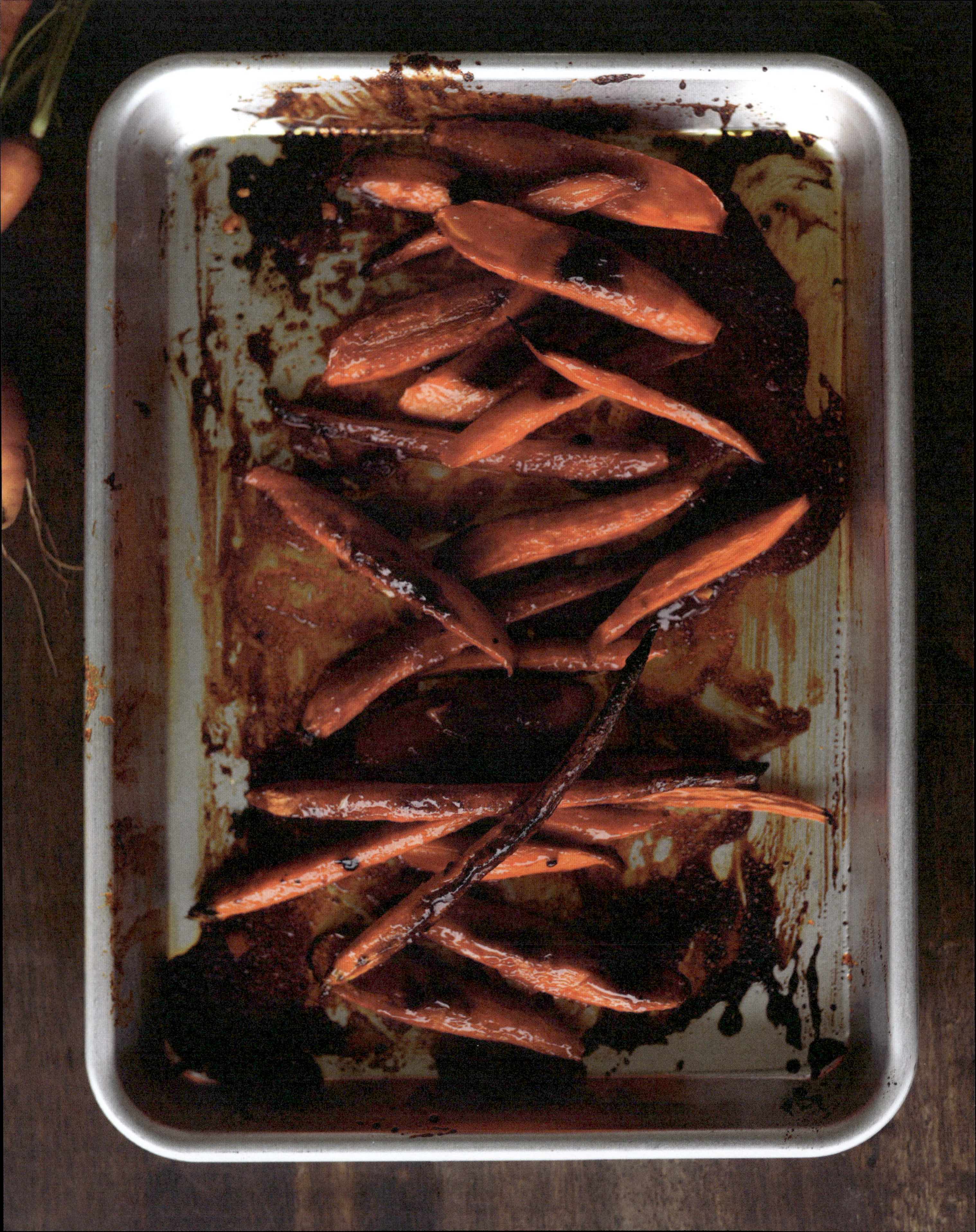

GOCHUJANG AND HONEY-GLAZED CARROTS

SERVES 4

Prep: 10 minutes
Cook: 35 minutes

Dairy Free
Follicular Phase

There's always a giant bag of organic carrots in my fridge—they're the ultimate essential. They're cheap, they never go bad, and I never get tired of them. We know they're full of fiber and vitamins, but cooking them makes their beta-carotene easier for us to metabolize. The body converts beta-carotene to vitamin A, which is great for hormone and skin health as well as immune function. Roasting carrots also brings out their sweetness, so eating these sweet carrots can help satisfy sugar cravings!

2 pounds (907 g) carrots
3 tablespoons avocado oil
1 teaspoon sea salt, or more to taste
½ teaspoon black pepper, or more to taste
¼ cup (100 g) gochujang
¼ cup (60 ml) honey
2 tablespoons liquid aminos or soy sauce
2 garlic cloves, crushed
Sesame seeds, optional

1. Preheat the oven to 425°F (220°C). Line a baking sheet with parchment paper.
2. Slice the carrots diagonally, about 1 inch (2.5 cm) thick. Place them in a large bowl and toss with the avocado oil, salt, and pepper.
3. Spread the carrots out evenly on the baking sheet. Roast for 15 minutes, or until fork-tender and slightly browned.
4. Meanwhile, combine the gochujang, honey, liquid aminos, and garlic in a small jar.
5. Remove the carrots from the oven, scrape them back into the large bowl you used earlier, drizzle with the glaze, and toss to coat.
6. Return the carrots to the baking sheet and roast for 15 to 20 more minutes, until browned and caramelized on the bottom.
7. Garnish with sesame seeds, if desired, and serve.

FOOD PREP ROAST VEGGIES

EACH RECIPE SERVES 4 TO 6

Dairy Free
Gluten Free

Sheet pan roast veggies are my weeknight go-to—easy to prep, endlessly versatile, and always delicious. I often use this as a quick food-prep method and make large batches of a chosen veggie or two to use in lots of ways through the week. You'll see these ones showing up in other recipes throughout the book!

Smoked Paprika Sweet Potatoes

Prep: 10 minutes
Cook: 40 minutes

2 pounds (907 g) sweet potatoes (3 large or 4 small)
3 tablespoons avocado oil
1 teaspoon smoked paprika
1 teaspoon sea salt
½ teaspoon black pepper
½ teaspoon garlic powder

1. Preheat the oven to 400°F (200°C). Line a baking sheet with parchment paper.
2. Peel and chop the sweet potatoes into ½-inch (1 cm) cubes.
3. Toss the sweet potato cubes with the oil, paprika, salt, pepper, and garlic powder in a large bowl until evenly coated.
4. Transfer to the baking sheet and roast for 35 to 40 minutes, stirring and flipping halfway through, until soft and caramelized on the edges.

Teriyaki Roast Broccoli

Prep: 5 minutes
Cook: 25 minutes

2 tablespoons avocado oil
2 tablespoons coconut aminos
1 tablespoon liquid aminos or low-sodium soy sauce
1 tablespoon sesame oil
1 tablespoon honey
1 teaspoon grated fresh ginger
½ teaspoon garlic powder
¼ teaspoon red pepper flakes, or more to taste
2 pounds (907 g) frozen broccoli florets
Sesame seeds (optional)

1. Preheat the oven to 425°F (220°C). Line a baking sheet with parchment paper.
2. Mix the avocado oil, coconut aminos, liquid aminos, sesame oil, honey, ginger, garlic powder, and red pepper flakes in a large bowl.
3. Add the broccoli, toss to coat in the sauce, and arrange on the baking sheet. Make sure the florets have plenty of space; if they are touching, divide them between two lined baking sheets so they can crisp up!
4. Roast the broccoli for 20 to 25 minutes, until it reaches your desired level of crispiness. Remove from the oven and sprinkle with sesame seeds if desired.

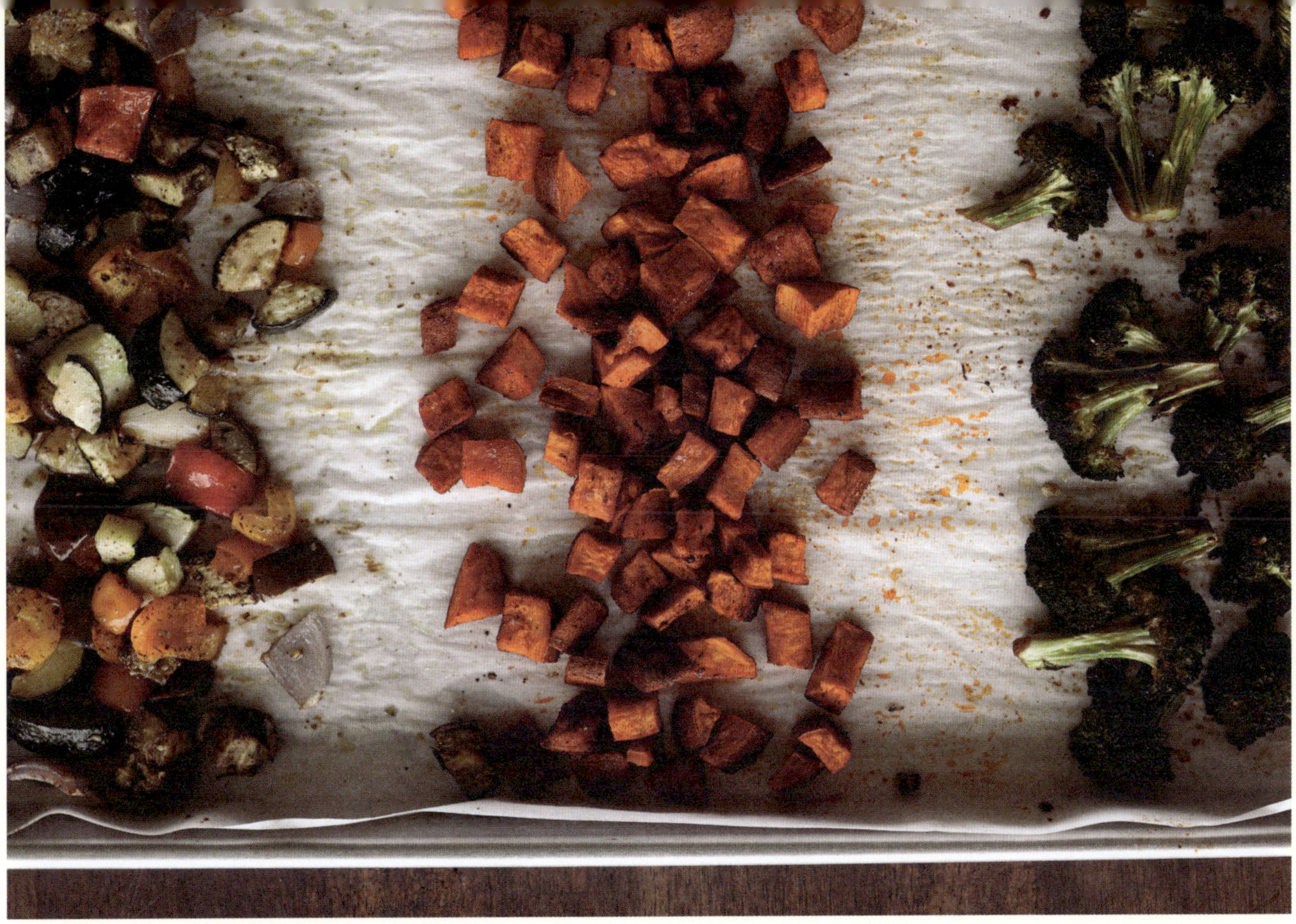

Mediterranean Summer Veg

Prep: 10 minutes
Cook: 40 minutes

3 zucchini (about 1 pound/454 g), chopped into 2-inch (5 cm) pieces
1 large eggplant (about 1 pound/454 g), chopped into 2-inch (5 cm) pieces
2 large bell peppers (about 1 pound/454 g), different colors, seeded and chopped into 2-inch (5 cm) pieces
1 medium red onion (about 140 g), chopped into 2-inch (5 cm) pieces
1 garlic bulb, top cut off to expose the cloves
2 tablespoons avocado oil
1 teaspoon dried basil
1 teaspoon dried oregano
1 teaspoon sea salt
1 teaspoon ground sumac (optional)
½ teaspoon ground cumin
¼ teaspoon red pepper flakes, or more to taste
1 tablespoon extra virgin olive oil
Juice of ½ lemon

1. Preheat the oven to 400°F (200°C). Line a baking sheet with parchment paper.
2. Place the zucchini, eggplant, bell peppers, and onion in a large bowl. Add the garlic bulb, avocado oil, basil, oregano, salt, sumac (if using), cumin, and red pepper flakes. Toss to coat the vegetables.
3. Arrange on the baking sheet. Make sure the vegetables have plenty of space; if they are touching, divide them between two lined baking sheets so they can crisp up!
4. Roast for 35 to 40 minutes, until tender and browned on the bottoms and edges.
5. Remove from the oven. Use tongs or a kitchen towel to hold the garlic bulb and squeeze the cloves into a small bowl. Combine with the olive oil and lemon juice, then drizzle over the veggies, toss, and serve.

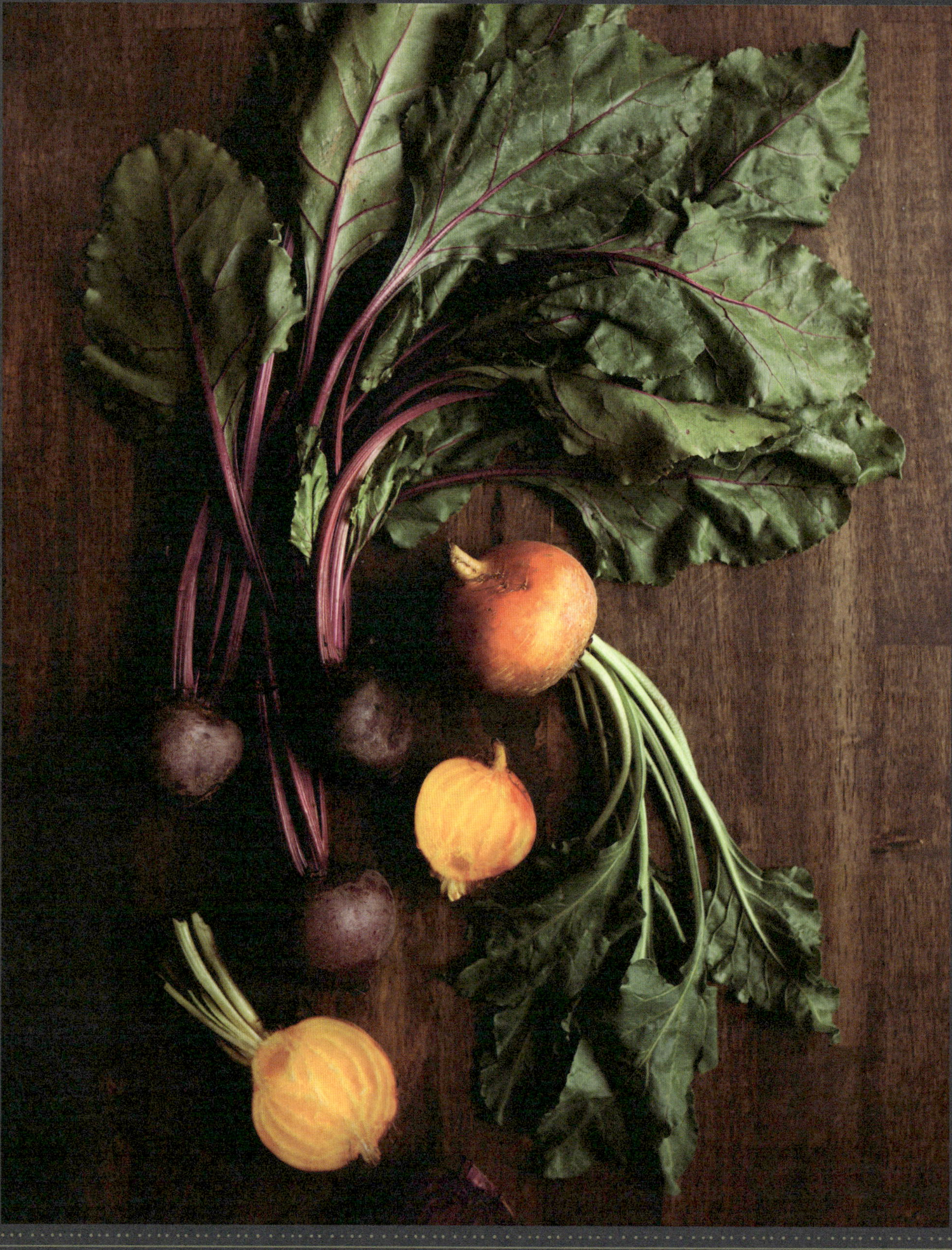

BEETS

Beets are the superfood we've all been overlooking. Humor me while I gush about them. They spring from the earth like little jewels, little bursts of color from the cold ground. Beets are tough, they grow easily, and they can be harvested well into December. When stored right, they can last for months, which makes them of great value. Plus, you get the two-for-one of the root and the greens, which are so delicious and should absolutely not be wasted. This alone puts them head and shoulders above other "superfoods," because they are actually cheap and accessible.

In cooking, beets are incredibly versatile. You can grate or chop them raw into salads and wraps, and they are incredible on a crudité platter! They make glorious baked goods, offering rich depth of flavor and moisture, and roasting them with just a little salt and oil brings out their gorgeous umami flavor. The greens are delectable raw or dry-sautéed with a dash of water and a sprinkle of balsamic vinegar. I could go on.

But to get down to the nitty-gritty: Nutritionally, beets are mind-blowing. Even though they are full of natural sugars, they have a superhigh fiber content and are very nutrient dense, which makes them a low-glycemic food. I particularly love them during my late luteal and menstrual phases, because they are a healthy cure for sugar cravings, but also because their earthiness is so grounding. I mean this energetically, as they have an earthy, rich, dark flavor, but also literally. They store tons of micronutrients and minerals, including some that are challenging to find elsewhere, like folate and other B vitamins, vitamin K, iron, and copper, making them super restorative. Their bright red color signals how packed full of antioxidants they are—and antioxidants are what fight cell decline and oxidative stress and neutralize free radicals (i.e., they combat aging and fight cancer). Don't skip those beet greens either because a lot of the nutrition is found there! They are powerful for heart, brain, and liver health and even boost stamina and athletic performance.

I could have written so many more recipes for beets, and in fact I had to cut some to make it fair to the other veggies. But I settled on the simple roast beets in the Honey Roast Beets with Labneh (page 141), which you can use in the Roasted Beet Dip (page 142), Beet and Farro Salad (page 138), and even the Beet-Berry Chia Pudding (page 77). You might as well just get a batch of them roasting right now—you're going to want a lot!

BEET AND FARRO SALAD

SERVES 8

Rest: 8 hours
Prep: 5 minutes
Cook: 30 minutes

Gluten Free
Menstrual Phase

This salad is hearty, earthy, good hot or cold, and great for food prep. It's also particularly grounding for women during the menstrual phase. The farro offers complex carbs as well as protein and minerals to support your energy and replenish your body during a phase that can be depleting. Beets, farro, and kelp are all iron-rich to support blood building and high in minerals to help manage symptoms and keep you feeling your best during a sensitive time.

1 cup (150 g) farro
5 cups (1.2 L) water, divided, plus more for soaking
2 cups (480 ml) broth
1 large piece dried kelp
½ teaspoon sea salt, plus more to taste
3 or 4 medium beets with greens
1 tablespoon avocado oil
2 tablespoons balsamic vinegar
¼ medium red onion, thinly sliced
¼ cup (37 g) crumbled feta

DRESSING

½ cup (120 ml) extra virgin olive oil
Juice of 1 lemon
2 garlic cloves, roughly chopped
2 tablespoons honey
1 teaspoon grated fresh ginger or ground ginger
1 teaspoon sea salt

1. Add the farro to a medium bowl and cover it with water by at least 1 inch (2.5 cm). Place a plate on top of the bowl, and let it rest for 8 hours or overnight.
2. The next day, drain and quickly rinse the farro and then transfer to a medium pot.
3. Add the broth, 1 cup (240 ml) water, kelp, and ½ teaspoon salt. Bring to a boil and cook until the farro is soft with a little chew, about 20 minutes. Drain, remove the kelp, and transfer the farro to a medium bowl.
4. Meanwhile, bring 4 cups (960 ml) of water to a boil in a medium pot with a generous pinch of salt. Remove and finely chop the beet greens and stems and set aside. Add the whole beets to the boiling water. Boil the beets until just fork tender, 20 to 40 minutes, depending on their size. Drain the beets, remove the skins if desired, and then quarter and slice them.
5. Heat the avocado oil in a large frying pan over medium heat. Add the sliced beets and a generous sprinkle of salt and sauté until they brown a little, 5 to 10 minutes. Add the balsamic vinegar and then immediately add the beet greens and cook, stirring quickly to soften the greens, about 3 minutes.
6. Add the beets, beet greens, onion, and feta to the bowl with the farro.
7. *Make the dressing:* Blend the olive oil, lemon juice, garlic, honey, ginger, and salt in a blender until creamy.
8. Dress the salad and serve warm or cold—it's great either way!

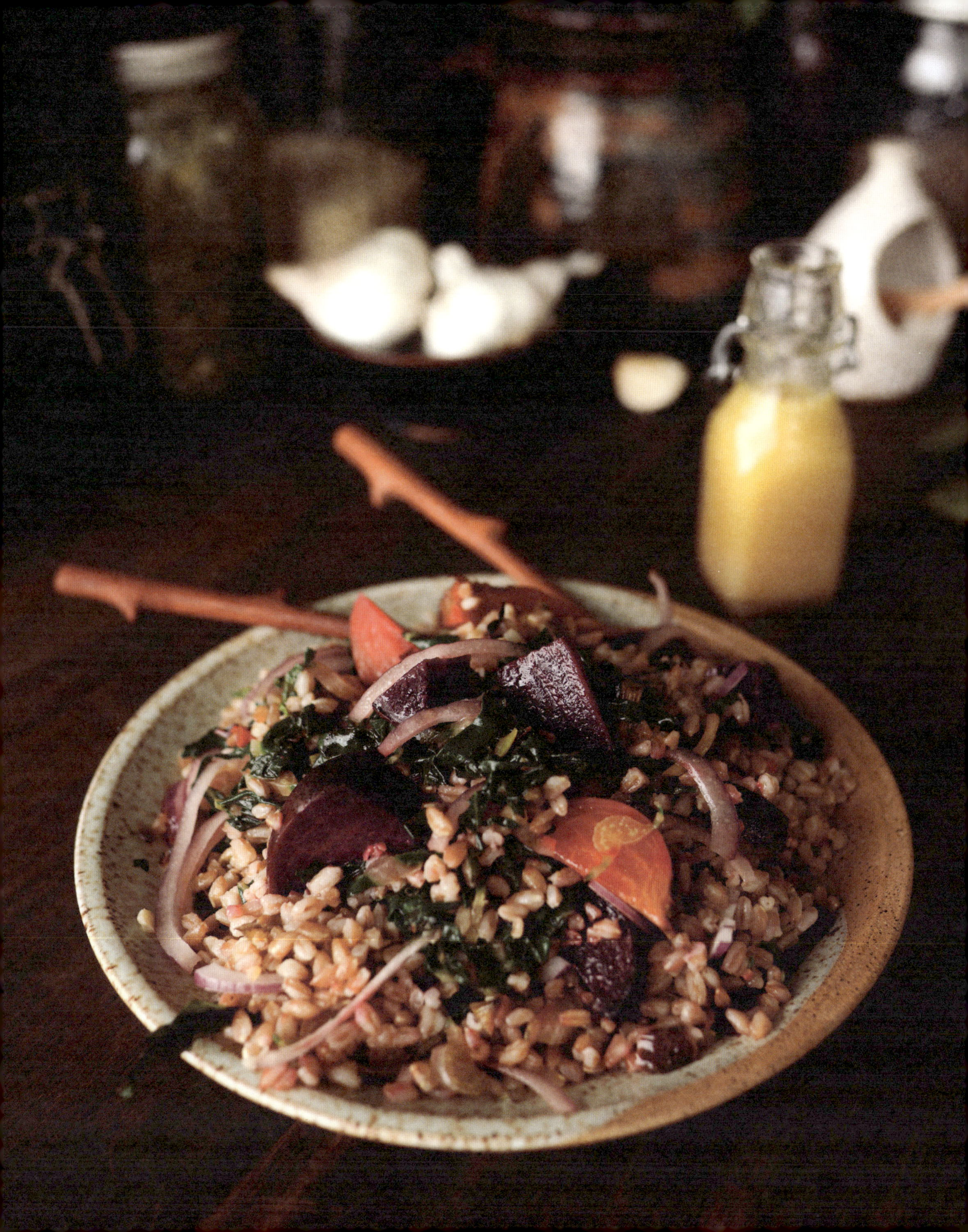

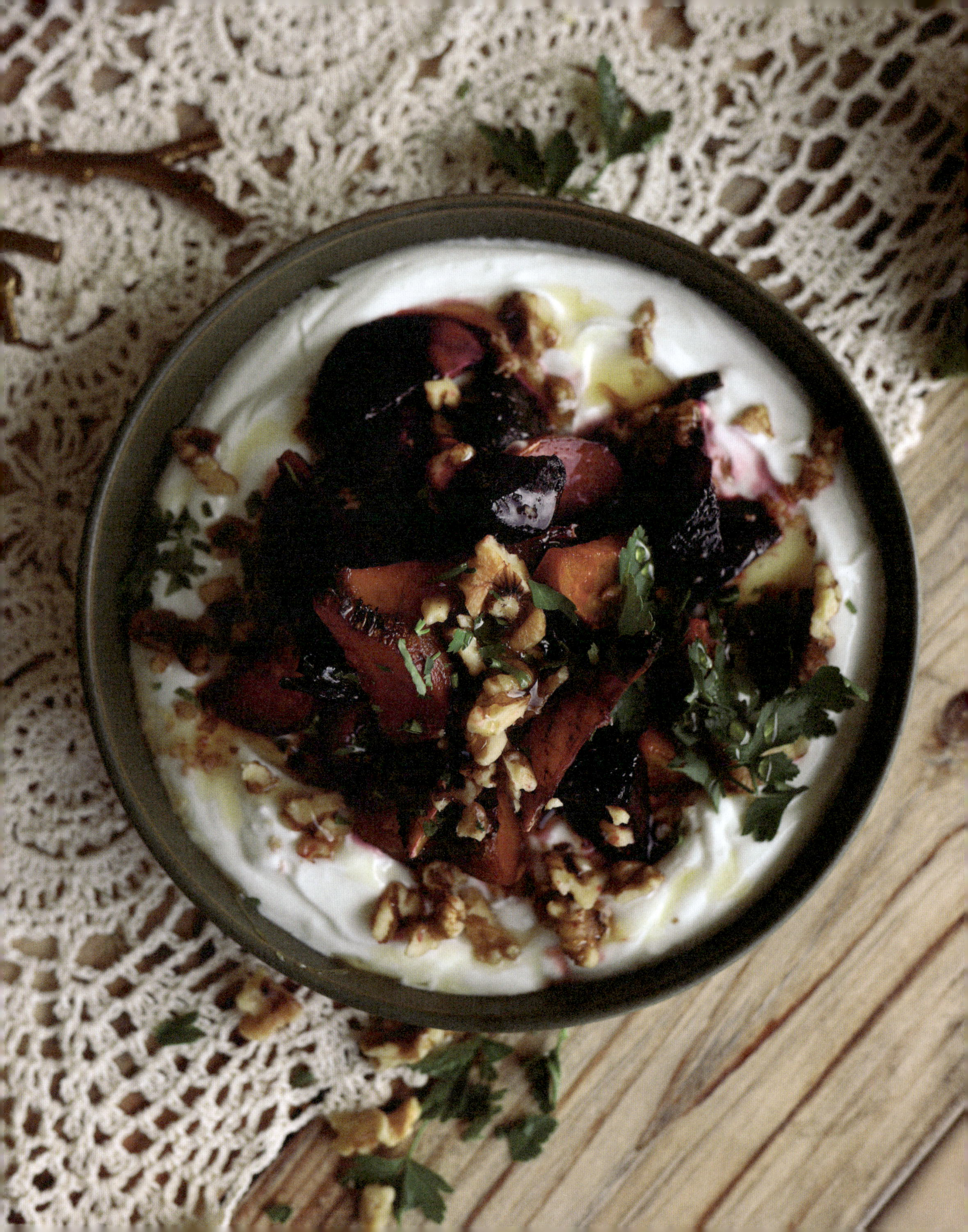

HONEY ROAST BEETS WITH LABNEH

SERVES 6

Prep: 5 minutes
Rest: 24 hours
Cook: 40 minutes

Blood Sugar Balancing

Gluten Free

Menstrual Phase

I firmly believe that if you don't like beets, you just aren't eating them right. Beets are such a powerful food ally: They are super sweet, but their high fiber and choline content makes them really beneficial for blood sugar balance. They can lower blood pressure, support digestive health, and increase blood flow to the brain and oxygen to the muscles. They're filling and sweet enough to satisfy a sweet tooth. With the additional fats from the labneh in this recipe, you get the most out of all the beets' vitamin and mineral content. This recipe is one of the best ways to eat beets, and I am so confident it will be a new favorite! If desired, you can make the garlic butter from the Crispy Smashed Taters (page 129) and spoon it over the top.

LABNEH

¼ teaspoon sea salt
4 cups (907 g) full-fat plain yogurt

BEETS

5 or 6 large beets
3 tablespoons avocado oil
3 tablespoons honey, divided
1 teaspoon sea salt
1 cup (100 g) walnuts

1. *Make the labneh:* Place a strainer in a medium bowl and line it with a fine cheesecloth. Stir the salt into the yogurt and pour the mixture into the cheesecloth. Twist the cheesecloth tightly around the yogurt and tie it with a string or secure it with a rubber band. Leave on the counter over the bowl for 24 to 72 hours.
2. *Make the beets:* Preheat the oven to 375°F (190°C). Line a baking sheet with parchment paper.
3. Wash the beets, cut off the tops and bottoms, and slice them into slender wedges or bite-size chunks.
4. Place the beets on the baking sheet and drizzle with the avocado oil and 2 tablespoons honey. Sprinkle with the salt and bake for 35 to 40 minutes, until soft.
5. Meanwhile, toast the walnuts in a dry pan over medium heat, stirring often, until they just start to brown, about 5 minutes.
6. Spread the labneh on a plate or platter. Top with the warm beets, sprinkle with the walnuts, and drizzle with the remaining honey.

ROASTED BEET DIP

MAKES 3 CUPS (720 ML)

***Prep:* 15 minutes**
***Cook:* 40 minutes**

Gluten Free
Menstrual Phase

In case you needed another reason to bow to beets, I present for your dipping pleasure this vibrant, complex, caramelized, and zesty dip. It's just as nourishing as it is moreish, and it's one of my favorite grounding foods for days when I need to cocoon. You can use leftover beets and labneh from the Honey Roast Beets with Labneh (page 141) and whip this up so easily!

3 medium beets, peeled and diced
2 tablespoons avocado oil
1½ teaspoons sea salt, divided, or more to taste
2 large garlic cloves
½ cup (120 ml) plain Greek yogurt or labneh (see page 141)
⅓ cup (80 ml) tahini (see Note on page 208)
Zest of 1 lemon
Juice of ½ lemon (about 1 tablespoon), or more to taste
1 teaspoon za'atar, plus more for garnish
½ teaspoon black pepper, or more to taste
¼ cup (60 ml) water, plus more as needed

YOGURT DRIZZLE

¼ cup (60 ml) plain Greek yogurt or labneh
Juice of ½ lemon, or more to taste
1 to 2 tablespoons water, plus more as needed
¼ teaspoon sea salt

GARNISH

Drizzle of extra virgin olive oil
Sprinkle of za'atar
Small handful of parsley, finely chopped

1. Preheat the oven to 375°F (190°C). Line a baking sheet with parchment paper and scatter the beets across it. Drizzle with the avocado oil and sprinkle with ½ teaspoon salt.
2. Roast for 35 to 40 minutes, until soft and browning on the edges.
3. About 15 minutes before the beets are done, add the garlic cloves to the baking sheet and quickly flip them to coat in the oil.
4. Transfer the beets and garlic to a food processor and add the yogurt, tahini, lemon zest, lemon juice, 1 teaspoon salt, the za'atar, and the pepper.
5. Blend until smooth, about 2 minutes, adding water a couple of tablespoons at a time until you get the texture you want. Taste the mixture and add additional salt, pepper, or lemon if you like.
6. Scoop the dip into a shallow bowl and swirl the surface a little to hold the toppings.
7. *Make the yogurt drizzle:* Combine the yogurt, lemon juice, 1 tablespoon water, and salt in a small jar. Put a lid on the jar and shake well to combine, adding the second tablespoon of water or more if needed until you have a consistency just loose enough to pour.
8. Swirl the yogurt drizzle on top of the beet dip, followed by a drizzle of olive oil, a sprinkle of za'atar, and a scattering of parsley.

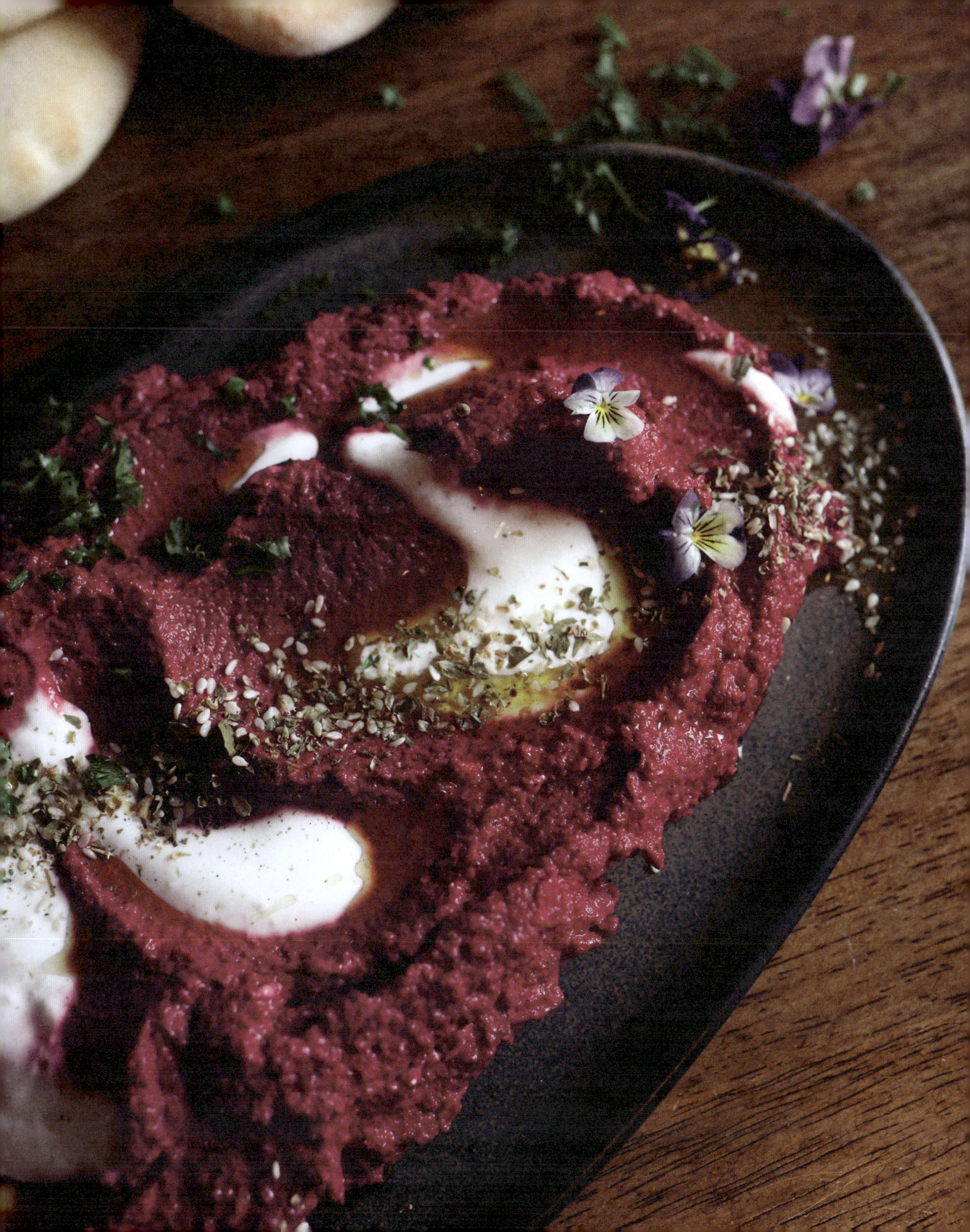

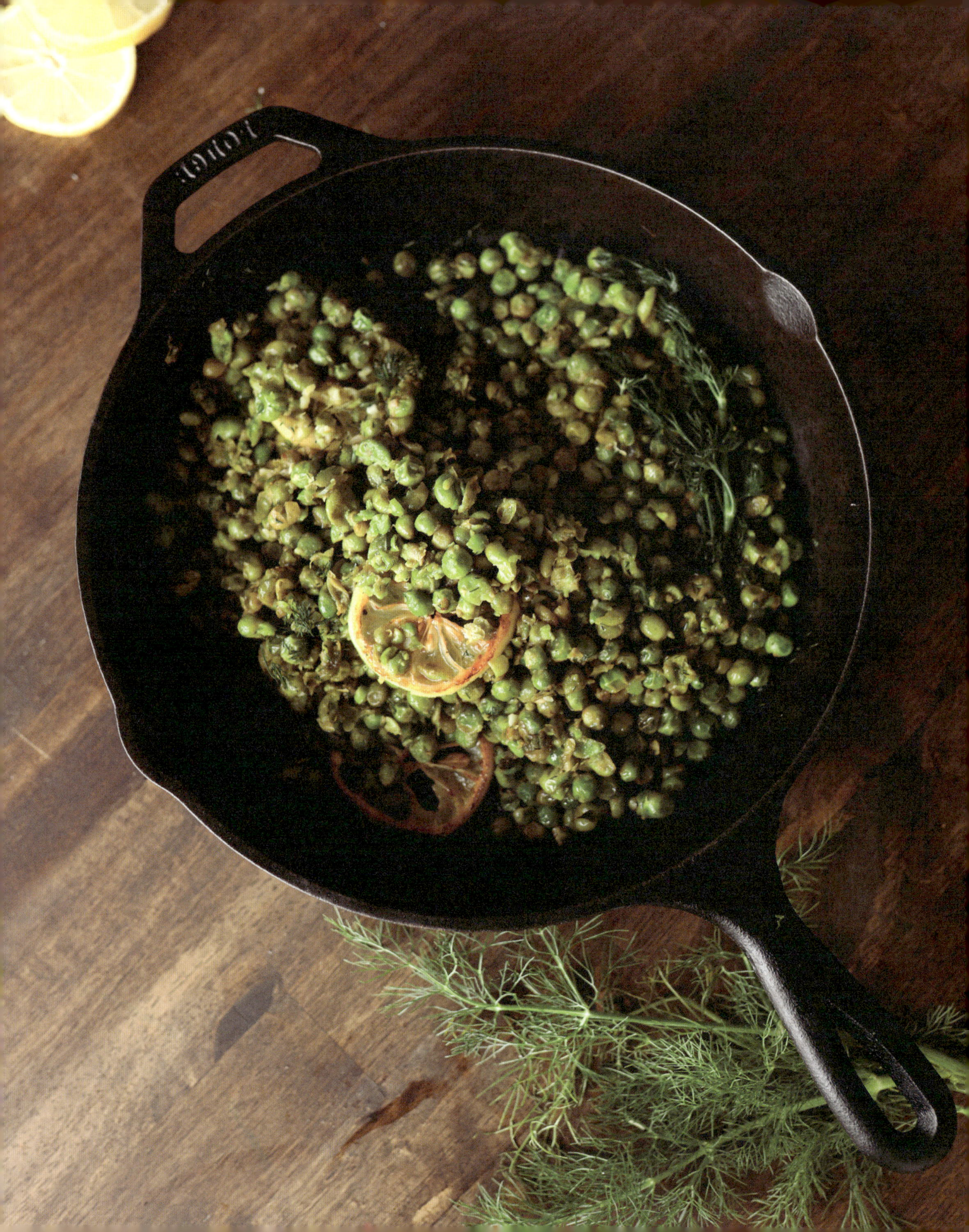
LODGE

HALF-SMASHED PEAS with LEMON AND DILL

SERVES 6

***Prep:* 10 minutes**
***Cook:* 30 minutes**

Follicular Phase
Gluten Free

When I was growing up in England, every fish and chip shop sold something called "mushy peas," and it was literally just that: mushy, smashed-up peas in a cup. I hated it. But I love peas! They are technically a superfood, high in fiber without being hard on digestion (unlike beans) and full of antioxidants. So yummy and fresh, this dish is an homage to the glorious pea with a little nod to my English heritage. It's the perfect side for a summer sunset dinner.

⅓ cup (75 g) salted butter
1 lemon, zested, then sliced
2 garlic cloves, minced
4 cups (535 g) frozen green peas
½ teaspoon sea salt
¼ cup (60 ml) water
1 tablespoon avocado oil
1 large bunch fresh dill, chopped, 1 sprig reserved

1. Melt the butter in a small pot over low heat. Add half of the lemon zest, two slices of the lemon, and the garlic. Cook gently, stirring occasionally and ensuring the butter doesn't begin to boil, 5 to 7 minutes. Remove from the heat.
2. Warm a large skillet over medium heat. Add the peas, then immediately sprinkle on the salt and add the water. Cover immediately and let steam until just softened, 5 to 8 minutes.
3. Remove the lid and allow any remaining water to evaporate. Pour in the avocado oil and increase the heat to medium-high.
4. Stir to coat the peas in the oil and sprinkle in half of the remaining lemon zest. Shift some peas aside, place two or three lemon slices flat against the pan, and throw in the reserved dill sprig. Cook, without stirring, until the peas and lemons begin to brown, 3 or 4 minutes.
5. Give the pan a good shake and stir. Then cook again without stirring to allow the peas and lemons to continue to brown, 2 to 3 more minutes.
6. Remove the browned lemon slices and dill sprig and set aside for garnish. Pour the butter mixture over the peas and add the chopped dill, reserving a tablespoon or so for garnish. Stir to combine.
7. Reduce the heat to low and use a potato masher to mash half of the peas. Choose your own adventure and leave lots of texture or make them really smooth.
8. Stir all the peas together and serve, garnishing with the remaining lemon zest and chopped dill, the reserved dill sprig, and the browned lemon slices.

HARISSA BAKED EGGPLANT

If your body does well with nightshades, eggplant can be an incredible source of prebiotic fiber and minerals. And the flavor of these well-roasted babies is unmatched. If you can get your hands on rose harissa (I buy it online, because I'm obsessed), I recommend using it instead of the standard variety for this recipe. This comes together in a few minutes and makes a great starter or side with fresh crusty bread.

SERVES 6

Prep: 5 minutes
Cook: 40 minutes

Dairy Free
Gluten Free
Ovulation Phase

2 tablespoons avocado oil, plus more for greasing
2 large Italian eggplants, halved
Sea salt
Black pepper
4 tablespoons rose harissa or harissa

FOR SERVING

Olive oil, to taste
Chopped herbs, such as parsley or cilantro (optional)
Pomegranate arils (optional)
Tahini Dressing (page 208; optional)
Labneh (see page 141; optional)
Crusty bread or flatbread

1. Preheat the oven to 450°F (230°C). Lightly grease a sheet pan with avocado oil.
2. Shallowly crosshatch the cut side of the eggplants and sprinkle with salt. Allow the eggplants to rest while the oven preheats, about 10 minutes; this will pull out some of the moisture.
3. Pat the eggplants dry, sprinkle with pepper, drizzle with the avocado oil, and generously slather with the rose harissa.
4. Place the eggplants, cut side down, on the baking sheet and bake for 35 to 40 minutes, until completely soft and browned on the bottom.
5. Transfer to a serving platter, cut side up, and drizzle with a generous glug of olive oil. Sprinkle with chopped herbs and/or pomegranate arils, and drizzle with Tahini Dressing or spoon some labneh on top (if using).
6. Serve with copious amounts of crusty bread or flatbread, ideally on a summer evening.

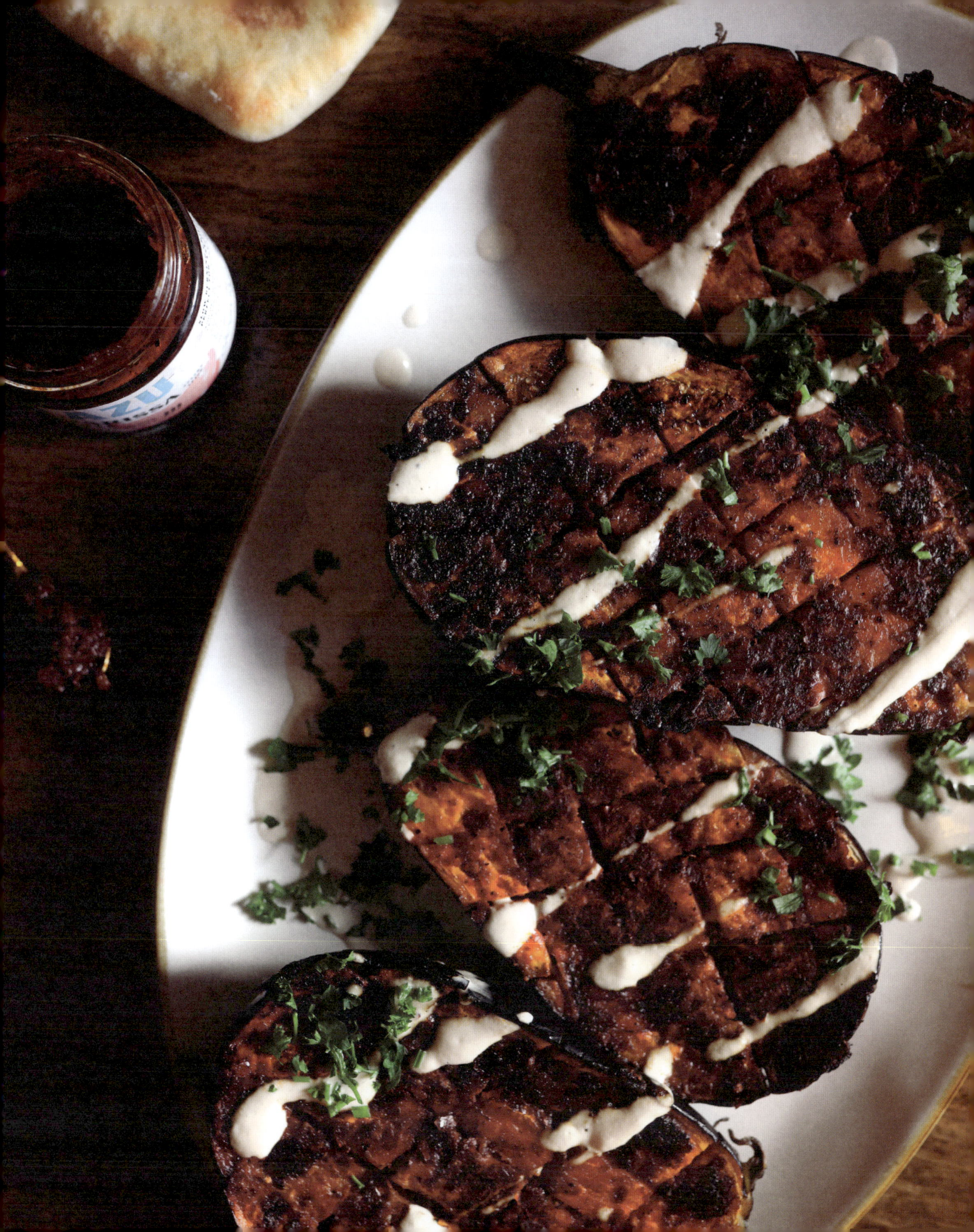

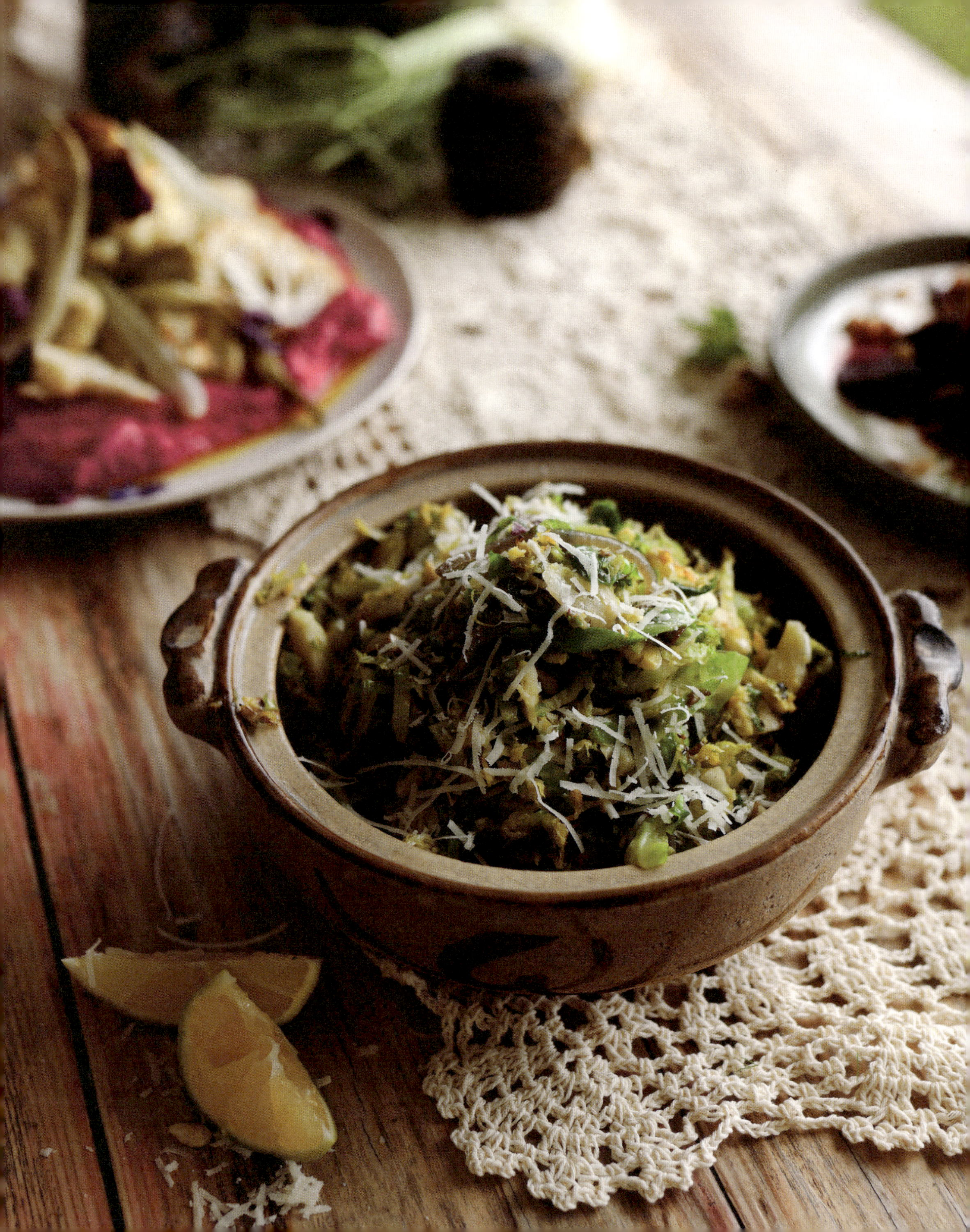

MAGIC BRUSSELS SPROUTS

SERVES 6

Prep: 15 minutes
Cook: 20 minutes

Blood Sugar Balancing
Dairy Free
Gluten Free
Hormone Supportive
Low FODMAP
Menstrual Phase
Ovulation Phase

Brussels sprouts get a bad rap, but cook them like this, and I promise it'll be an effort not to eat the whole batch. Which is great, because brussels are kind of an enigma—they contain a compound called indole-3-carbinol (I3C) which can reduce estrogen production and improve its metabolism, while their insoluble fiber makes them great for the body's elimination systems. That fiber content also helps balance blood sugar, further supporting hormone balance. In small servings (½ cup/45 g), brussels sprouts are low FODMAP and easy to digest while still feeding your gut bacteria tons of prebiotics. Also, that ½ cup serving contains almost all of your recommended intake of vitamin K, which promotes blood clotting and can ease excessive menstrual bleeding. And that, I think, is all pretty magical.

3 tablespoons avocado oil, plus more as needed
1½ pounds (680 g) brussels sprouts, finely shredded
½ large red onion, thinly sliced
4 garlic cloves, thinly sliced or crushed
¼ cup (35 g) raw sunflower seeds
Sea salt and black pepper, to taste
½ cup (50 g) freshly grated Parmesan
Olive oil, for drizzling
Juice of ½ lemon

1. Heat a large skillet over medium heat.
2. Add the avocado oil to the pan, followed by the brussels sprouts. Stir to coat the brussels in the oil and sauté until they turn bright green, about 2 minutes.
3. Toss the onion into the pan. Stir, cover with a lid, and reduce the heat to medium-low. Cook for 3 or 4 minutes before removing the lid, stirring, and covering again for another 5 minutes.
4. Uncover the pan and push the brussels sprouts to the edges to make a space in the middle. Add the garlic to the center and sauté for about 1 minute, adding a little more avocado oil if it sticks.
5. Scoot the garlic to the side and add the sunflower seeds to the center. Toast them for 1 or 2 minutes, stirring occasionally, then combine with the sprouts.
6. Increase the heat to medium and cook until the sprouts are soft and beginning to brown, 3 to 5 more minutes. Sprinkle with salt and pepper and stir to combine, then remove from the heat.
7. Add the Parmesan, a drizzle of olive oil, and the lemon juice. Toss together and serve warm.

MISO BRAISED CABBAGE

SERVES 6

Prep: 5 minutes
Cook: 25 minutes

Gluten Free
Luteal Phase

This dish is a twist on a childhood favorite of mine. It has a gorgeous umami flavor, and it's become one of my go-to recipes, as I almost always have a cabbage around these days. Cabbage is coming up in the world; it's the most underrated vegetable, and I'll stand by that. It's cheap, it lasts forever in the fridge, it's so simple to cook with, and it's the easiest thing to ferment. But it's also shockingly nutrient rich, with tons of vitamin K, vitamin C, folate, and minerals. Brassicas can be hard to digest, but when cooked, they're easy on the stomach while still retaining tons of fiber and prebiotic goodness. Eat more cabbage!

1 to 2 tablespoons salted butter
1 large head cabbage (red, green, or a mixture), thinly sliced (about 2½ pounds/1.1 kg)
1 large white onion, thinly sliced
¼ teaspoon sea salt
⅔ cup (160 ml) water
3 tablespoons apple cider vinegar
2 bay leaves (optional)
2 tablespoons honey
¼ cup (60 ml) heavy cream
2 tablespoons red or white miso

1. Heat a large skillet over medium heat. Make sure you have a lid that fits!

2. Add 1 tablespoon butter, then immediately add the cabbage and onion. Sprinkle with the salt, stir, and sauté until the onion softens, 3 to 4 minutes.

3. Add the water, vinegar, and bay leaves (if using). Stir, cover, and let simmer for 1 to 2 minutes. Stir again, then reduce the heat to medium-low, cover, and cook until the cabbage is significantly softened, 8 to 10 minutes.

4. Remove the lid. Stir in the honey and 1 more tablespoon of butter if desired. Cook, stirring occasionally, until the cabbage is super soft and tender and most of the liquid has evaporated, about 10 minutes.

5. Remove from the heat and let cool slightly. Just before serving, remove and discard the bay leaves (if using), then gently stir in the heavy cream and miso. Serve warm.

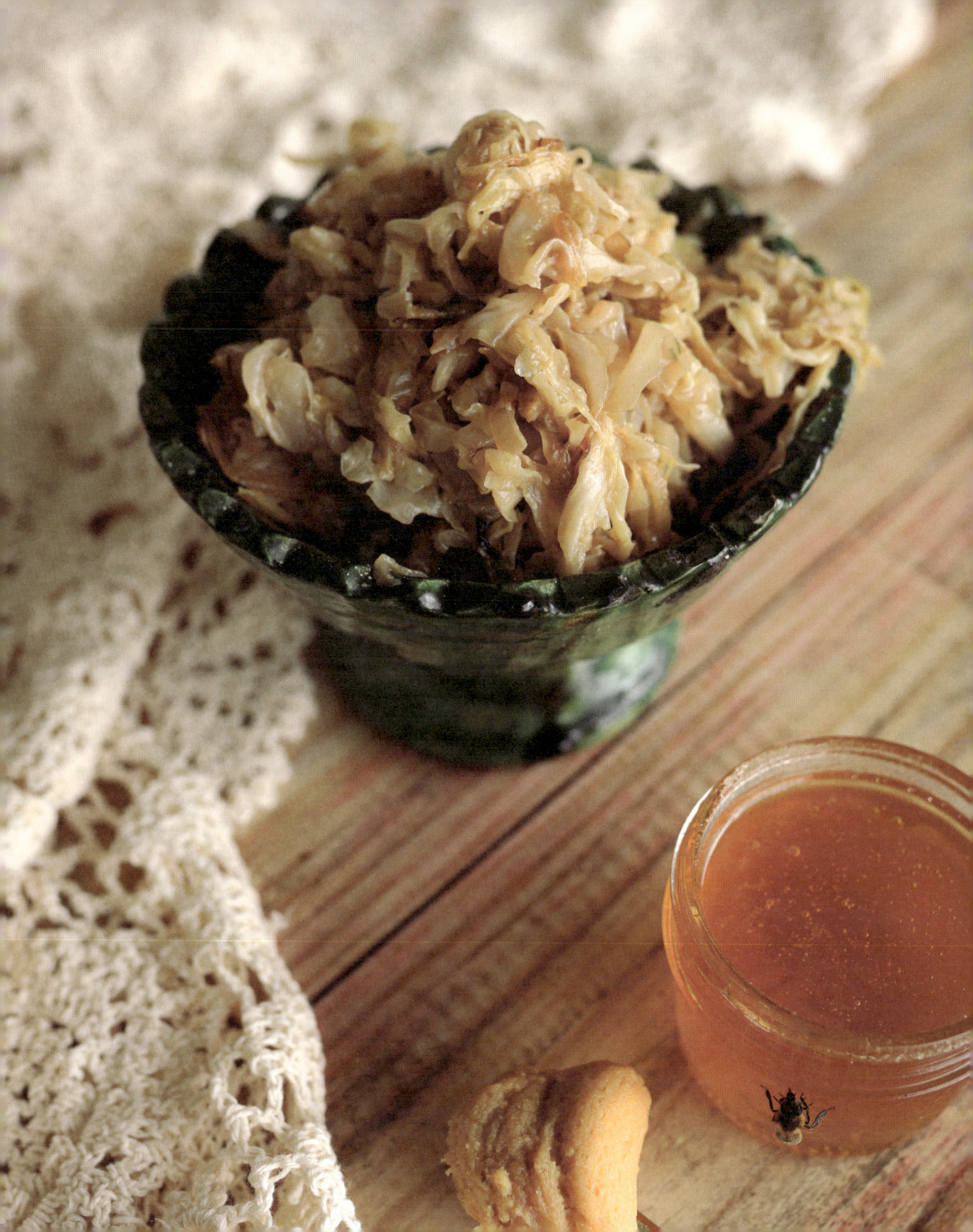

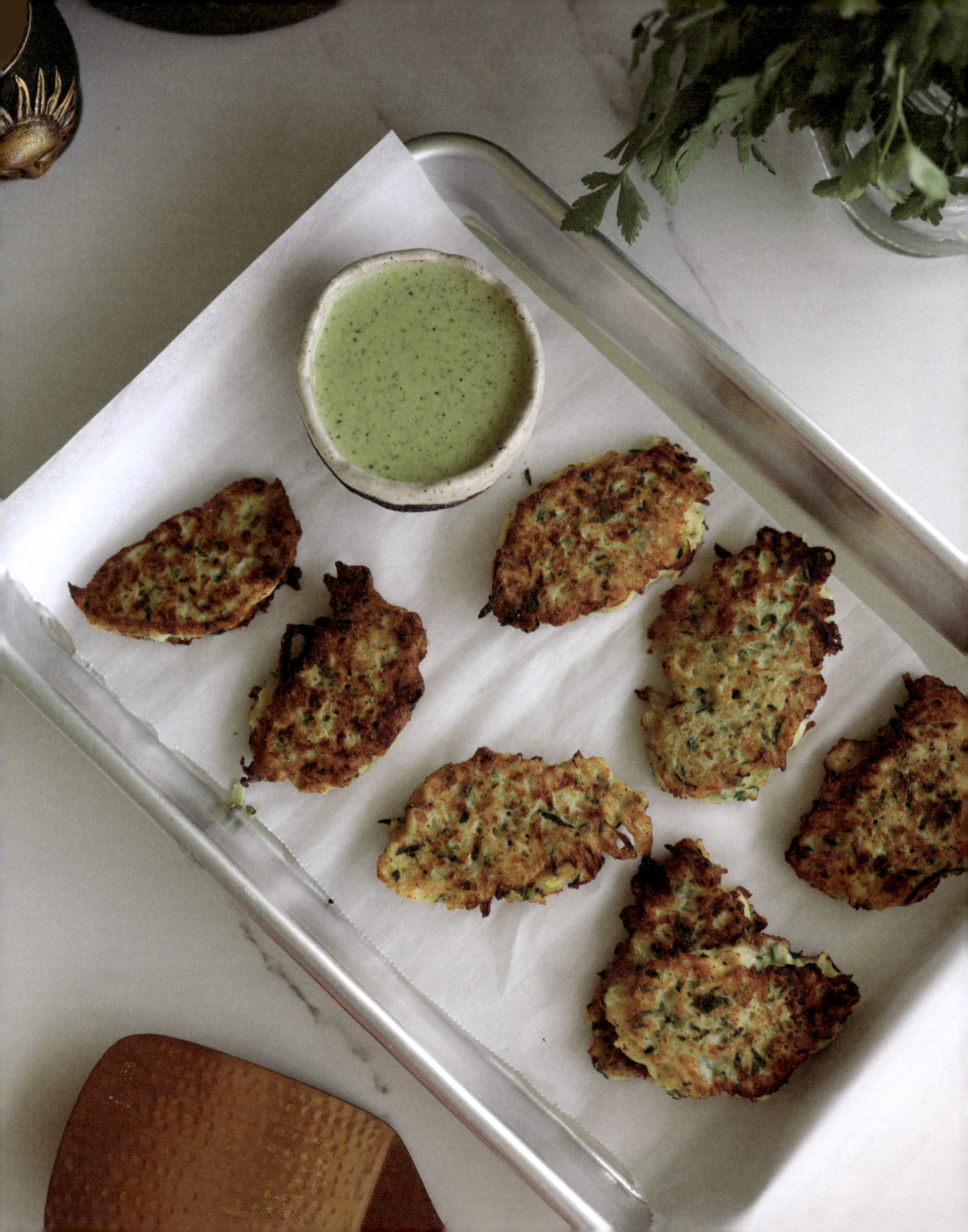

ZUCCHINI FRITTERS

MAKES 16 FRITTERS

Prep: 20 minutes
Cook: 25 minutes

Follicular Phase
Menstrual Phase

I will eat these any time of day, but they are a great breakfast if you're tired of eggs. They're also an excellent way to get a picky toddler to eat some extra greens and a really good meal prep recipe. A little more prep time to get the excess water out of the zucchini makes all the difference here, so don't skimp on that step. These are so good with a little sriracha mayo or Herbaceous Green Dressing (page 210)!

2 large zucchini, grated (3 to 4 cups/350 to 500 g; see Tip)
¼ teaspoon sea salt, plus more for sprinkling
2 large eggs
½ cup (60 g) all-purpose flour
Black pepper, to taste
½ cup (75 g) crumbled feta, or more to taste
Handful of fresh dill or parsley, finely chopped (optional)
3 tablespoons avocado oil, ghee, or tallow

1. Place the zucchini in a large bowl, sprinkle with salt, and toss to coat. Transfer to a fine strainer and set over the bowl for about 15 minutes, to allow the salt to draw out the moisture from the zucchini.
2. Dump the zucchini into a cheesecloth or cotton tea towel, or even pile it on a few layers of paper towels with more paper towels on top. Squeeze it as hard as you can to get out as much liquid as possible—don't go easy on it.
3. Dump the liquid out and wipe the bowl dry. Add the eggs to the bowl and beat, then return the zucchini to the bowl, followed by the, flour, salt, and pepper. Stir to combine.
4. Mix in the the feta, adding more to taste if you like, adding more to taste if you like—the more, the better, in my opinion—and some fresh herbs if you like.
5. Heat a skillet over medium-high heat and add the avocado oil. Test the heat by adding a drop of the zucchini mixture to the skillet. Does it immediately sizzle without the oil smoking? If so, you're good to go!
6. Add the zucchini mixture to the skillet in 2-tablespoon portions. Cook until the edges begin to lose their shine and the fritters hold their shape, 3 to 4 minutes, then flip and cook 3 to 4 more minutes, until golden on each side. Serve warm.

TIP

I like to use a food processor to grate the zucchini.

CHAPTER FIVE

SOUPS & STEWS

SOUPS ARE THE ULTIMATE HEALING FOODS.

They're what we take to a postpartum mama's house, the first foods we eat after surgery, and what we crave when we have the flu. They're traditionally a recovery food, and for good reason: They're nutritional powerhouses and very easy to metabolize. Soft cooked foods are really easy to break down and digest, enabling the body to conserve energy for healing instead of using it for digestion. Usually, a soft-boiled vegetable or meat loses lots of its nutritional value, but in a soup or stew any nutrients that come out of the ingredients hang around in the broth, so you end up getting the most out of them. Just put a ton of goodness in one big cauldron, let it literally stew in its own juices for a while, and reap the nutritional and medicinal benefits in one savory bowl. Add healing spices and herbs to the pot, allow them to simmer for a while, and you're basically a potion master—my Spiced Beef Stew (page 160) has added warming spices like star anise and clove for exactly this reason. The star anise adds digestive support for that red meat as well as strong immune support and antibacterial properties, and the clove helps with nausea, bloating, pain, and inflammation. The long stewing time draws most of those properties out into the stew, so alongside great nutritional support, you get targeted medicinal benefits when you need them.

I love to make a pot of soup at the start of the week as food prep—it's a one-and-done, super-quick meal. I particularly love eating soup for breakfast, as it means starting the day with a great energy source and lots of fiber and protein, while spending little energy on digestion. It's also a great way to clean out the fridge and use up leftovers and vegetable scraps. I've thrown spare rice, leftover burgers, floppy celery, and anything you could imagine into soups with great results, so feel free to experiment with what's in your fridge!

BROTHS

Broth nourishes us at the deepest level; we all know it intuitively. We eat chicken noodle soup when we're sick, and there are countless stories of languishing ladies being nursed to health with a bowl of broth. The reason is simple: Broth is like a bone tea, with all the goodness—minerals, vitamins, proteins—sucked out from bones and meat and concentrated into an easy-to-digest form. It's incredibly healing for the gut due to its high levels of gelatin, collagen, and the amino acids glutamine, glycine, and proline. So not only is it easy to digest for those of us with digestive issues, but it actually repairs our gut lining. It is anti-inflammatory, stimulates digestive juices, and feeds our good gut bacteria. And the cherry on top is that it's super easy to make. Making your own broth will help you reduce kitchen waste and stretch your food budget, too.

Bone broth in particular is the more nutrient-dense broth we are aiming for; where a standard meat stock simmers for 2 to 6 hours, bone broth cooks for 12 to 24 hours, allowing time for the bones, marrow, and cartilage to break down, releasing the amino acids, collagen, and nutrients—the magic makers.

The most accessible broths for many are beef and chicken broth. They have slightly differing health benefits and cooking methods; I'll show you how to make both.

Chicken broth is lighter and easier to digest. It's great for healing from a cold or flu, full of type II collagen (which makes it great for joints), and soothing for sensitive tummies. Any time you cook bone-in chicken, save the bones and store them in the freezer until you have a pot full to make broth.

Beef broth is richer and contains more minerals. It's great for long-term nutrition and deep healing. It contains more type I and III collagen, which makes it great for gut lining, skin, and deep-tissue repair. You can buy bones for this broth at most butchers, even butchers in large grocery stores.

The best bones for broth are joint bones that contain lots of connective tissue and cartilage. Chicken bones will typically create a less gelatinous broth; add chicken feet if you're looking for more collagen. Beef knuckles and other joint bones are perfect for beef bone broth; you can ask the butcher for help sourcing them.

Beef bones have more "impurities"—things like blood, fat, and connective tissue that can give the broth a gamier flavor and murkier appearance. These impurities can also make the bones pretty stinky to boil. For this reason, I always blanch beef bones first. Blanching is a very quick boil that will bring these impurities out (you'll see foam and other bits floating to the top of the water). You'll discard this water and rinse the bones before roasting and boiling them for the broth. There is no need to blanch chicken bones, as they have far fewer impurities.

If you can get into the habit of making a batch of broth a week, it will serve you so well! In seasons of extra stress or when I need to jump start good eating habits and improve my gut health, I try to start each day with a cup of warm broth. I usually make my broth very plain and then season it with some sea salt and maybe a squeeze of lemon when I warm it to drink. Of course, you can also use these broths in soups, stews, curries, or for cooking grains to add extra nutrition everywhere.

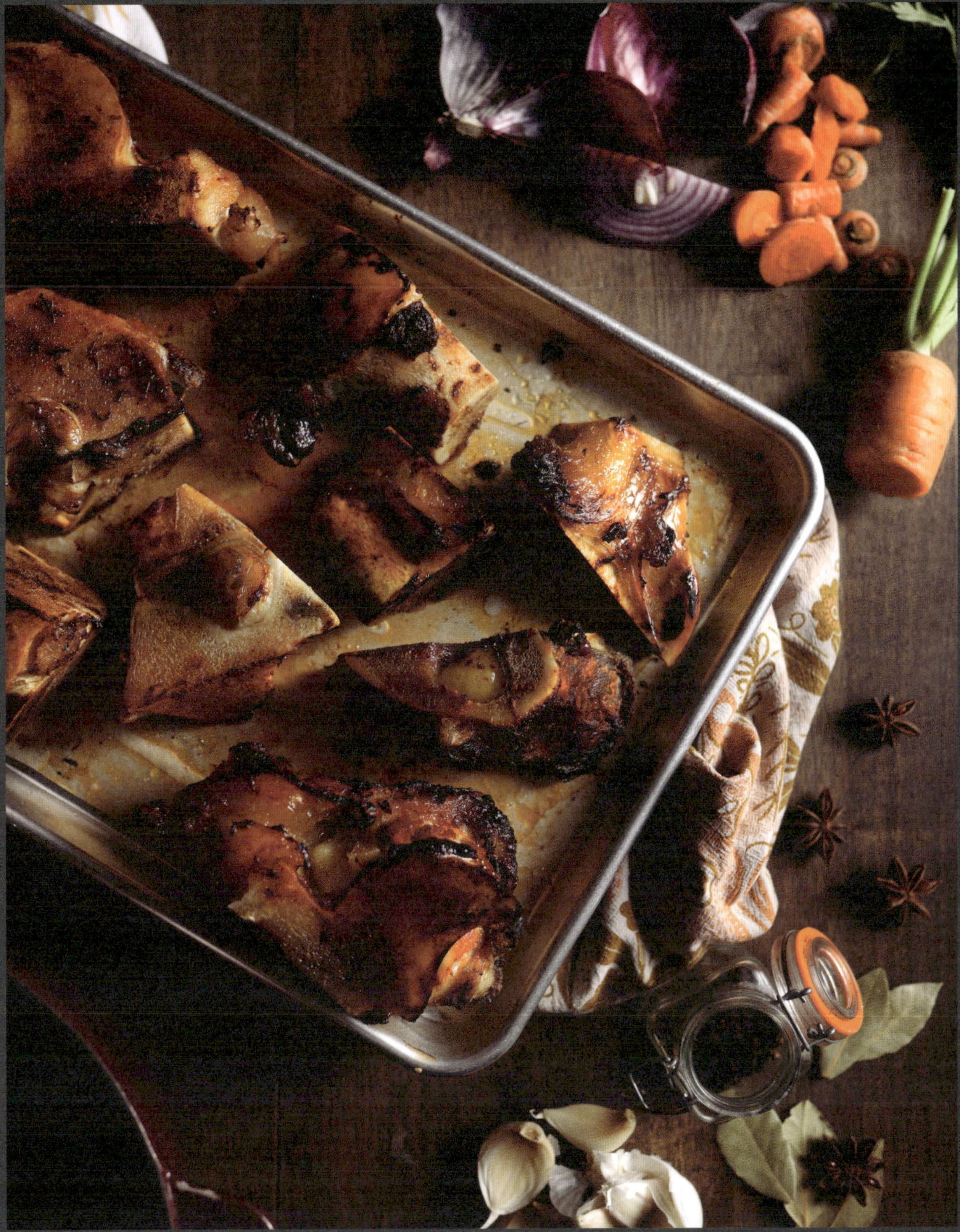

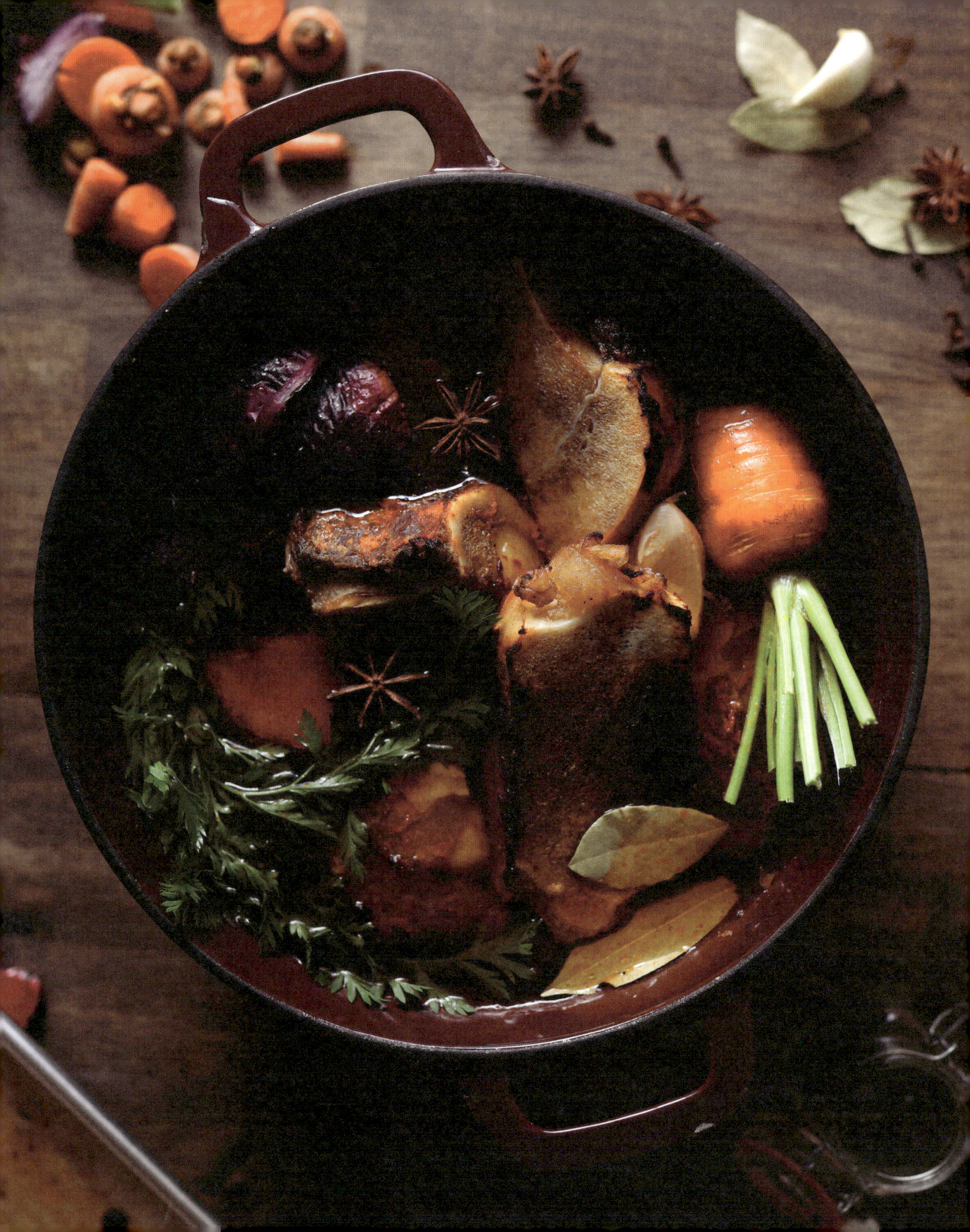

BONE BROTH

Don't be daunted: If you have a pot and some bones, you can whip this up while you sleep and reap all the benefits of this mineral-rich, gut-soothing, deeply nourishing ancestral food. I love that it really gets the most out of your animal products, because good meat is expensive and eating nose-to-tail is one of the best ways we can be more sustainable with our consumption of it!

MAKES
1/2 TO 1 GALLON
(1.9 TO 3.8 L)

***Prep:** 15 minutes*
***Cook:** 14 hours*

Anti-Inflammatory
Dairy Free
Gluten Free
Gut Healthy
Hormone Supportive
Low FODMAP

2 to 3 pounds (907 g to 1.3 kg) beef knuckle bones or assorted chicken bones and feet
2 to 3 cups (480 to 720 ml) leftover veggie scraps, such as celery stalks, onions and onion skins, carrots and carrot tops, and kale stems
One 6-ounce (170 g) can tomato paste (if making beef broth)
Handful of herbs, such as parsley, cilantro, rosemary, sage, or thyme (optional; see Note)
Small handful of aromatics, such as garlic, turmeric, ginger, star anise, cloves, black pepper (optional)
1 gallon (3.8 L) filtered water
2 tablespoons apple cider vinegar

1. If using chicken bones, skip to step 3. If using beef bones, blanch them to remove impurities: Place the bones in a large stockpot. Fill the pot with water and bring it to a rolling boil over high heat. Simmer for about 30 minutes, periodically skimming off any impurities (the brownish-grey scum that floats to the surface) with a slotted spoon.
2. Drain and rinse the beef bones, then arrange on a baking sheet. Coat the bones with the tomato paste, if using (no need to be perfect) and then roast in the oven at 450°F (230°C) for 1 hour, or until browned.
3. Place the bones in a large stockpot along with the veggie scraps and any herbs and aromatics, if using (see Note).
4. Fill the pot with the filtered water to cover the bones by about 2 inches (5 cm). Add the vinegar. Bring to a boil and then reduce the heat to a low simmer.
5. Cover and simmer for 12 to 24 hours, depending on how rich you want the flavor to be (the longer it simmers, the deeper the flavor). Make sure the ingredients stay mostly covered with liquid (it will reduce and they will peek out). The water should be hot enough for a few bubbles to simmer up regularly—ideally between 180 and 205°F (80 and 95°C)—but not at a rolling boil.
6. Remove from the heat, let cool slightly, and then strain through a large colander into another large pot. Discard the bones and veggie scraps and use a funnel to decant the broth into a large mason jar.
7. Leave the lid off and refrigerate to let it cool as quickly as possible. The fat will rise to the top of the jar; you can skim it off (beef broth will create a pretty thick layer that can be taken off and used in recipes like Spiced Beef Stew; page 160).
8. Cover and store for up to 1 week in the fridge or up to 6 months in the freezer.

NOTE

For a mild, all-purpose broth that you can use in recipes with different flavor profiles (like my Bone Broth Hot Cocoa on page 254), don't add any aromatics or spices. For a sipping broth, or if you're making broth for a specific recipe (like my Quick Ramen on page 169), you can add whatever your heart desires. Avoid adding salt, as this is better added after you've added the broth to the recipe.

SPICED BEEF STEW

SERVES 8

***Prep:** 25 minutes*
***Cook:** 3 hours, 30 minutes*

Blood Sugar Balancing

Dairy Free

Gluten Free

Gut Healthy

Menstrual Phase

Stew is personal. Everyone's mama has their own recipe. I love a thick broth, a rich, umami flavor profile, and lots of vegetables. This is a great recipe to use up whatever is in your fridge, although it's hard to beat root veggies. It's a great meal for recovery, as everything is slowly cooked, creating a broth that's full of nutrients and easy to digest. The added spices give this an extra healing boost with antiviral, antibacterial, and anti-inflammatory properties.

2 tablespoons avocado oil or beef fat (see Bone Broth; page 159)
2 pounds (907 g) chuck roast or stew steak
Sea salt and black pepper, to taste
2 celery stalks, diced
1 medium yellow onion, diced
3 garlic cloves, minced
4 to 5 medium carrots, cut into bite-size pieces
3 cups (450 g) chopped red potatoes or halved mini red potatoes
2 tablespoons tomato paste
¼ cup (30 g) cornstarch
½ cup (120 ml) red wine (see Note 1)
8 cups (1.9 L) beef Bone Broth (page 159)
2 bay leaves, fresh or dried
1 fresh rosemary sprig
1 fresh thyme sprig
3 star anise pods
3 to 5 whole cloves
1 tablespoon brown sugar
1 teaspoon Worcestershire sauce

1. Heat the oil in a Dutch oven over medium-high heat.
2. Meanwhile, chop the roast into 1-inch (2.5 cm) cubes and sprinkle with salt and pepper. Add the meat to the pan. It should sizzle loudly (if it doesn't, the oil isn't hot enough).
3. Sear the cubes on each side, quickly browning them but not cooking them through, about 2 minutes per side. Transfer the cubes to a plate while you cook the vegetables.
4. Reduce the heat to medium-low and add the celery and onion to the pan with a generous sprinkle of salt. Sauté gently, stirring occasionally until the vegetables begin to soften, about 5 minutes (see Note 2).
5. Add the garlic and sauté until fragrant, 1 or 2 minutes. Add the carrots and potatoes and cook, stirring occasionally, until browned, 1 to 2 minutes.
6. Return the beef to the Dutch oven, add the tomato paste, and stir to coat. Stir in the cornstarch. Add the wine and scrape the pan to deglaze.
7. Add the broth, bay leaves, rosemary, thyme, star anise, and cloves (see Note 3), then add the brown sugar, Worcestershire sauce, and salt and pepper to taste.
8. Bring to a boil and then immediately reduce to a low simmer. Cook for at least 3 hours, or all day if possible—the longer it cooks, the more tender the meat will be. Partially cover with a lid to keep the liquid from evaporating. If the liquid reduces too much, add some extra broth or water.

NOTES

1. You can substitute ¼ cup (60 ml) extra broth mixed with 2 tablespoons of balsamic or red wine vinegar for the red wine.

2. If meat residue causes the onions to stick, deglaze with 3 to 4 tablespoons red wine, red wine vinegar, or beef broth.

3. For a rustic stew, throw the whole spices and herbs straight in, but be aware of them when eating. You can also make a small sachet with a bit of cheesecloth and some string, loosely tied to keep the spices and herbs inside.

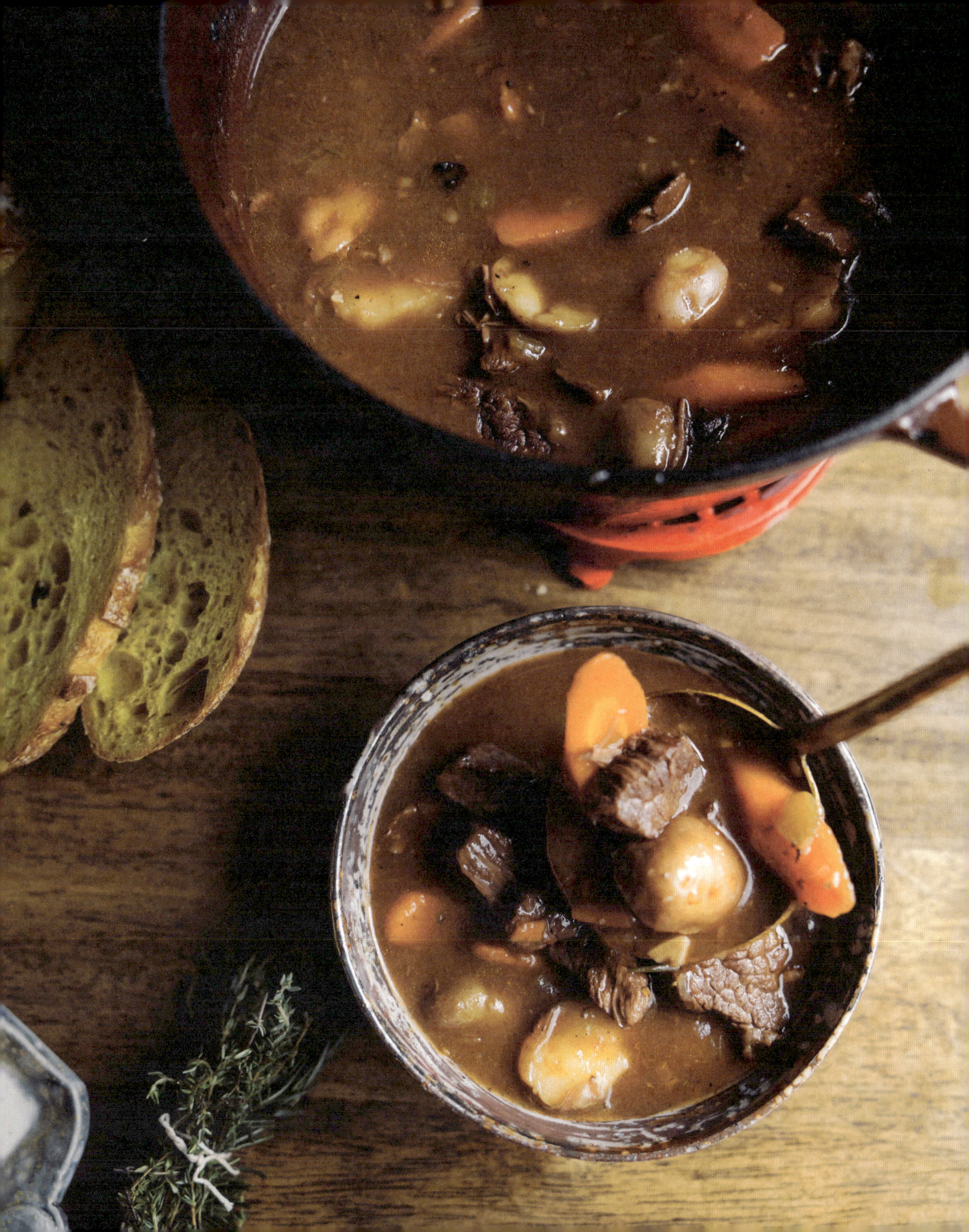

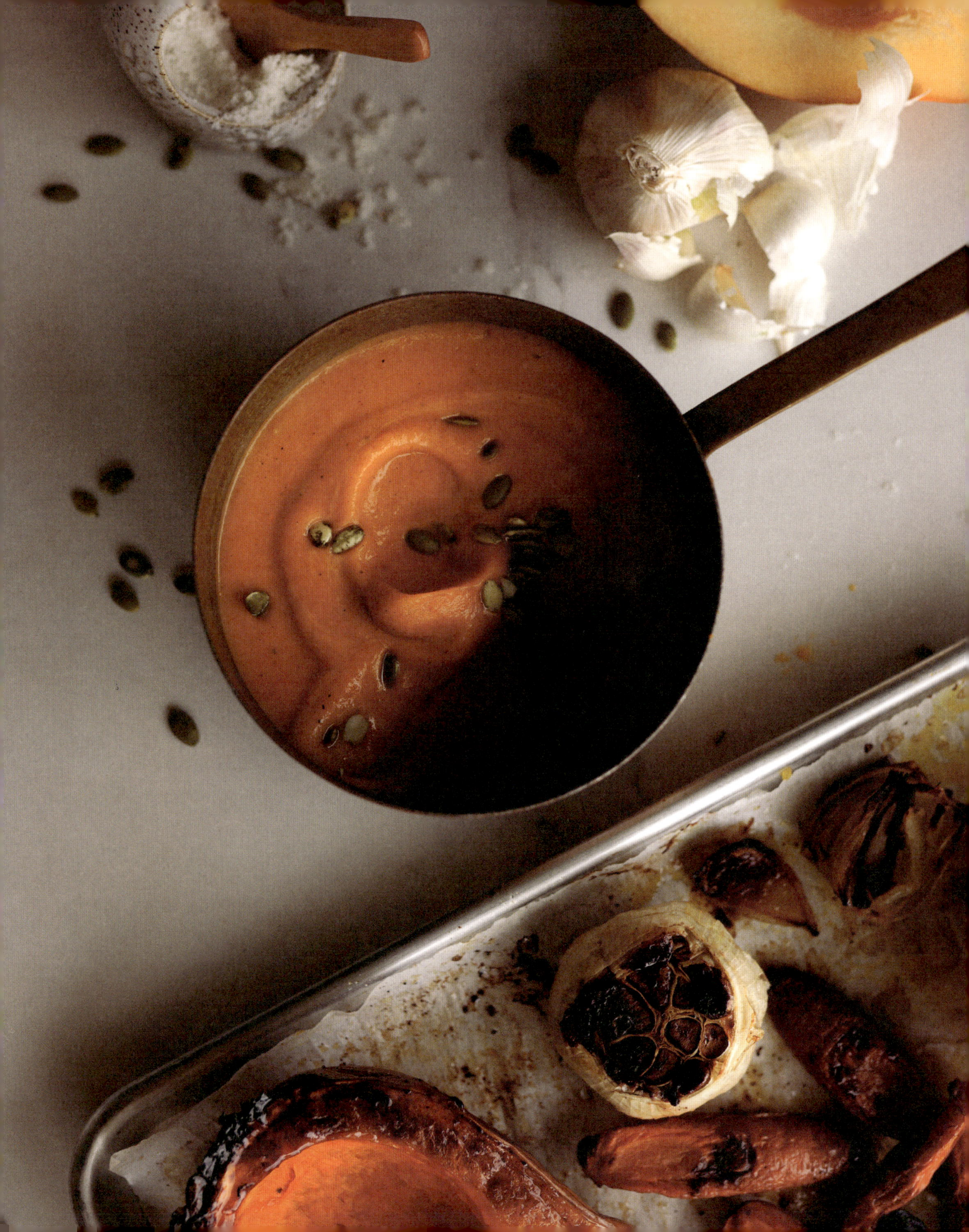

EASY PEASY ROASTY SQUASH SOUP

SERVES 8

Prep: 15 minutes
Cook: 1 hour, 10 minutes

Anti-Inflammatory
Blood Sugar Balancing
Dairy Free
Gluten Free
Hormone Supportive
Luteal Phase

This is what to cook when you don't feel like cooking. It's an easy one to pull out of the hat on a day when you're tired, postpartum, or sick and need a good nourishing meal with little effort. Ingredient-wise, it's very flexible: You can use any combination of winter squash, carrots, or sweet potatoes. Theoretically you could roast up any vegetables and use the same method to turn them into soup!

3 medium or 4 large carrots (about 1 pound/454 g), roughly chopped

1 medium (2 to 3 pounds/907 g to 1.3 kg) butternut squash, halved

½ medium (1 to 2 pounds/454 g to 907 g) acorn squash, halved

1 large white or yellow onion, peeled and quartered

3 tablespoons avocado oil

2½ teaspoons sea salt, divided, plus more to taste

1 teaspoon black pepper

1 garlic bulb, top cut off to expose the cloves

4 to 5 cups (960 ml to 1.2 L) broth (any kind)

½ teaspoon ground ginger

½ teaspoon ground turmeric

¼ teaspoon ground allspice

½ cup (120 ml) coconut cream, plus another ½ cup (120 ml) for garnish

¼ cup (35 g) pumpkin seeds, for garnish

1. Preheat the oven to 375°F (190°C). Line a baking sheet with parchment paper.
2. Place the carrots, butternut squash, acorn squash, and onion on the baking sheet. Toss with the avocado oil, about 1 teaspoon of the salt, and the pepper.
3. Roast the vegetables in the oven for 20 minutes and then add the garlic bulb, cut side down, rubbing it on the oiled pan to grease it a little. Roast for 40 more minutes, or until the butternut squash is soft throughout. Remove from the oven and allow the vegetables to cool to the touch.
4. Remove the seeds from the butternut and acorn squashes. Then, scoop the squash flesh into a blender along with the carrots and onions. Discard the skins. Squeeze the garlic cloves from the skins into the blender.
5. Add 4 cups (960 ml) broth, the remaining salt (or more to taste), and the ginger, turmeric, and allspice. Blend until smooth. Add the remaining broth if desired for a thinner consistency.
6. Transfer the mixture to a large pot and cook over medium heat until warmed through, about 10 minutes. Stir in the coconut cream.
7. Serve with a drizzle of coconut cream and a sprinkle of pumpkin seeds.

THAI VIBE CHICKEN SOUP

If you want a refreshing twist on a sick-day chicken soup, this is the one. Cilantro helps cleanse the body's elimination pathways while aiding digestion and combating inflammation, and the ginger and garlic bolster all-around wellness. This soup is comforting and savory without being heavy, and it's super nourishing if made with a good-quality broth.

SERVES 6

Prep: 25 minutes
Cook: 50 minutes

Anti-Inflammatory
Blood Sugar Balancing
Dairy Free
Gut Healthy
Ovulation Phase

6 garlic cloves, divided
2 jalapeños, deseeded and divided
Juice of 1½ limes, divided
1 large bunch cilantro, divided
One 3-inch (7.5 cm) chunk fresh ginger or 3 teaspoons ground ginger
¼ cup (60 ml) water, plus more if needed
4 chicken breasts (about 2 pounds/907 g), cut into 2-inch (5 cm) chunks
2 tablespoons coconut oil, divided
2 tablespoons rice vinegar, for deglazing
½ medium white or yellow onion, finely chopped
2 teaspoons sea salt
4 large carrots, diagonally sliced
1 large bell pepper, any color, sliced
5 cups (1.2 L) chicken broth
1 tablespoon soy sauce or coconut aminos
1½ teaspoons fish sauce
One 13.5-ounce (400 ml) can coconut cream

1. Place 4 garlic cloves, 1 jalapeño, the juice of 1 lime, half of the cilantro, the ginger, and the water in a blender. Blend on high until mostly smooth, adding more water 1 tablespoon at a time if necessary, up to 30 seconds.
2. Place the chicken in a large bowl. Scoop or pour the blender contents over the chicken. Toss to coat and then let the chicken marinate for at least 20 minutes (or longer in the fridge).
3. Slice the remaining jalapeño and chop the remaining garlic and cilantro. Set aside.
4. Heat a large pot over medium-high heat and add 1 tablespoon coconut oil. Lift the chicken out of the bowl and add it to the pot, setting aside the marinade. Quickly sear the chicken on each side without cooking the center of the meat, about 2 minutes per side. Transfer the chicken to a large plate.
5. Deglaze the pan with the rice vinegar, scraping up any stuck-on flavor goodness. Reduce the heat to medium and add the remaining 1 tablespoon coconut oil.
6. Add the onion, sprinkle with the salt, and sauté until translucent, about 5 minutes. Add the carrots, bell pepper, sliced jalapeño, and chopped garlic. Sauté until fragrant, 5 to 10 more minutes.
7. Pour the leftover marinade over the veggies, stir to incorporate, and cook until fragrant, 1 to 2 more minutes.
8. Return the chicken to the pot and pour in the broth, soy sauce, fish sauce, and the juice of ½ lime. Reduce the heat to medium-low and simmer, until the chicken cooks through and the veggies soften, about 20 minutes.
9. Reduce the heat to low and add a handful of the chopped cilantro (reserve about ¼ cup for garnish) and the coconut cream from the top of the can (use the remaining coconut water for another purpose).
10. Stir and cook for 10 more minutes, or until you're ready to eat. Serve with the rest of the cilantro on top.

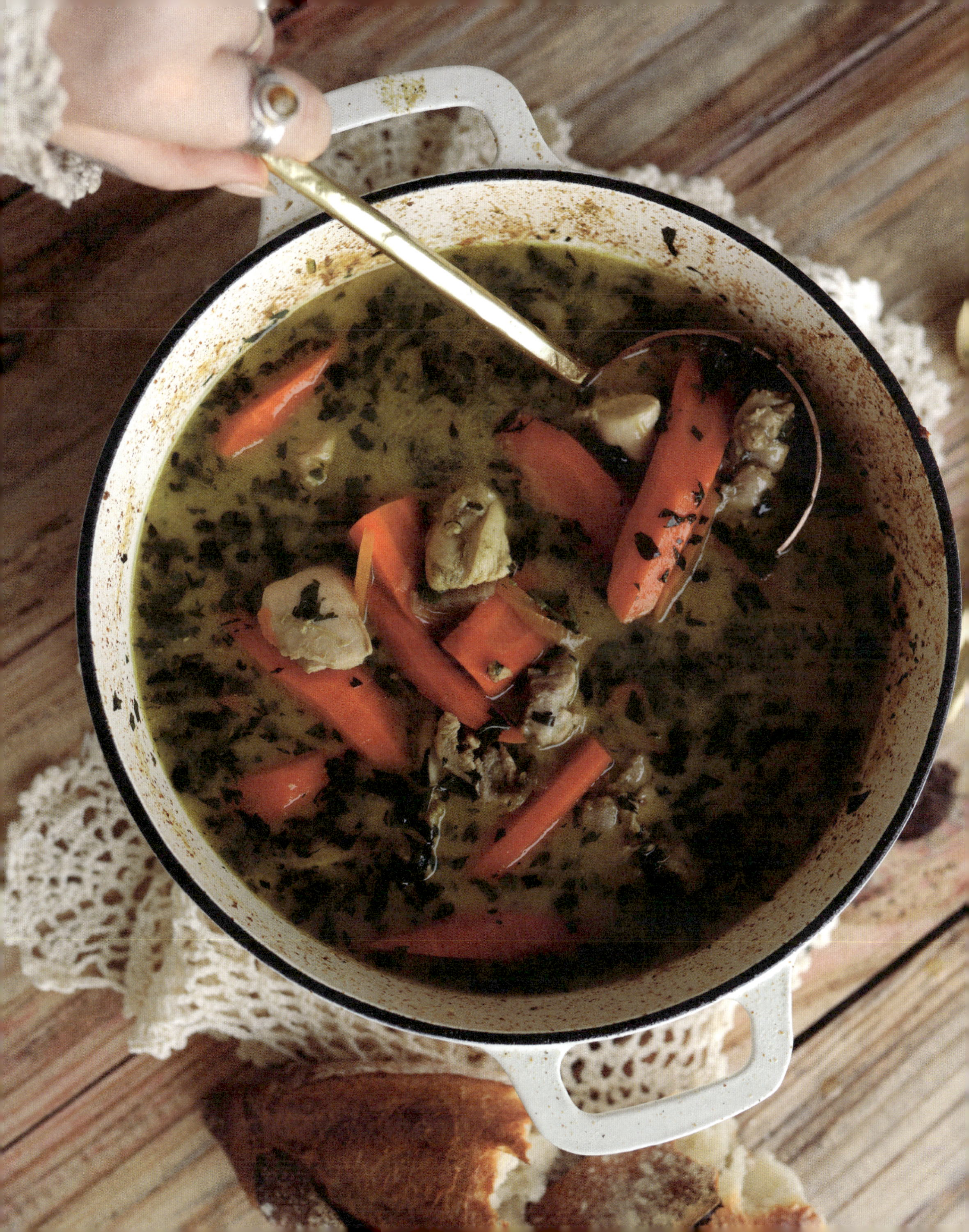

CURRIED TURKEY MEATBALL SOUP

SERVES 8

***Prep:* 15 minutes**
***Cook:* 50 minutes**

Anti-Inflammatory
Dairy Free
Gluten Free
Luteal Phase
Ovulation Phase

This is one of my favorite comforting concoctions. I love eating it soup-style with some crusty buttered sourdough but it's also great served over rice or quinoa. It's a textbook luteal phase recipe with lots of fiber, magnesium, and natural sugars to satisfy a little sweet tooth, but it can work really well for the ovulation phase, too. It's particularly helpful during ovulation if you make the meatballs with lamb, which I highly recommend; lamb has a super-rich flavor and is full of B vitamins and folate (which also makes this a favorite pregnancy and postpartum recipe!).

MEATBALLS

1 pound (454 g) ground turkey or lamb
½ medium white onion, grated
⅓ cup (27 g) quick oats
Small handful of cilantro (including the stems!), chopped
2 teaspoons garam masala
1 teaspoon garlic powder
1 teaspoon onion powder
1½ teaspoons fine ground sea salt divided
1 teaspoon black pepper
2 tablespoons avocado oil

SOUP

2 to 3 tablespoons ghee or coconut oil
2 leeks, scrubbed and finely chopped
2 medium celery stalks, finely chopped
1 large carrot, finely chopped
1 medium yellow, white, or red onion, finely chopped
4 to 6 garlic cloves, roughly chopped
1 heaping teaspoon sea salt, plus more to taste
2 tablespoons mild Indian curry paste or 2 teaspoons garam masala and 1 teaspoon curry powder
2 tablespoons tomato paste
2 inches (5 cm) fresh ginger, grated
1 teaspoon ground coriander
1 teaspoon ground cumin
½ teaspoon ground turmeric
Black pepper, to taste
6 cups (1.4 L) beef, chicken, or vegetable broth
1 tablespoon brown sugar (optional)
1 large sweet potato, cubed
One 15-ounce (425 g) can chickpeas, drained and rinsed
2 to 3 cups (70 to 95 g) packed chopped spinach, tatsoi, or other leafy greens
One 13.5-ounce (400 ml) can coconut cream

FOR SERVING

Coconut cream
Cilantro, chopped
Bread and butter or steamed rice

1. *Make the meatballs:* Combine the turkey, onion, oats, cilantro, garam masala, garlic powder, onion powder, salt, and pepper in a large bowl. Use your hands to mix thoroughly.

2. Shape into rough balls, about 1½ inches (3.5 cm) in size. Don't worry about making them perfectly smooth; any little funky edges just make more space for the meatballs to develop that yummy umami flavor!

3. Heat a large pan over medium heat, add the oil, and then gently add the meatballs. They should sizzle when they hit the pan! Cook, turning the meatballs until they are browned on all sides, about 3 minutes per side. Transfer to a towel-lined plate.

4. *Make the soup:* Melt the ghee in a large pot over medium heat. Add the leeks, celery, carrot, onion, and garlic. Add a pinch of salt and stir to combine. Reduce the heat to low and sauté, stirring occasionally, until the vegetables soften, about 10 minutes.

5. Add the curry paste, tomato paste, ginger, coriander, cumin, turmeric, the remaining salt, and the pepper. Stir well, reduce the heat to medium-low, and cook until the spices are fragrant and everything is well coated, 2 to 3 minutes.

6. Scoop the veggie mix into a blender and add as much broth as will fit. Blend until smooth, return the mixture to the pot, and add any remaining broth. Taste the soup. Add

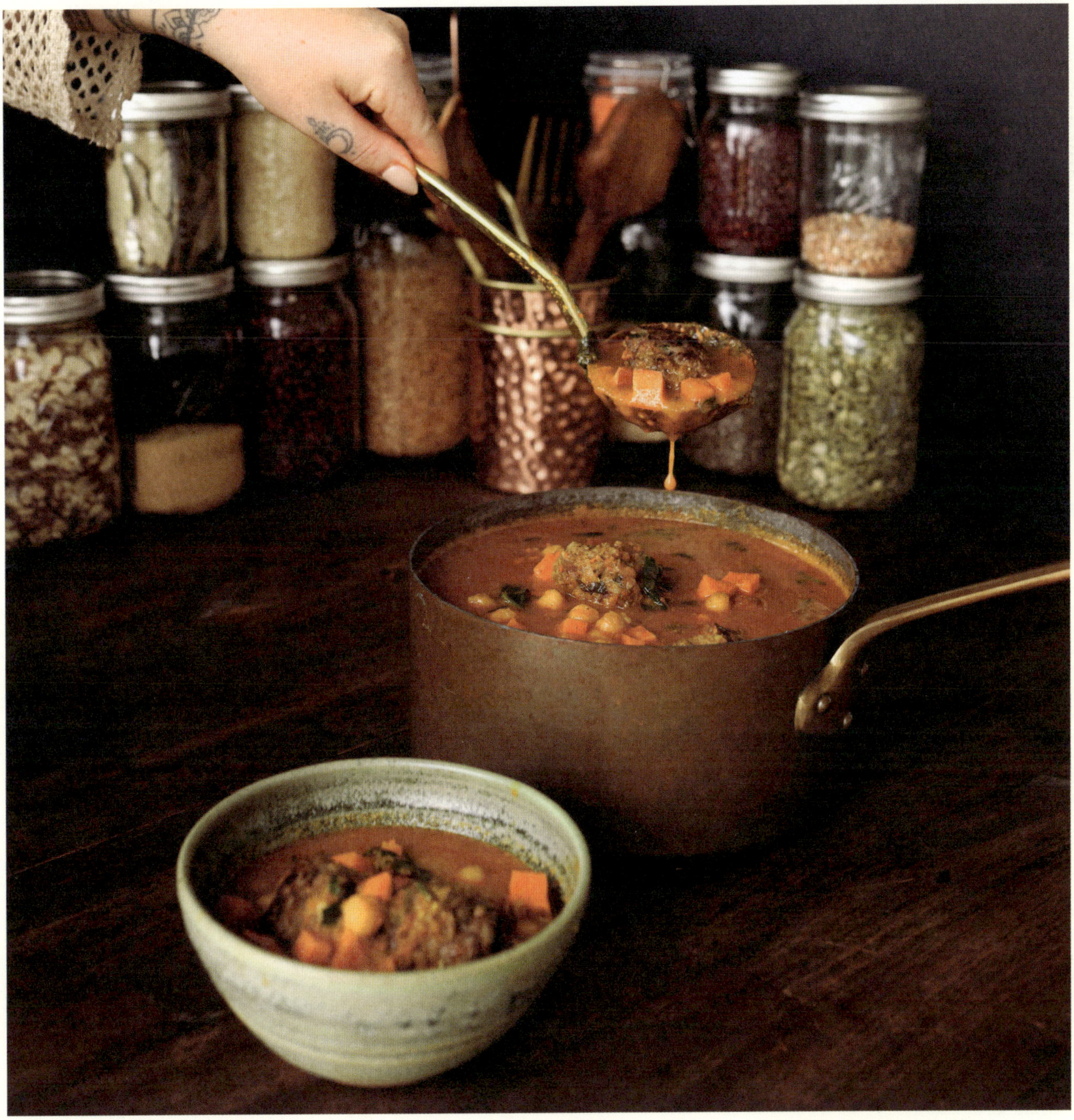

salt and pepper if needed and, if you like, the brown sugar (I like).

7. Plop the meatballs, sweet potato, and chickpeas into the soup pot and bring to a simmer. Cook until the sweet potato is cooked through, about 20 minutes.

8. Remove from the heat. When the mixture stops simmering, stir in the spinach and coconut cream (if you add coconut cream to boiling liquid, the mixture won't be as creamy). Cover with a lid and let sit until the spinach softens, 2 to 3 minutes.

9. Garnish with a little coconut cream and cilantro. Serve with bread and butter or over rice.

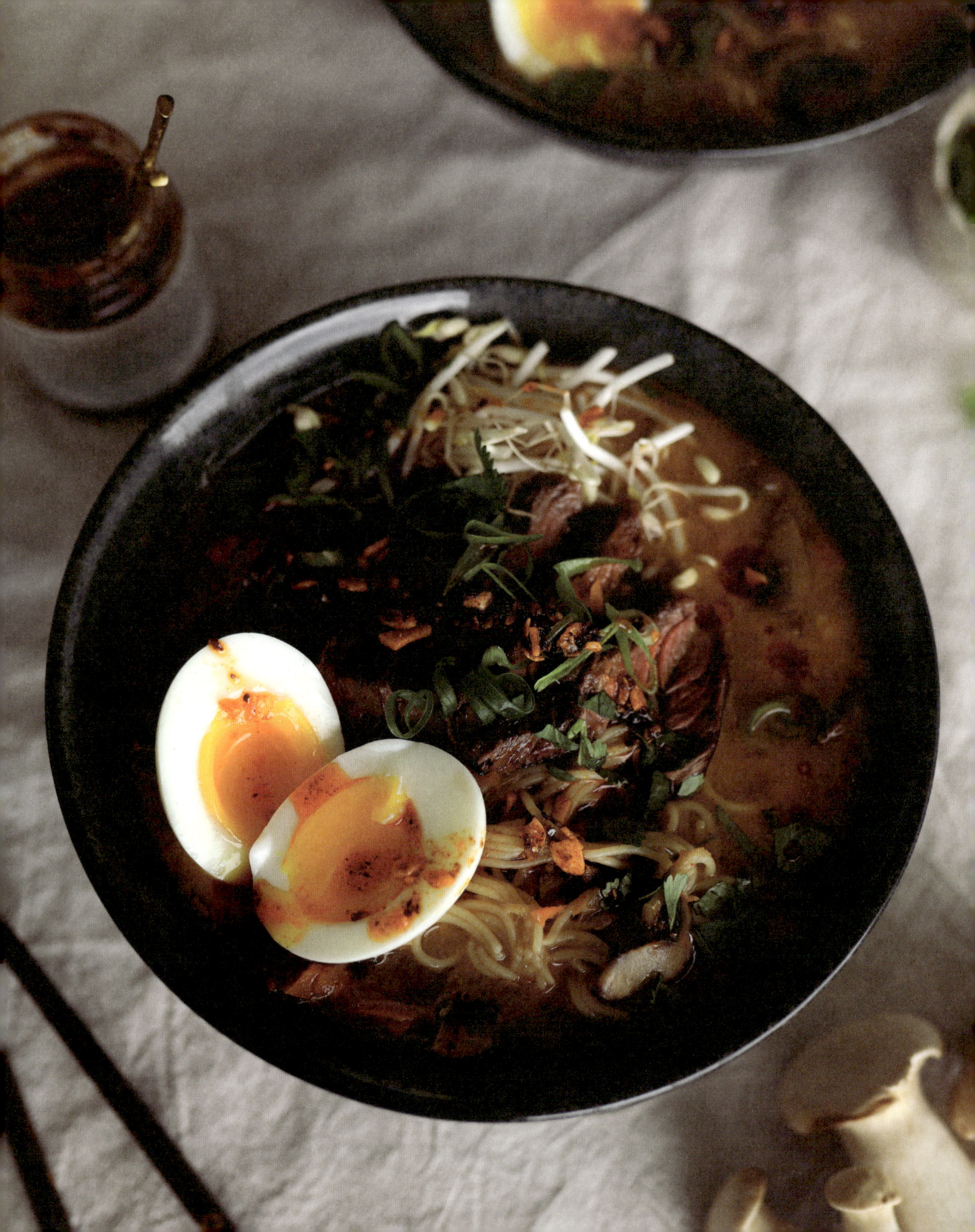

QUICK RAMEN

This "quick ramen" is my Western-ified, fast version of the Japanese dish—but it's definitely slower than making Maruchan instant noodles. But whereas those have hardly any nutritional value, this ramen is mineral-rich, good for your gut lining, and a healing comfort food. I like to use rice ramen noodles here, as they tend to be easier to digest than wheat noodles for many and they make this recipe lower FODMAP and more broadly supportive.

SERVES 2 TO 4

Prep: 10 minutes
Cook: 40 minutes

Anti-Inflammatory
Dairy Free
Gut Healthy
Hormone Supportive
Menstrual Phase

1 tablespoon sesame oil
1 medium shallot or ¼ medium yellow onion, finely chopped
3 garlic cloves, sliced
1-inch (2.5 cm) piece fresh ginger, grated
1 cup (70 g) button or oyster mushrooms, sliced
6 cups (1.4 L) chicken Bone Broth (page 159)
2 to 4 large eggs
Handful of dulse or other edible seaweed
3 to 4 tablespoons white or red miso, to taste
2 to 3 tablespoons soy sauce or liquid aminos, to taste
1 to 2 tablespoons gochujang, to taste
1 tablespoon honey
One 10-ounce (283 g) pack rice ramen or 4 ramen cakes (I like Lotus Foods)
½ cup (55 g) grated carrots

TOPPINGS
1 tablespoon chili crisp
½ small bunch cilantro, chopped
½ cup (100 g) mung bean sprouts
½ small bunch scallions, chopped
6 to 8 ounces (170 to 198 g) cooked chicken or steak, thinly sliced

1. Heat the sesame oil in a medium pot over medium-low heat. Add the shallot and sauté until softened, about 2 minutes. Stir in the garlic and ginger and sauté until the fragrance mellows, 2 to 3 minutes.
2. Throw in the mushrooms and stir until they soften and take on a little color, 2 to 3 minutes. Pour in the broth, raise the heat to medium-high, and bring to a boil.
3. Drop in the whole eggs (don't crack them), and boil for exactly 6 minutes and 30 seconds. Remove the boiled eggs with a slotted spoon and immediately transfer to a small bowl of cold water to cool. Peel the eggs while holding them under the cold water.
4. Reduce the heat to low and throw in the seaweed. Cover and gently simmer the broth for 20 minutes or so (you could also leave it cooking gently on low heat all afternoon, until you are ready to eat).
5. Scoop out ½ cup (120 ml) broth into a small jar. Add the miso, soy sauce, gochujang, and honey to the jar. Mix and then pour the mixture into the pot of broth.
6. Add the ramen noodles and carrots. Cook the noodles according to the package directions, about 6 minutes.
7. Divide the ramen among large bowls. Halve the eggs and place them on top along with the chili crisp, cilantro, bean sprouts, scallions, and meat.

NOTE

If you have veggie scraps on hand (like onion or celery butts, turnip tops, or carrot peels), you can add them to the simmering broth in step 4 and fish them out before step 6.

CHAPTER SIX

ONE-POT WONDERS

THESE ARE THE MEALS TO GATHER AROUND,

the comfort food that is made to be shared, with more focus on connection than presentation. Most of the recipes in this chapter are easy weeknight dinners, but all of them are full of flavor and packed with whole-body-healthy ingredients!

Food has always brought my people together. Growing up, we always had extra people at the dinner table, and even though we didn't necessarily have a lot to spare ourselves, there was always enough food—a little more water in the soup or a few more potatoes in the oven to fill extra bellies. My mom was frugal and knew how to stretch resources, but even still we never felt a lack. And our food reflected that—it was simple, healthy, and always delicious. That's probably why our dear friend Max always happened to show up at dinnertime (often also happening to come bearing homemade tiramisu). Feasting with friends was an integral part of my family's life. Every Saturday night, we'd have at least 20 people around my parents' table—sometimes around an extravagant spread and sometimes sharing a big vat of beans and rice.

All that to say, even if you are on a tight budget, even if cooking from scratch and for health feels overwhelming, you absolutely can make simple, delicious, healthy food a part of life, with more than enough to share.

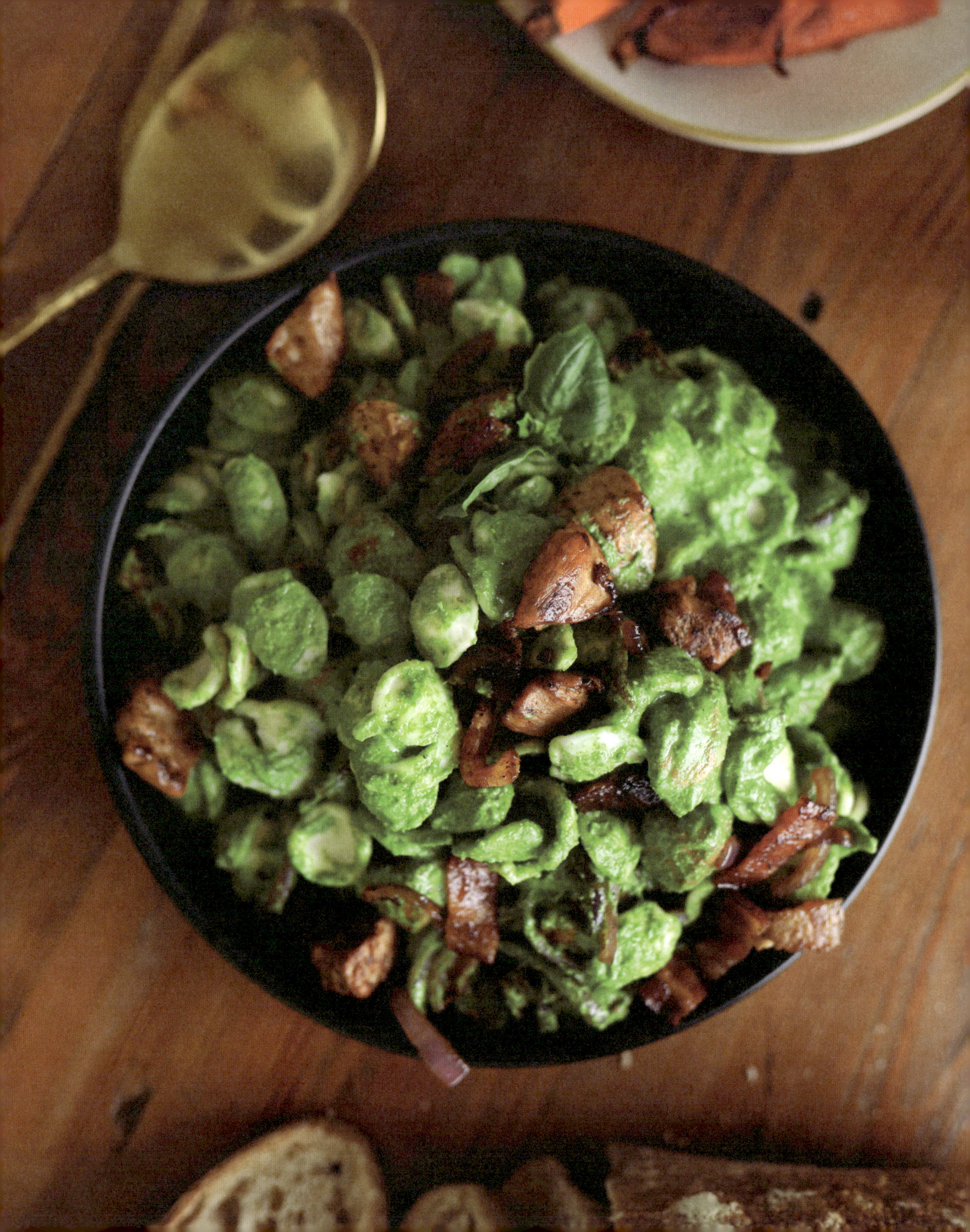

KALE PESTO PASTA

SERVES 4 TO 6

Prep: 5 minutes
Cook: 30 minutes

Menstrual Phase

This was one of the only ways I could eat fresh greens during my first trimester of pregnancy, and it's one of the few ways I can get my toddler to eat them, too! It comes together so quickly, especially if you have some leftover roast chicken or a rotisserie chicken from the store. This recipe is also great for seed cycling! Switch out the pumpkin seeds for sunflower seeds during the second half of your cycle.

1 tablespoon plus 1 teaspoon sea salt, divided, plus more to taste

16 ounces (454 g) pasta (I like orecchiette)

1 tablespoon avocado oil

4 ounces (113 g) bacon, roughly chopped

½ medium red onion, thinly sliced

2 large chicken breasts, roughly chopped

½ teaspoon black pepper, plus more to taste

1 tablespoon balsamic vinegar

SAUCE

1 bunch kale (6 to 8 stems)

6 to 8 basil sprigs

1 cup (100 g) freshly grated Parmesan, plus more for topping

½ cup (120 ml) extra virgin olive oil, plus more as needed

¼ cup (60 ml) lemon juice

¼ cup (30 g) hemp seeds, plus more for topping

¼ cup (35 g) pumpkin seeds, plus more for topping

4 garlic cloves

1. Bring a large pot of water to a boil and add 1 tablespoon salt. Add the pasta and cook according to package instructions.
2. Heat the avocado oil in a large pan over medium-low heat. Add the bacon and cook for 5 minutes, stirring often, then add the onion and sauté until the bacon is crispy, 3 to 5 more minutes.
3. Increase the heat to medium-high, add the chicken, and season with 1 teaspoon salt and the pepper. Sear the chicken, about 3 minutes per side.
4. Deglaze the pan with the balsamic vinegar. Reduce the heat to medium-low and cover, lifting the lid and stirring occasionally, until the chicken is cooked through, about 5 more minutes. The chicken should break apart easily and the juices should run clear. Remove from the heat and cover while you prepare the sauce.
5. *Make the sauce:* Remove the stems from the kale by grabbing the stem with one hand and stripping the green leaves down and off both sides with the other. Place the leaves in a blender. Add the basil (stems and all), reserving 1 sprig for garnish. Add the Parmesan, olive oil, lemon juice, hemp seeds, pumpkin seeds, and garlic. Blend until smooth, adding a few more tablespoons of oil (or water) if needed to help the mixture come together. Stop and scrape down the sides of the blender if needed—the mixture should be thick.
6. Add the sauce to the pan with the chicken and warm over medium heat stirring occasionally, until the flavor mellows and the color darkens a tad, about 5 minutes. Remove the leaves from the remaining basil sprig and slice into thin ribbons.
7. Drain the pasta and return it to the pot, then pour in the sauce and stir to coat. Serve topped with the basil ribbons, extra cheese, and seeds to taste.

NOTE

Blending and gently heating kale gives you the benefits of its nutrients and fiber while making it way easier to digest.

CREAMY ZUCCHINI PASTA

SERVES 6 TO 8

Prep: 10 minutes
Cook: 1 hour

Follicular Phase
Ovulation Phase

This pasta is fresh and light while also feeling indulgent and creamy. Zucchini is such a water-rich vegetable (it's technically a fruit, but shhh), making this a great option if you're feeling bloated or struggling with gut health. The dairy ingredients can be eliminated or subbed for dairy-free alternatives. This goes great with the meatballs from my Curried Turkey Meatball Soup (page 166) or some leftover roast chicken!

2 tablespoons butter or avocado oil
1 medium yellow onion, finely chopped
3 or 4 medium zucchini, grated (6 to 7 cups/680 to 790 g)
1 tablespoon plus 2 teaspoons sea salt, divided, plus more to taste
4 garlic cloves, grated or minced
16 ounces (454 g) egg noodles, tagliatelle, or other long pasta noodles
⅓ cup (33 g) grated Parmesan or 3 tablespoons nutritional yeast
1 teaspoon chicken or vegetable bouillon
1 teaspoon stone-ground mustard
1 teaspoon Worcestershire sauce
⅓ cup (80 g) sour cream, nondairy yogurt, or coconut cream
2 teaspoons to 1 tablespoon lemon juice
Black pepper, to taste

FOR SERVING

Basil leaves
Lemon zest
Grated Parmesan

1. Heat the butter or oil in a large saucepan over medium heat. Add the onion and sauté until it begins to soften, 3 to 5 minutes.
2. Add the zucchini and 2 teaspoons salt. Stir, then sauté until the zucchini begins to soften, 1 or 2 minutes. Add the garlic and sauté until fragrant, 1 or 2 more minutes.
3. Reduce the heat to medium-low and cook until the zucchini breaks down and everything begins to mush together into a thick, chunky, saucy texture. This will take about 45 minutes; check and stir regularly, reducing the heat if the vegetables begin to stick or brown.
4. When the zucchini is almost done, make the noodles. Bring a large pot of water to boil and add 1 tablespoon of salt, then add the pasta and cook according to the package instructions.
5. Transfer the sauce to a blender along with the Parmesan, bouillon, mustard, and Worcestershire sauce. Blend until smooth.
6. Transfer the sauce back to the saucepan and reheat over medium-low heat for about 5 minutes. Add the sour cream, lemon juice, and pepper to taste.
7. Drain the noodles and toss in the sauce, then serve with a sprinkle of basil, lemon zest, and Parmesan.

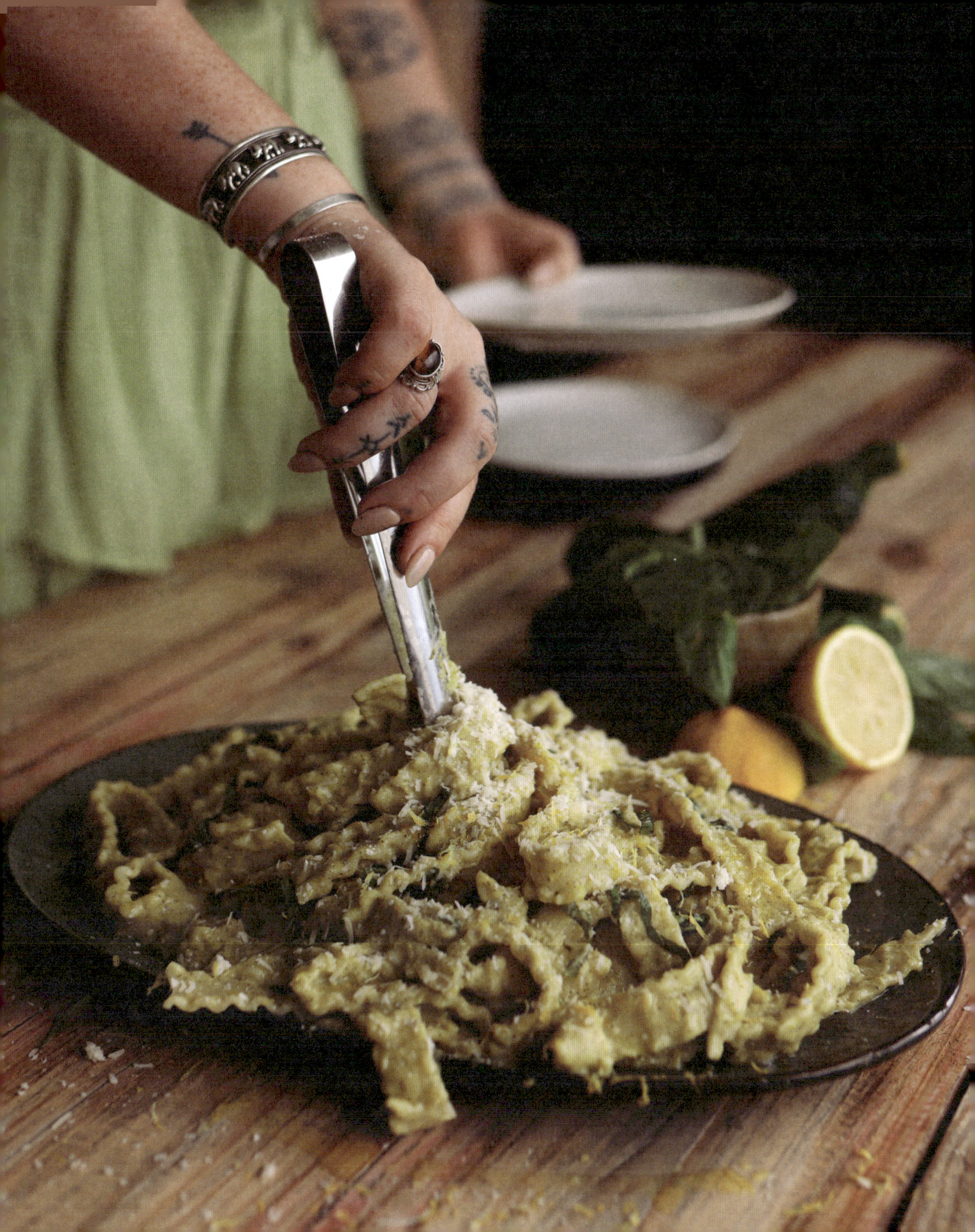

KABOCHA SQUASH BUTTER CHICKEN

SERVES 10

***Rest:* 30 minutes**
***Prep:* 15 minutes**
***Cook:* 2 hours**

Dairy Free
Follicular Phase
Gluten Free
Hormone Supportive
Luteal Phase

Butter chicken (murgh makhani) is a classic Indian recipe (I spent time in India as a kid and have been chasing those flavors ever since). It's full of flavor but mild enough for the whole family, and my nontraditional addition of kabocha squash makes this recipe nutrient rich and full of extra fiber. Serve over fluffy white jasmine rice with lots of garlic naan!

1 cup (130 g) cashews
½ large kabocha squash (see Note) or other winter squash
1 cup (240 ml) warm water
2½ pounds (1.1 kg) boneless, skinless chicken thighs, cut into rough chunks
½ cup (250 g) full-fat plain yogurt
¼ cup (75 g) plus 3 tablespoons curry paste (I recommend Patak's), divided
Juice of 1 lemon
1 teaspoon sea salt, divided, plus more to taste
¼ teaspoon black pepper
3 tablespoons ghee or coconut oil, divided, plus more if desired
1 medium yellow onion, finely chopped
1 large red pepper, finely chopped
1 jalapeño, deseeded and chopped
4 or 5 garlic cloves, to taste, finely chopped
2 inches (5 cm) fresh ginger, grated
One 6-ounce (170 g) can tomato paste
Four 14.5-ounce (411 g) cans crushed tomatoes
1 to 2 tablespoons coconut sugar or brown sugar
1 cup (240 ml) coconut cream or heavy cream

FOR SERVING
Steamed rice and/or garlic naan
Handful of cilantro

1. Soak the cashews in a small bowl of hot water for at least 30 minutes or in cold water overnight.
2. When you're ready to make the curry, preheat the oven to 400°F (200°C).
3. Place the squash, cut side down, on a baking sheet and roast for about 1 hour, until soft. Remove the seeds.
4. Once the cashews are soft, place them in a blender with the warm water and blend on medium-high for about 60 seconds to make a super smooth cream.
5. While the squash roasts, marinate the chicken. Place the chicken, yogurt, ¼ cup (75 g) curry paste, lemon juice, ½ teaspoon salt, and the pepper in a large bowl. Mix thoroughly, cover, and set aside for at least 30 minutes, or place in the fridge for up to 1 day.
6. Heat a large pot or Dutch oven over medium heat and add 2 tablespoons of ghee, allowing it to melt. Scoop the chicken out of the bowl with a slotted spoon to let some of the excess marinade drain (if any is still left).
7. Add the chicken to the pot, in batches if necessary, and sear on all sides, about 10 minutes total. Ensure your heat is high enough for a really good sizzle as soon as the chicken hits the pan. Remove the chicken.
8. Add the onion, bell pepper, jalapeño, 1 tablespoon ghee, and ½ teaspoon salt to the pot. Stir and sauté until the vegetables are soft and the onions are becoming translucent, about 5 minutes.
9. Add the garlic and ginger and stir until fragrant, about 3 more minutes. Stir in the remaining 3 tablespoons curry paste. Cook until fragrant and darkened in color, 1 or 2 minutes.
10. Add the tomato paste, stirring until everything is coated. Cook until the color deepens, about 1 or 2 minutes. Stir in the crushed tomatoes until fully incorporated. Simmer the mixture until slightly reduced and darkened in color, 10 to 15 minutes.
11. Blend the sauce: Ladle the vegetable mixture into a blender and blend until completely smooth, 1 to 2 minutes. Scoop the roasted squash flesh from its skin and add to the mixture, blending for another 30 seconds until smooth.

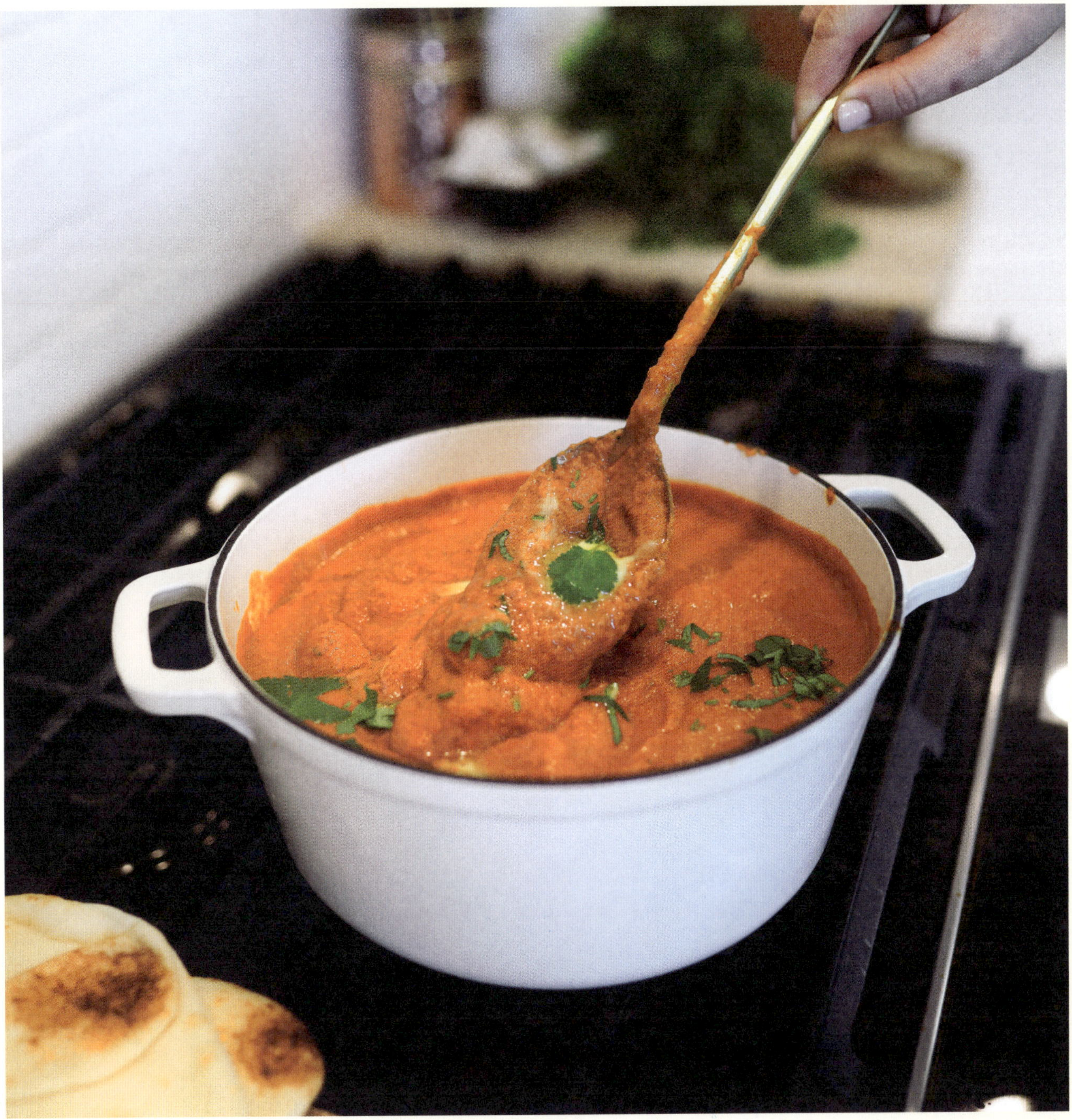

12. Pour the sauce back into the pot and add the chicken, then reduce the heat to low. Stir in the cashew cream, taste, and add more salt if needed. Add the coconut sugar to taste.

13. Simmer for 20 more minutes or up to 1 hour, until the chicken is cooked and the sauce has reduced a little and thickened. Before serving, stir in the coconut cream. Serve over steamed rice and garnish with cilantro.

✦ NOTE ✦

Kabocha squash is rich in hormone-and-thyroid supportive vitamin A, which also aids metabolism of the copper in the cashews, which in turn helps with iron abosrption.

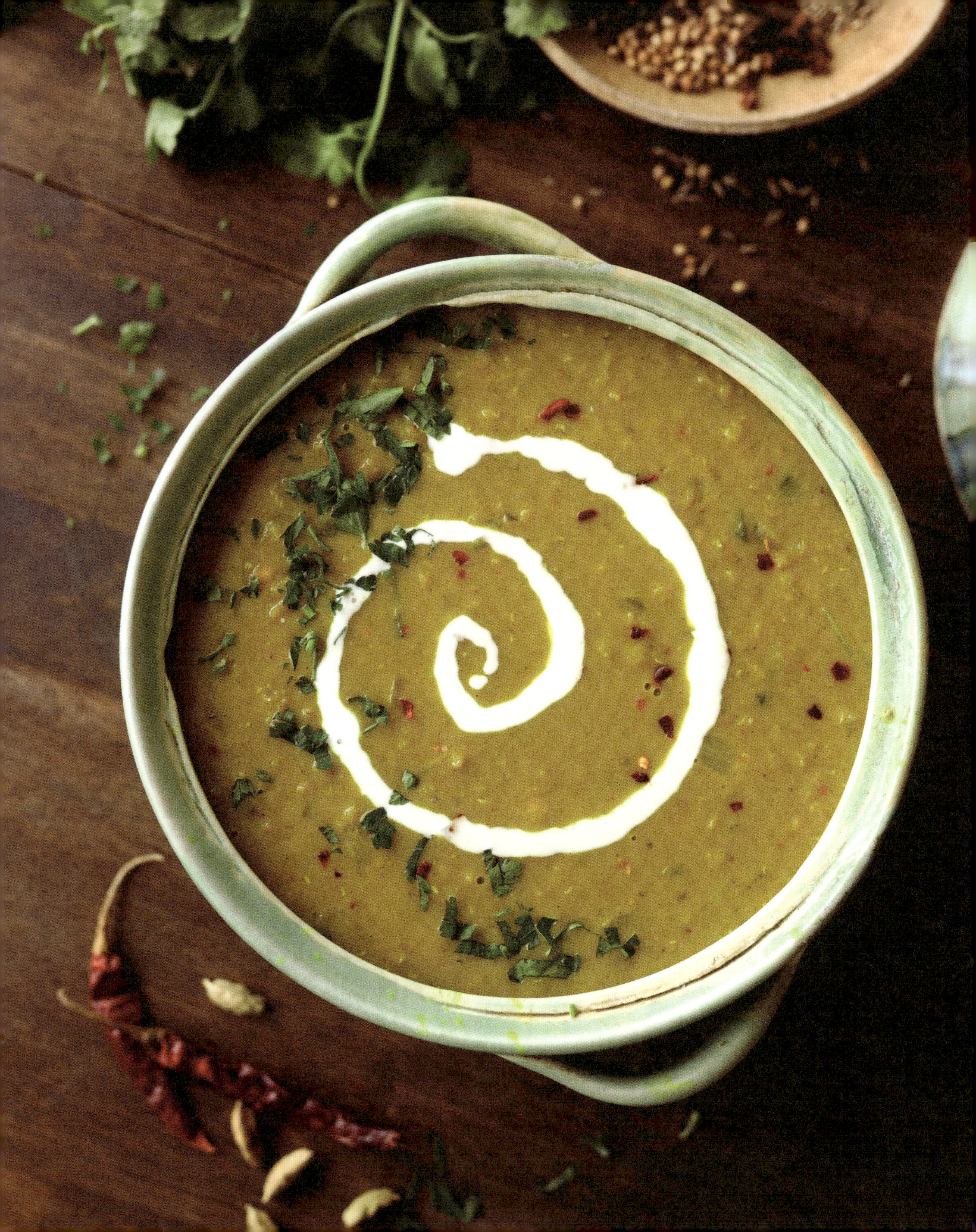

LENTIL DAL

SERVES 8

***Rest:* 30 minutes**
***Prep:* 15 minutes**
***Cook:* 45 minutes**

Dairy Free
Gluten Free
Ovulation Phase

My love for dal bhat (lentils and rice) began during a three-month stay in Nepal, the country that runs off lentils and rice. It's an incredibly cheap meal, made from shelf-stable ingredients that can take on so much flavor! On top of that, the combination of lentils and rice provides all the essential amino acids we need, creating a complete protein. Combine that with its high fiber content, minerals like iron, folate, potassium, copper, and magnesium, and tons of aromatics that support overall health, and it's no wonder this food fuels nations. This recipe is dairy free if you don't use the butter, but I like the richness it adds. I serve it over rice with a generous dollop of ghee or butter and a big sprinkle of fresh cilantro.

2 cups (400 g) dried red lentils, rinsed
6 cups (1.4 L) water, plus more for soaking
2 teaspoons ground turmeric
One 2-inch (5 cm) cinnamon stick, broken into pieces
2 small dried red chiles, seeded
6 black peppercorns
4 whole cloves
1 teaspoon coriander seeds
1 teaspoon cumin seeds
2 cardamom pods
4 tablespoons ghee or coconut oil
1 medium yellow or white onion, finely chopped
1 small jalapeño, seeded and chopped
Sea salt, to taste
1½ to 2 inches (4 to 5 cm) fresh ginger, finely grated
4 garlic cloves, finely chopped or crushed
One 13.5-ounce (400 ml) can coconut cream
1 small bunch of cilantro, chopped

FOR SERVING

Butter or ghee, optional
Steamed rice

1. Place the lentils in a medium bowl, cover in cold water, and soak overnight, or soak in hot water for 30 minutes to 1 hour. Drain and rinse thoroughly.
2. Use a spice grinder to grind up the cinnamon stick, chiles, peppercorns, cloves, coriander, cumin, and cardamom into a fine powder.
3. Melt the ghee in a large, heavy-bottomed pot or Dutch oven over low heat, and throw the ground spices into the pot, stirring to combine. Cook until the spices are fragrant, 3 to 4 minutes.
4. Add the onion, jalapeño, and a pinch of salt. Sauté, stirring occasionally, until softened and translucent, 7 to 10 minutes. Add the ginger and garlic and cook, stirring continuously, until fragrant, 1 to 2 minutes.
5. Add the soaked lentils to the pot with the aromatics and stir to coat them in the goodies. Sauté for 2 to 3 minutes before adding 6 cups (1.4 L) of water.
6. Bring to a boil and then reduce to a low simmer. Cook for about about 20 minutes, or until the lentils have softened and are losing their shape (see Note).
7. Once fully cooked, add a generous amount of salt—start with ½ teaspoon and keep adding a little at a time until the dish tastes good. You'll need about 1 teaspoon.
8. Gently simmer for 5 to 10 minutes, to allow the flavors to develop.
9. Remove from the heat and stir in the coconut cream and chopped cilantro, reserving some of each for garnish if you like. Serve over steamed rice with a dollop of butter or ghee.

NOTE

Cook time for lentils can vary depending on the age of your dried lentils, anywhere from 10 to 30 minutes, so keep an eye on them!

BUTTERNUT SAGE RISOTTO

SERVES 8

Prep: 15 minutes
Cook: 45 minutes

Gluten Free
Luteal Phase

Risotto takes such humble ingredients and turns them into decadent, warming-from-the-inside-out comfort food. All it requires is a little patience and time. The butternut squash and sage give this dish distinctly fall vibes, but I first made this on a warm spring evening, and it hit the spot. It's a relatively easy recipe; it doesn't have to take forever, but it shouldn't be rushed either. This dish is best enjoyed with some good music and a cup of something yummy in your hand.

1 tablespoon avocado oil
½ medium butternut squash, peeled, seeds discarded, and flesh grated
1 small yellow onion, finely chopped
½ teaspoon sea salt, divided, plus more to taste
4 garlic cloves, minced
4 tablespoons salted butter
4 or 5 fresh sage sprigs or 1 teaspoon ground sage
2 cups (400 g) Arborio rice (see Note)
½ cup (120 ml) white wine or splash of white wine vinegar
8 cups (1.9 L) chicken Bone Broth (page 159)
Black pepper, to taste
½ cup (50 g) finely grated Parmesan

1. Heat a large, deep skillet or cast-iron pan over medium-low heat. Add the avocado oil and then the squash and onion. Sauté until softened and beginning to brown, 3 to 5 minutes, then add ¼ teaspoon of salt.
2. Scoot all the onions and squash to the edges of the pan, making a large open space in the center. Add the garlic and sauté, stirring occasionally, until fragrant, about 1 minute.
3. Add the butter to the center, allow it to melt, and then add the sage. Brown the butter, being careful not to burn it, 2 to 3 minutes. Pour in the rice and stir quickly to coat. Cook, stirring often, until the outer layer of the rice grains begins to look translucent, about 5 minutes. Pour in the wine and stir until it evaporates, 1 or 2 minutes.
4. Meanwhile, pour the broth into a medium saucepan, sprinkle in ¼ teaspoon of salt, and gently warm over low heat (don't bring to a boil).
5. Slowly add the broth to the rice, ½ to 1 cup (120 to 240 ml) at a time. Stir constantly for about 5 minutes as the rice soaks up the broth, adding more when the broth stops pooling on the bottom of the pan.
6. Continue adding the broth slowly, stirring until the rice is soft but not mushy, the broth becomes a thick, creamy sauce that coats the back of a spoon, and the texture is porridgy and thick, 20 to 30 minutes. You may not use all the broth; or you may need to add a little extra at the end, but trust the process, because the rice will likely soften right when you least expect it. Pay attention here, and just enjoy the experience.
7. Remove from the heat and remove the sage. Stir in the Parmesan, then taste and add more salt and pepper accordingly—without fear! It wants a good amount of salt. Serve.

NOTE

Traditionally, risotto is made with Arborio rice, a short-grain, starchy variety. Sushi rice can be a good substitute, but I have also made great risotto with jasmine or other standard long-grain varieties; you'll just find that it takes longer and you'll most likely need a little extra liquid.

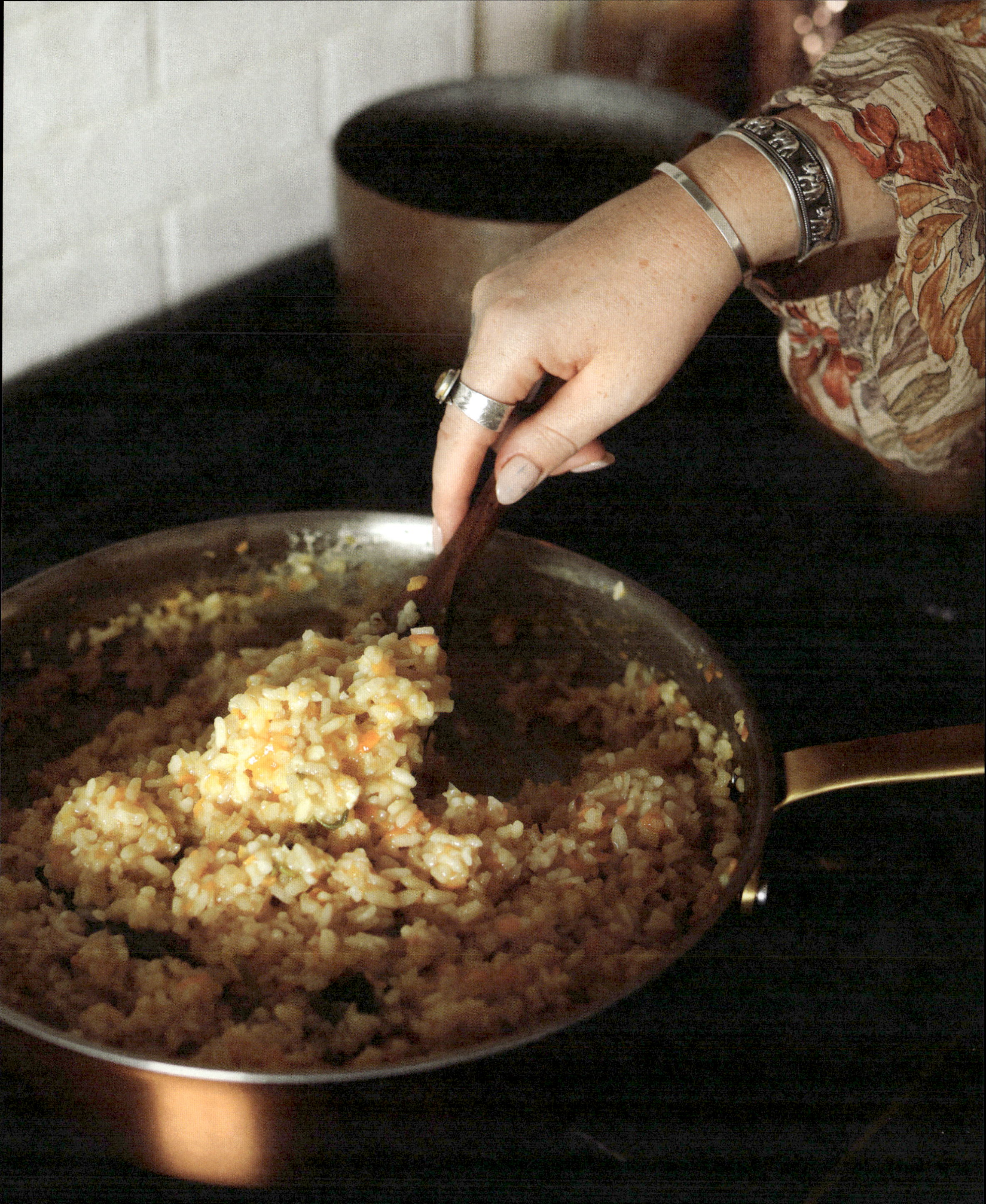

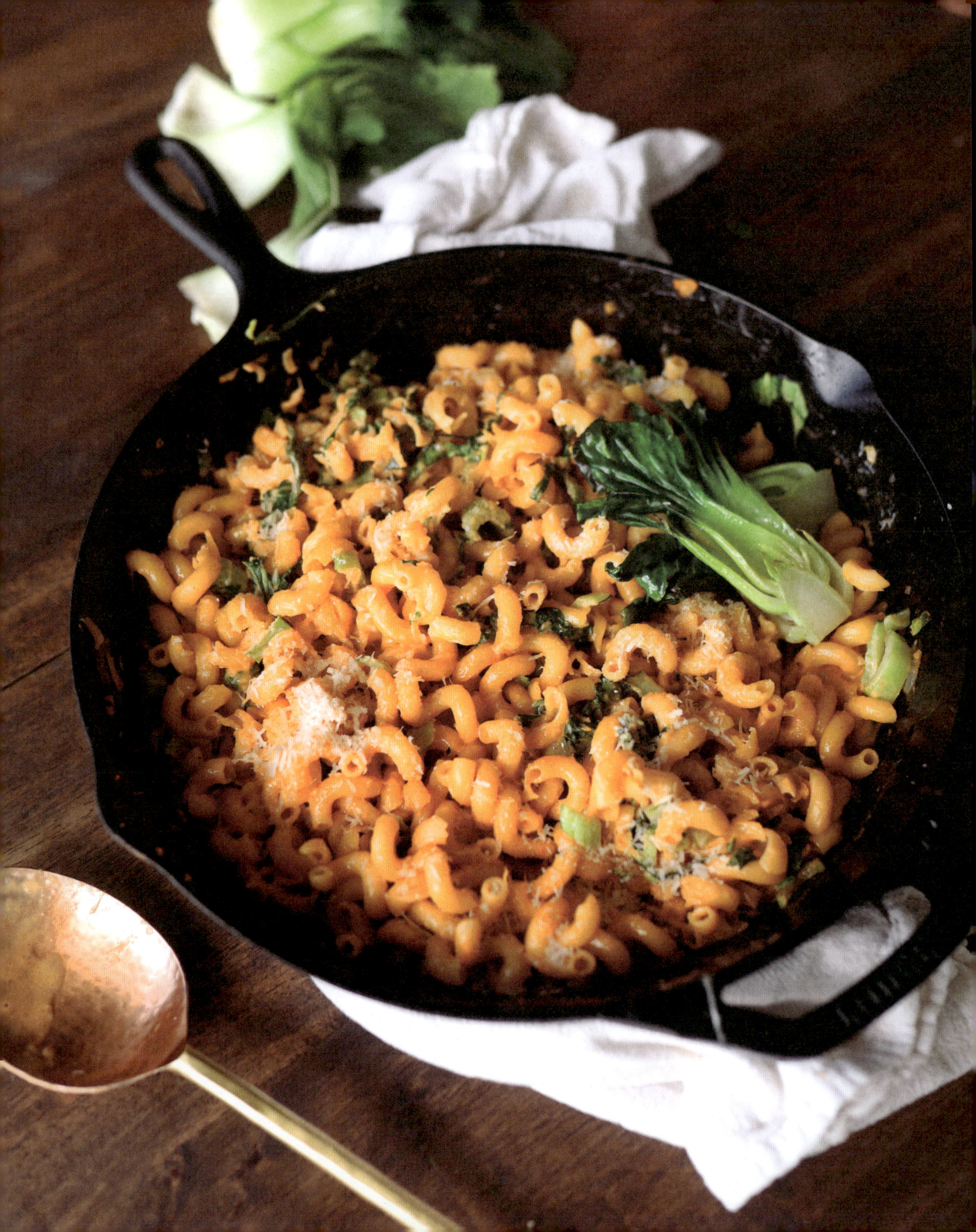

GOCHUJANG PASTA with BOK CHOY

SERVES 4

***Prep:** 10 minutes*
***Cook:** 20 minutes*

Menstrual Phase
Ovulation Phase

Say it with me: ***I don't fear carbs. I don't fear carbs.*** Carbs are necessary for energy production and hormone function—particularly thyroid hormones and cortisol! In the past, I had totally brainwashed myself against pasta, but let's be real, if you use good pasta—especially any of the cool brands made with powerhouse ingredients like quinoa or chickpeas—it can be such a great source of fiber and even protein. Plus, it's easy, epic comfort food, which your body needs sometimes. Whip this up during your next menstrual phase or on a chill evening—the added spice is just enough to warm you from the inside out!

Sea salt, to taste
12 ounces (340 g) cavatappi or rotini (I love Banza and Ancient Harvest)
4 tablespoons salted butter
2 medium shallots, thinly sliced
4 garlic cloves, grated
2 to 3 tablespoons gochujang, to taste
5 baby bok choy, sliced
2 teaspoons soy sauce or liquid aminos
½ cup (120 ml) heavy cream or full-fat coconut milk
½ cup (50 g) freshly grated Parmesan, plus more for serving
1 small bunch scallions or cilantro, chopped, for serving

1. Bring a large pot of salted water to a boil. Add the pasta and cook just until al dente, according to the package directions (it will finish cooking in the sauce). Reserve 1 cup (240 ml) of the pasta water and then strain the pasta and rinse in cold water.
2. Meanwhile, heat a large saucepan over medium heat. Add the butter and allow it to melt, then add the shallots and cook until softened, 2 to 3 minutes.
3. Add the garlic and stir consistently until the fragrance begins to mellow, 2 to 3 more minutes.
4. Reduce the heat to medium-low to ensure nothing burns or browns too quickly, and then, plop in the gochujang. Stir quickly to incorporate and allow the flavor to bloom, 30 to 60 seconds, then pour in the reserved pasta water. Stir quickly again, scraping the bottom to deglaze and get all the good flavor incorporated.
5. Add the drained pasta to the pan, stir to coat it fully, and cover.
6. Allow the mixture to bubble gently for 1 or 2 minutes before adding the bok choy and soy sauce. Stir until the bok choy wilts, 1 to 2 minutes.
7. Remove from the heat and stir in the heavy cream and Parmesan. Serve, garnished with an extra sprinkle of Parmesan and the scallions.

CHAPTER SEVEN

PROTEINS

I EAT MEAT, I DO.

If you don't, that is totally okay. But for me, it is a healthy part of a balanced diet, and a great source of protein, heme iron, and fat-soluble vitamins A, D, E, and K. Quality does matter when it comes to meat, and while quality meat quickly gets expensive, try to go for the highest quality cuts you can afford, and eat less of them. Filling out the rest of the meal with grains, veggies, and plant proteins is an easy way to make the most of your meat.

A NOTE ON SOURCING MEAT: For chicken, the ideal is organic, pasture-raised chicken. This means the birds have had an idyllic, free-roaming life, eating grubs and other delights. Their meat will be healthier and more nutrient-rich, and it's the most sustainable and ethical option. Organic, free-range chicken will be the next best, followed by cage-free. Neither of those monikers really means much, but they're better than conventionally raised chicken, where birds are very inhumanely kept, usually in cages that completely restrict movement. Air-chilled chicken is another thing to look for; it is more quickly and cleanly preserved, with less opportunity for bacterial contamination. And whole chickens will always be the healthier birds compared to pre-cut breasts, thighs, and other chicken parts, as processors usually choose the best looking (and healthiest) to keep whole. Armed with this information, just do your best with what you have.

For beef, the specifics don't matter quite as much, as there is generally less contamination throughout the beef production process. The highest quality beef will always be grass-fed and finished, as it has the highest amount of those fat-soluble vitamins. Otherwise, look for organic prime or choice grades when possible. Meat should be a vibrant red color, firm with clean white or soft yellow fat marbling. Look for the most recently packaged option with the least amount of liquid in the container. When choosing ground beef, avoid the very lean 90/10 blends and head more towards 80/20 to get the most flavor and moisture—remember, natural fats are not the fats you need to worry about.

When possible, look for local sources: farm shops and ranch stores, stands at local farmers markets, or butchers. They will often have the highest quality meat, with clear sourcing and information. This will also be a great way to find bones and carcasses for broth (see page 159).

CAST-IRON CHICKEN with SAFFRON RICE

SERVES 5

Prep: 25 minutes
Cook: 1 hour

Follicular Phase
Gluten Free
Ovulation Phase

Nothing beats an oven-baked skillet dish: deep flavor, minimal cleanup, and major hobbit vibes. The rice soaks up all that delicious chicken flavor. This dish works as a simple dinner on its own but would be great with the Sprouted Hummus (page 214), Roast Cauliflower and Fennel (page 130), or Harissa Baked Eggplant (page 146). Turn it into a feast with warm pita, olives, and any other goodies you can think up!

CHICKEN

2 pounds (907 g) bone-in, skin-on chicken thighs
¼ cup (60 ml) olive oil
Juice of 1 lemon
4 garlic cloves, crushed
3 teaspoons dried oregano
1½ teaspoons sea salt
¾ teaspoon ground allspice
3 to 4 tablespoons avocado oil

RICE

10 to 15 strands saffron
¼ teaspoon sugar
2 tablespoons hot water
½ medium yellow onion, diced
½ teaspoon sea salt, plus more as needed
2 or 3 garlic cloves, finely chopped
1 cup (195 g) basmati or white rice, rinsed
1 teaspoon smoked paprika
2½ cups (600 ml) chicken or vegetable broth
Juice of ½ lemon (about 1 tablespoon)
1 or 2 bay leaves, fresh or dried

SAUCE

⅔ cup (160 ml) mayonnaise
½ cup (120 g) Greek yogurt
Zest of ½ lemon, plus more to taste
Juice of ½ lemon (about 1 tablespoon)
1 garlic clove, crushed
1 tablespoon white vinegar
2 teaspoons honey
Sea salt and black pepper, to taste

FOR GARNISH

Handful of pomegranate arils
Chopped fresh parsley, to taste

1. *Make the chicken:* Place the chicken in a medium bowl and add the olive oil, lemon juice, garlic, oregano, salt, and allspice. Let marinate for 15 to 20 minutes.
2. Meanwhile, preheat the oven to 350°F (175°C).
3. Heat the avocado oil in an oven-safe skillet over medium heat until sizzling hot.
4. Place the chicken in the skillet, skin side down, and sear until crispy, about 10 minutes. Transfer to a plate.
5. *Make the rice:* Place the saffron strands and sugar in a mortar and use a pestle to grind until the saffron and sugar have blended into a powder. (You can also use scissors to cut the strands as small as possible.) Add the hot water to the saffron, either in the mortar or in a small cup. Let sit for about 3 minutes to bring out the color and flavor.
6. Reduce the heat to medium-low. Add the onion to the skillet with a little salt and sauté until the onion begins to soften, about 5 minutes. Then, add the garlic and sauté until fragrant, 1 to 2 more minutes.
7. Add the rice and paprika to the skillet. Stir and cook, allowing the rice to heat and sizzle a bit, about 3 minutes.
8. Add the bloomed saffron in its water, the broth, lemon juice, bay leaves, and ½ teaspoon salt, and stir. Place the chicken back into the pan on top of the rice, skin side up.

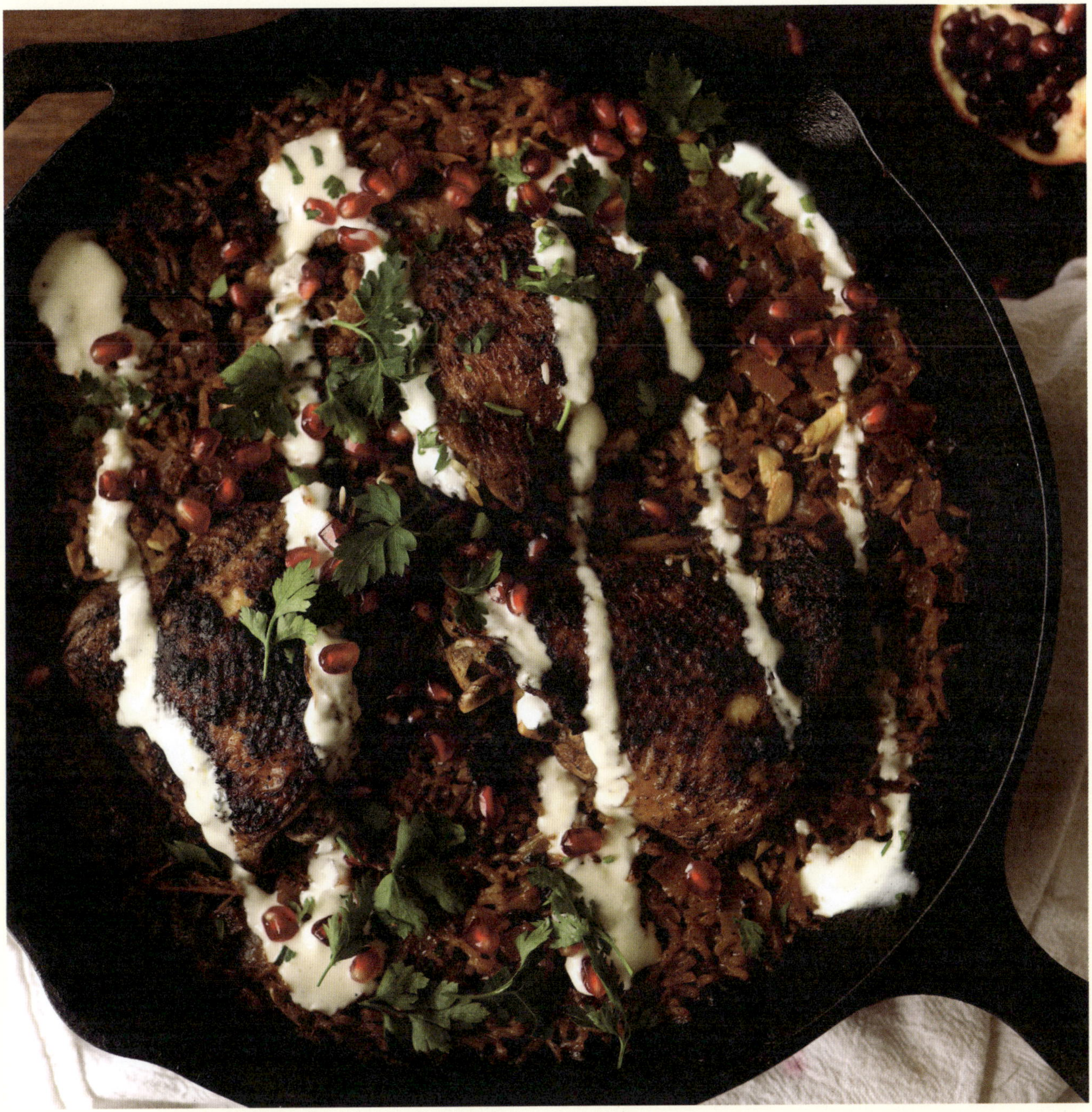

9. Cover the pan with an oven-safe lid or foil and cook in the oven for 40 to 45 minutes, until the liquid is absorbed and the chicken is cooked through: either 175°F (80°C) with a meat thermometer or when the juices run clear and there is no pink in the thickest part of the thigh.

10. *Meanwhile, make the sauce:* Whisk together the mayonnaise, yogurt, lemon zest and juice, garlic, vinegar, honey, salt, and pepper in a small bowl or jar. Set aside.

11. Remove the lid from the pan and set the oven to broil on high for 5 minutes to crisp the chicken skin.

12. Remove the pan from the oven. Drizzle the yogurt sauce on top of the chicken and rice and serve with extra on the side. Garnish with the pomegranate arils and parsley.

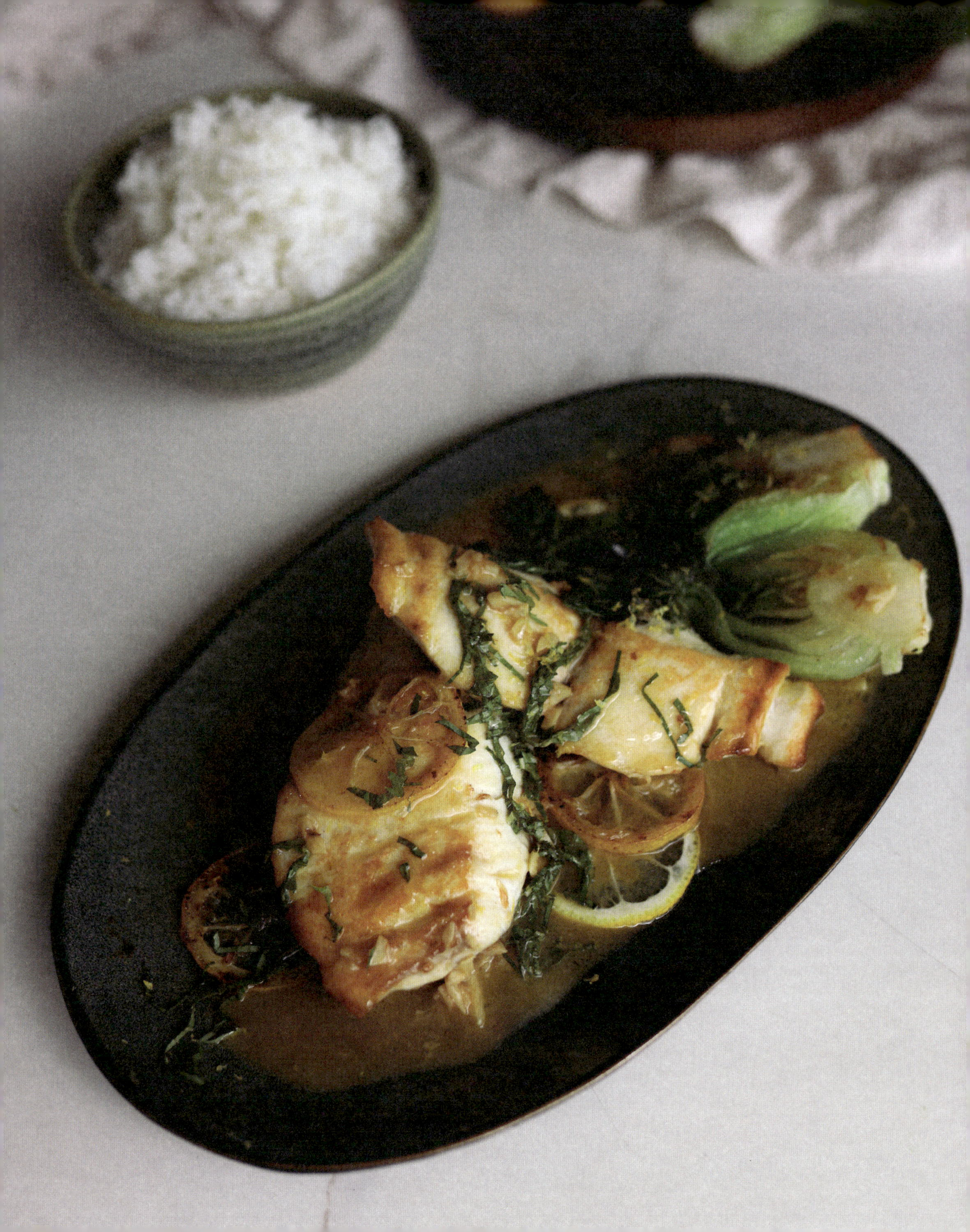

PAN-SEARED SEA BASS with LEMON BUTTER SAUCE

SERVES 4

Prep: 10 minutes
Cook: 20 minutes

Follicular Phase
Gluten Free
Ovulation Phase

This fancy-tasting fish dish feels super posh but comes together so fast and is one of the simplest things you'll ever cook. You can sub the sea bass for cod, tilapia, or a similar white fish, although you may have to adjust the cooking time for thinner fillets. Serve with any of your favorite veggie sides; I would go for a fresh green veggie and some rice.

Four 4- to 6-ounce (113 to 170 g) center-cut sea bass or other flaky white fish fillets (see Note), fresh or thawed from frozen

Sea salt and black pepper, to taste

2 tablespoons avocado oil

4 tablespoons salted butter, divided

Juice of 1 lemon, divided, plus 3 or 4 slices

4 garlic cloves, crushed, divided

¼ cup (5 g) basil, thinly sliced, divided

¼ cup (60 ml) dry white wine

1. Thoroughly pat dry the sea bass fillets and sprinkle both sides with salt and pepper.
2. Heat a large stainless steel or cast-iron skillet over medium-high heat. Add the oil and 1 tablespoon of butter to the pan to melt.
3. When the butter has melted, add the fillets to the pan, skin-side down. Do not move them for 3 to 5 minutes; you will know they are ready to flip when they easily unstick from the pan. If they are stuck, try again in 20 seconds or so, then flip.
4. Add another tablespoon of butter to the pan, along with half of the lemon juice, the lemon slices, and half of the garlic. When the butter melts, use a spoon to baste the fish as it cooks.
5. Cook the fish, until the second side unsticks from the pan and the fish easily flakes with a fork, another 3 to 5 minutes. (You can check for doneness with a thermometer; the fish should be between 140 and 145°F (60 and 63°C). Transfer to a plate.
6. Reduce the heat to medium-low. Add the remaining butter and garlic and half the basil. Stir until the garlic is fragrant and the lemon slices are browned, about 3 minutes.
7. Pour in the wine and quickly stir to deglaze, allowing the alcohol to cook off, about 2 minutes.
8. Pour the butter mixture over the fish, add the remaining lemon juice on top, and garnish with the rest of the basil and the browned lemon slices. Serve immediately.

COCONUT-CRUSTED FISH TACOS

SERVES 4

Prep: 15 minutes
Cook: 30 minutes

Dairy Free
Gluten Free
Luteal Phase
Ovulation Phase

These crispy fish tacos are super quick, super fresh, and super kid-friendly. Serve them with Good Gut Coleslaw (page 111) and you have a high-fiber, relatively low-carb (depending on your taco shells) meal that will feed your gut bacteria and fuel you without feeling heavy. Switch up the sauces depending on your mood, but this would slay with Kefir Ranch (page 211) or salmon bite sauce (see page 192).

1 pound (454 g) white fish (like tilapia or cod), ideally fresh
1 teaspoon sea salt, divided, plus more to taste
¾ teaspoon black pepper, divided, plus more to taste
4 tablespoons cornstarch
Juice of 1 lime
3 tablespoons coconut aminos
¾ cup (65 g) shredded unsweetened coconut
½ cup (55 g) fine ground cornmeal or almond flour
1 teaspoon garlic powder
½ teaspoon ground ginger
½ teaspoon ground turmeric
Avocado oil spray, as needed

FOR SERVING

6-inch (15 cm) corn or almond flour tortillas
Good Gut Coleslaw (page 111)
Sliced avocado
Chopped cilantro
Kefir Ranch (page 211) or salmon bite sauce (see page 192)

1. Preheat the oven to 375°F (190°C). Set a wire rack over a baking sheet.
2. Slice the fillets against the grain into small strips. Sprinkle with ½ teaspoon salt and ½ teaspoon pepper and dust each side thoroughly with the cornstarch. Squeeze the lime juice over them, add the coconut aminos, and let sit for 3 to 5 minutes.
3. Toast the shredded coconut in a dry, medium pan over medium-low heat, stirring consistently until golden brown, about 5 minutes.
4. Combine the toasted coconut, cornmeal, garlic powder, ground ginger, ½ teaspoon salt, turmeric, and ¼ teaspoon pepper in a shallow dish.
5. Coat the fish in the breading mixture one strip at a time, flipping and gently pressing each side to coat, shaking off any excess.
6. Lay the fish on the wire rack to ensure it cooks evenly and gets nice and crispy. Spray all over with avocado oil.
7. Bake for 20 minutes, until golden, crisp, and easily breaking apart, then flip each piece, spray with a little more avocado oil, and broil for 3 to 5 more minutes, or until the fish is crispy to your liking.
8. Warm the tortillas. Heat them one at a time in a small pan over medium heat for 30 seconds on each side, or stack about 10 tortillas, wrap them in foil, and place them in the oven while the fish cooks, about 10 minutes.
9. Divide the fish among the tortillas, add the coleslaw, top with avocado and cilantro, and drizzle with sauce.

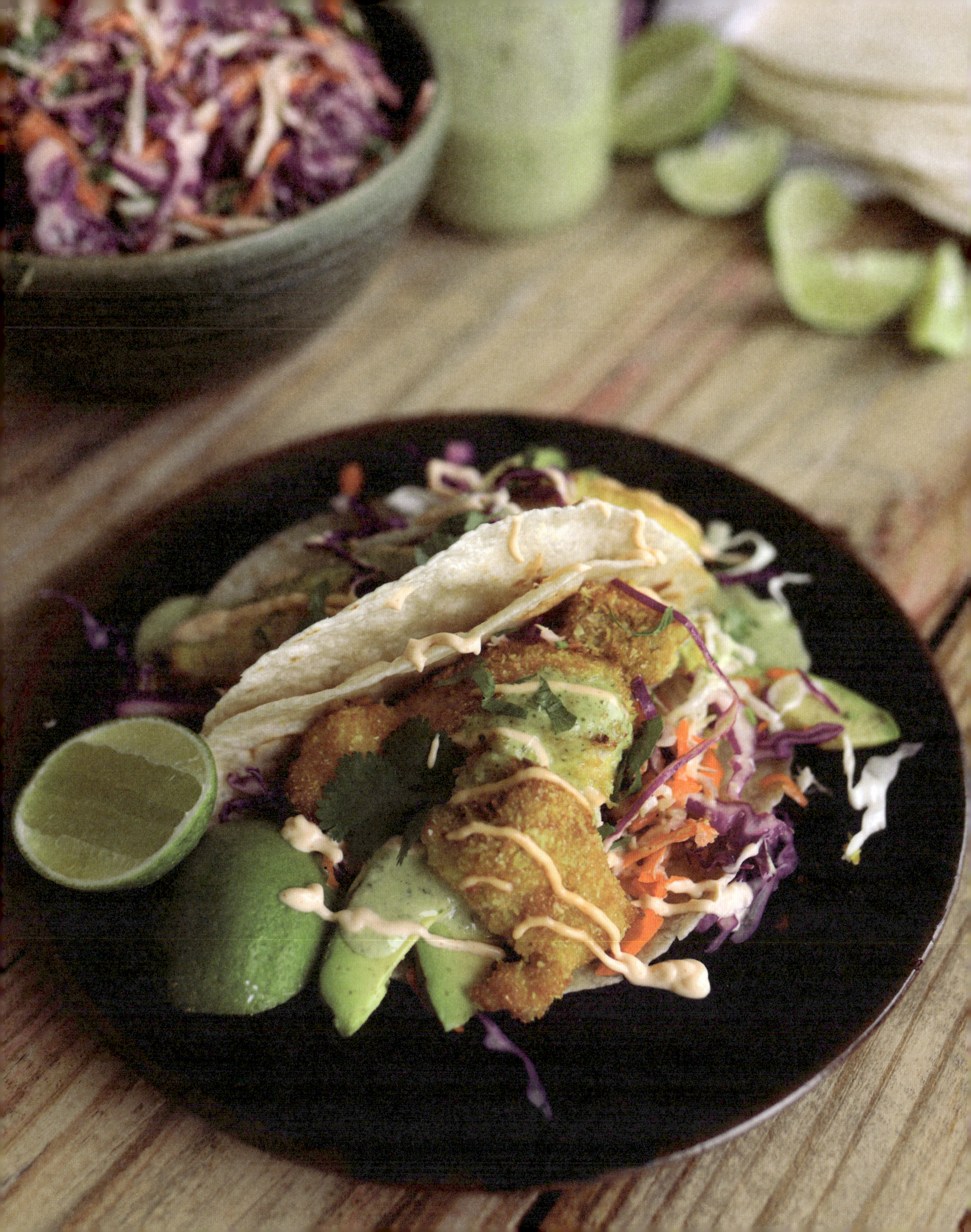

SMOKY SALMON BITES with COCONUT RICE

SERVES 6

Prep: 10 minutes
Cook: 20 minutes

Dairy Free
Follicular Phase
Ovulation Phase

This is my favorite way to get omega-3s, and it's one of the only ways I get my toddler to eat fish! It's such a quick dinner—I love to serve it up with my Teriyaki Roast Broccoli (page 134) and any other fresh green veggies I have around. Salmon skin is protein- and collagen-rich, has high levels of omega-3s, and gets nice and crispy when pan fried! You can remove it if you like, but I beg you not to.

RICE

1½ cups (290 g) white rice, rinsed (jasmine or other long-grain varieties are my go-tos)
3 cups (720 ml) water
3 tablespoons coconut oil

SALMON BITE SAUCE

¾ cup (180 ml) Avocado Oil Mayo (page 212)
3 tablespoons honey
2 tablespoons soy sauce or liquid aminos
2 tablespoons sriracha, or to taste
1 tablespoon avocado oil
1 tablespoon rice vinegar
2 teaspoons smoked paprika

SALMON BITES

4 skin-on salmon fillets (about 2 pounds/907 g)
5 tablespoons avocado oil, divided
2 teaspoons cornstarch
1 teaspoon garlic powder
1 teaspoon onion powder
1 teaspoon smoked paprika
½ teaspoon ground ginger
½ teaspoon sea salt
Black pepper, to taste

FOR SERVING

1 avocado, sliced
Teriyaki Roast Broccoli (page 134)
1 small bunch cilantro, chopped
½ large cucumber, chopped
4 tablespoons sesame seeds
Drizzle of sriracha, to taste

1. *Make the rice:* Place the rice and water in a medium pot. Add the coconut oil, bring to a boil, and then cover and reduce the heat to medium-low. Simmer for 15 minutes and then remove from the heat. Let the rice sit, covered, for another 10 minutes, or until ready to serve.
2. *Mix up the sauce:* Whisk the Avocado Oil Mayo, honey, soy sauce, sriracha, avocado oil, rice vinegar, and paprika together in a small jar.
3. *Make the salmon:* Cut the salmon fillets into bite-size chunks and very thoroughly pat them dry. Place in a medium bowl and drizzle with 2 tablespoons avocado oil.
4. Combine the cornstarch, garlic powder, onion powder, paprika, ground ginger, salt, and pepper in a small jar or bowl. Sprinkle onto the salmon and gently toss to coat.
5. Heat a large skillet over medium-high heat and add the remaining 3 tablespoons avocado oil (see Tip). Tumble the salmon bites into the hot oil, turn them skin-side down, and sear, until they easily release from the pan before flipping, 2 to 3 minutes. Sear on the second side for another 1 to 2 minutes.
6. Pour half of the sauce into the pan and toss the salmon quickly to coat. Let the sauce bubble and reduce for 1 minute, then remove from the heat.
7. Divide the rice among bowls and top with salmon. Serve with the avocado, broccoli, cilantro, cucumber, and sesame seeds. Drizzle with the remaining sauce and sriracha to taste.

TIP

For a less hands-on approach, bake in the oven at 425°F (220°C) on a foil-lined sheet pan for 10 minutes, removing after 5 minutes to toss with half of the sauce. Finish with a few minutes under the broiler for extra crispiness!

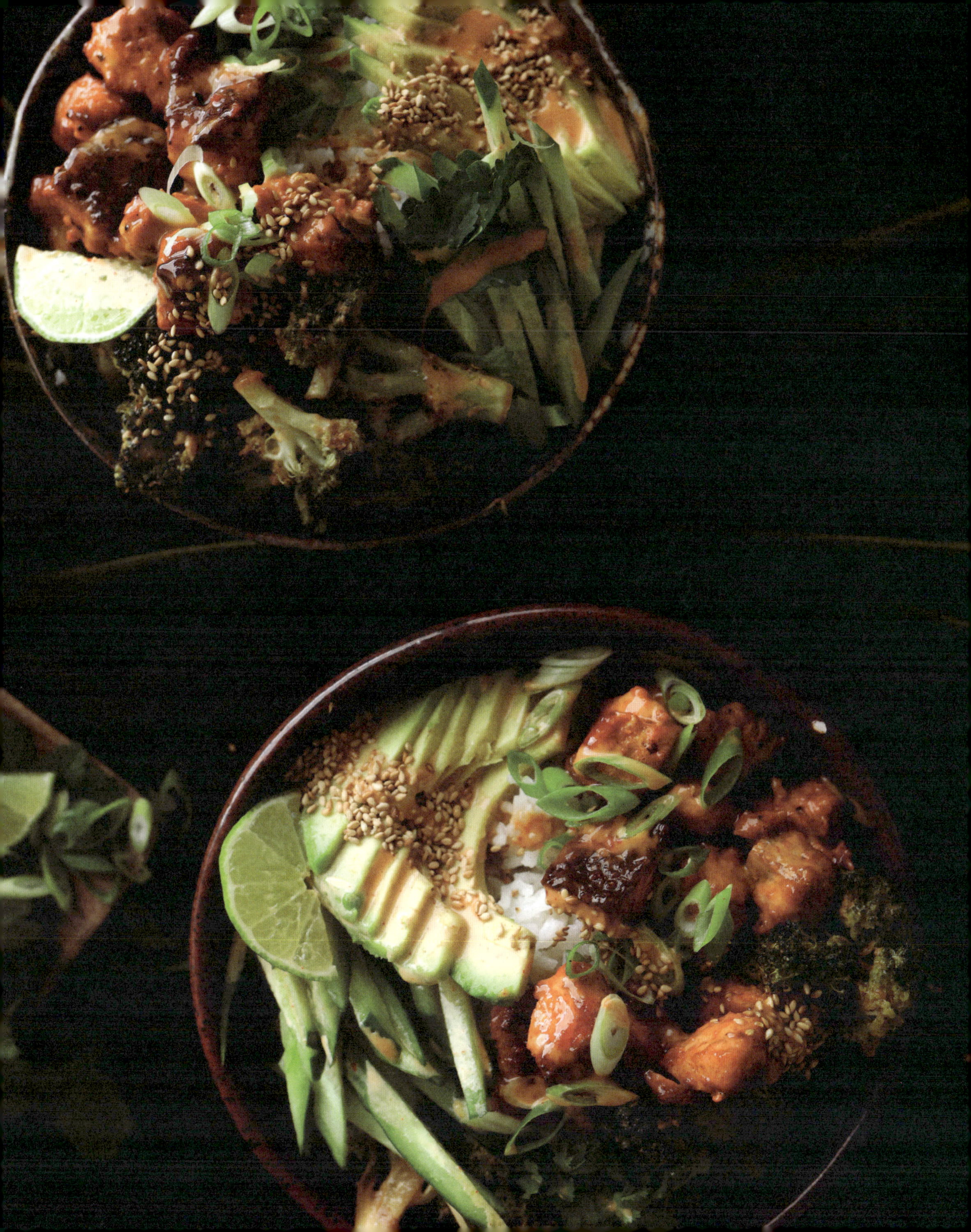

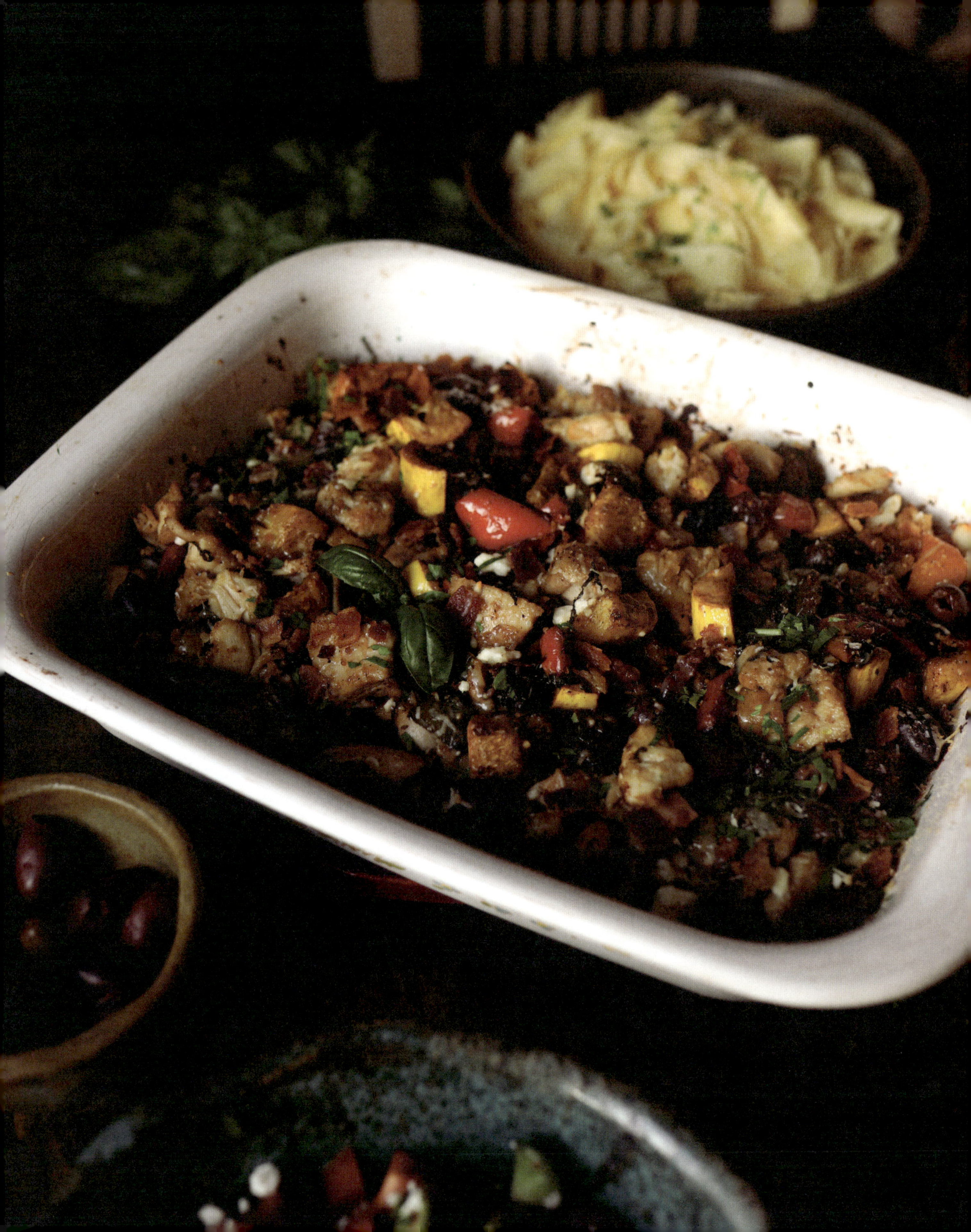

MEDO-CHICK (MEDITERRANEAN CHICKEN)

SERVES 8

***Prep:* 10 minutes**
***Cook:* 1 hour**

Dairy Free
Gluten Free
Follicular Phase
Ovulation Phase

This is a classic Papa Gillespie recipe. It's rich, delicious, and soul-nourishing (he definitely doesn't pull any punches when it comes to the glories of bacon and cheese, so this is in no way low-fat, but that's okay!). It's the perfect meal for your follicular or ovulation phases, and since you might feel more social during those times, you might as well make it for a dinner party. Serve over pasta (I like tagliatelle) or with Sprouted Hummus (page 214), pita bread, and a good salad!

1 tablespoon avocado oil, ghee, or beef tallow, plus more for greasing
8 slices uncured bacon, chopped
2 pounds (907 g) boneless, skinless chicken thighs, cut into bite-size pieces
1 teaspoon sea salt, divided, plus more to taste
½ teaspoon black pepper, plus more to taste
1 medium red onion, diced
1 medium green bell pepper, cut into bite-size pieces
1 medium red bell pepper, cut into bite-size pieces
1 medium yellow bell pepper, cut into bite-size pieces
½ cup (120 ml) white wine, divided
4 garlic cloves, finely diced
2 medium summer squash, cut into bite-size pieces
½ teaspoon dried oregano
¼ teaspoon ground allspice
10 large basil leaves or a handful of tarragon, thinly ribboned
⅔ cup (66 g) grated Parmesan or mature cheddar, or more to taste
Sprinkle of crumbled feta (optional)
½ to 1 cup (67 to 135 g) whole pitted kalamata olives, to taste

1. Preheat the oven to 350°F (175°C).
2. Heat the avocado oil in a large skillet over medium heat. Add the bacon and cook, stirring once or twice, until rendered and crispy, 15 to 20 minutes. Transfer to a plate, leaving the bacon fat in the skillet.
3. Toss the chicken with ½ teaspoon of the salt and the pepper in a medium bowl. Then plop the chicken into the skillet and raise the heat to medium-high. Cook the chicken, searing each side but not cooking through, about 5 minutes per side. Transfer to the plate with the bacon.
4. Reduce the heat to medium-low. Add the onion and peppers to the pan and deglaze with 2 tablespoons of the white wine, mixing and scraping up all of the goodness stuck on the pan. Sauté slowly, until the onions are translucent and everything begins to brown, 5 to 7 minutes.
5. Add the garlic, stir, and cook until fragrant, about 1 more minute. Increase the heat to medium, then move everything to the edges of the pan. Add the squash, and sear until it begins to brown, 2 to 3 minutes, then sprinkle with the remaining ½ teaspoon of salt and stir again.
6. Add the oregano, the allspice, and pepper to taste. Deglaze the pan with the remaining white wine, scraping up any bits stuck to the pan. Add the basil.
7. Dump all the veggies into a lightly oiled, oven-safe casserole dish and pile the chicken and bacon on top.
8. Sprinkle liberally with the Parmesan, add a little feta if you like, and move things around a bit to get the cheese into the cracks. Scatter the olives across the top—as many as you like!
9. Bake for 30 minutes, or until the chicken is cooked through (easily tearing apart with clear juices and no pink remaining) and the top is golden brown.

KOREAN-STYLE BBQ BEEF BOWLS

SERVES 4

Prep: 20 minutes
Cook: 30 minutes

Dairy Free
Luteal Phase

This recipe is a weeknight go-to or quick-fix crowd-pleaser that makes its rounds at our table pretty regularly. The beef-and-rice base can be seasoned in so many different ways and zhuzhed up with endless combos of toppings, but this is by far my favorite. All the greens make this really fresh and fiber-rich while still being filling and comforting.

BROCCOLI

1 medium head broccoli, cut into bite-size pieces
2 tablespoons soy sauce or coconut aminos
1 tablespoon avocado oil
1 tablespoon sesame oil

RICE

1½ cups (290 g) white or brown long-grain rice
3 cups (720 ml) water

BEEF

2 tablespoons coconut oil
½ medium white or yellow onion, finely chopped
4 garlic cloves, finely chopped
1 inch (2.5 cm) fresh ginger, grated, or 2 teaspoons ground ginger
1 pound (454 g) ground beef
½ teaspoon sea salt
1 tablespoon tomato paste
¼ cup (60 ml) honey
¼ cup (60 ml) soy sauce or coconut aminos
2 teaspoons sesame oil
2 tablespoons rice vinegar
1 to 2 teaspoons red pepper flakes, to taste
Black pepper, to taste

MISO MAYONNAISE

¼ cup (60 ml) mayonnaise
2 tablespoons red or white miso
1 tablespoon honey
1 tablespoon rice vinegar

FOR SERVING

Two large avocados, sliced
1 small cucumber, chopped
Small bunch scallions, thinly sliced
Sesame seeds, for sprinkling
Sriracha, for drizzling

1. Preheat the oven to 400°F (200°C). Line a baking sheet with parchment paper.
2. *Make the broccoli:* Spread the broccoli onto the baking sheet. Drizzle with the soy sauce, avocado oil, and sesame oil. Gently toss the broccoli with your hands. Roast in the oven for 15 to 20 minutes, until browned on the bottom.
3. *Make the rice:* Rinse the rice in a sieve until the water runs clear. Transfer to a medium pot, add the water, and bring to a boil. Stir, cover, and reduce the heat to low. Simmer for 15 minutes and then remove from the heat. Let sit, covered, for 10 minutes or until serving.
4. *Meanwhile, make the beef:* Heat a large cast-iron skillet or pan over medium heat and add the coconut oil. Add the onion and sauté until translucent, 3 to 5 minutes. Then, add the garlic and fresh ginger and cook until fragrant, 1 or 2 more minutes. (If you're using ground ginger, add it in step 6 instead.)
5. Add the beef. Sprinkle with the salt and sauté, breaking it up with a spatula as it cooks, until almost fully cooked through (crumbled completely and mostly browned), about 7 minutes.
6. Reduce the heat to medium-low, add the tomato paste, and stir until it coats the beef. Add the honey, soy sauce, sesame oil, vinegar, red pepper flakes, and black pepper. Reduce the heat to low, stir, and let simmer for 2 to 3 minutes while you prep the sauce.
7. *Make the miso mayonnaise:* Combine the mayonnaise, miso, honey, and vinegar in a small jar. Adjust the amount of each to taste.
8. Serve the beef and broccoli over the rice, topped with avocado, cucumber, scallions, a sprinkle of sesame seeds, and a drizzle of sriracha.

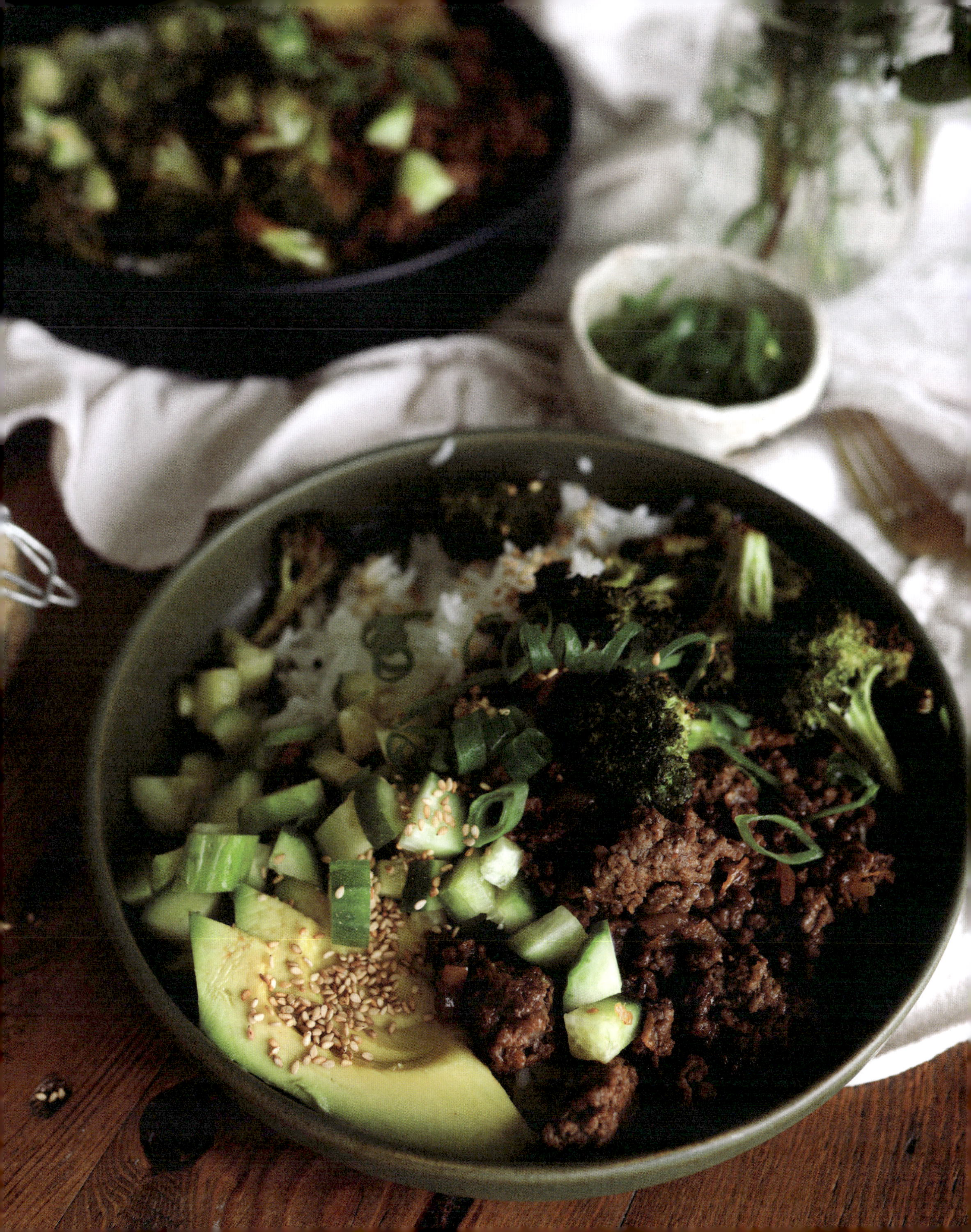

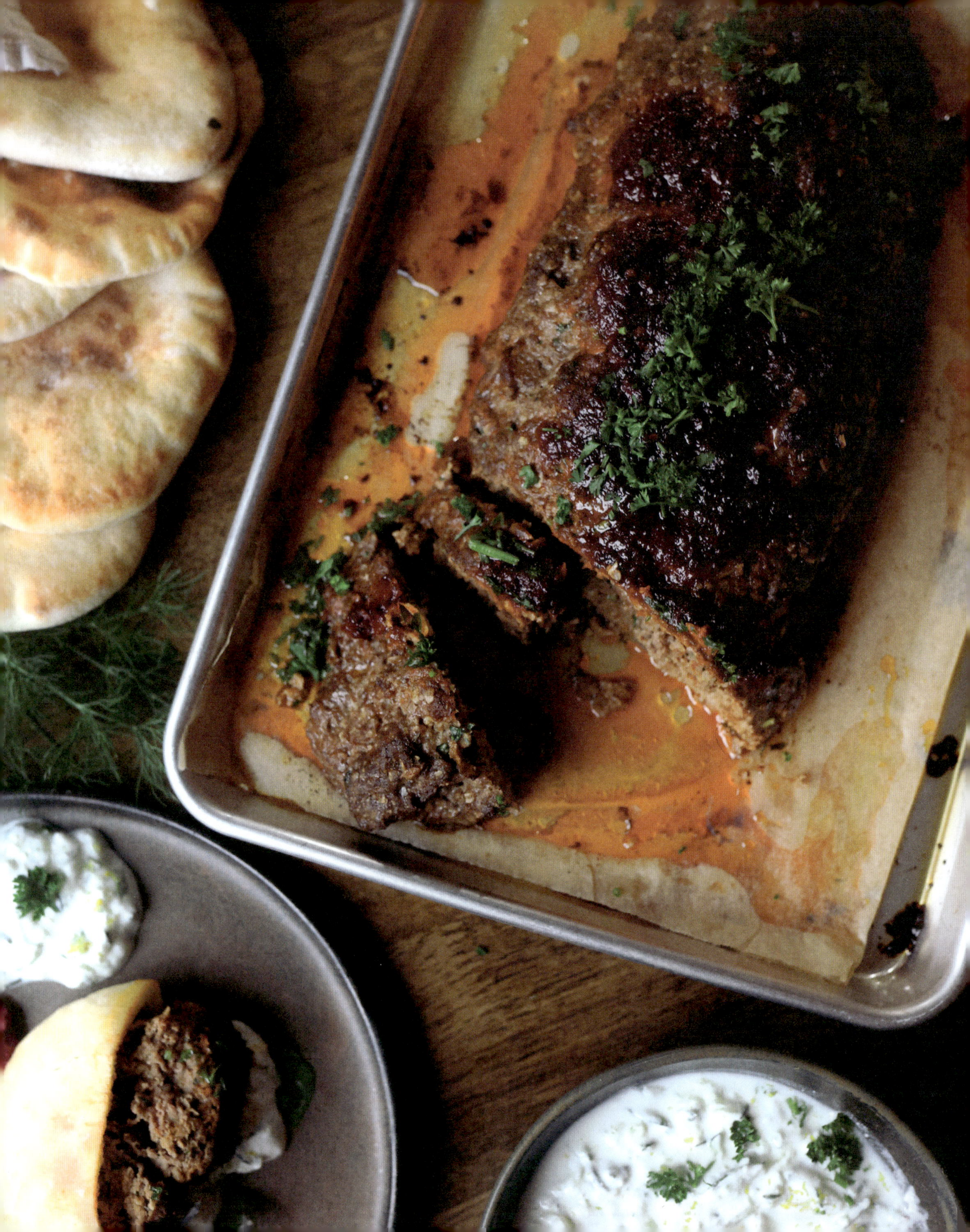

KOFTA-STYLE MEATLOAF with TZATZIKI

SERVES 6

Prep: 15 minutes
Cook: 40 minutes

Gluten Free
Luteal Phase
Ovulation Phase

This is another souped-up classic that is definitely not your grandma's meatloaf. It's a quick, simple dinner with so much flavor and a ton of moisture thanks to the grated onion and oats (the oats are like little juice collectors). The little swap of ketchup on top for a honey-harissa blend is divine. I love this sliced generously and served in a fresh warm pita bread with tzatziki, and I would also add some Roasted Beet Dip (page 142) or Sprouted Hummus (page 214) into the mix and serve with the Quinoa Salad (page 107) and Harissa Baked Eggplant (page 146)—a feast!

MEATLOAF

1 pound (454 g) ground beef
1 pound (454 g) ground lamb
1 cup (80 g) quick oats
¾ medium white onion, grated
Large handful of fresh parsley, finely chopped
2 teaspoons paprika
1½ teaspoons sea salt
1 teaspoon ground allspice
1 teaspoon dried oregano
½ teaspoon ground coriander
½ teaspoon ground nutmeg
½ teaspoon black pepper
½ teaspoon ground sumac
⅓ cup (80 g) mild harissa
2 tablespoons honey

TZATZIKI

½ large cucumber
Sea salt, to taste
1 cup (225 g) full-fat plain Greek yogurt
Zest and juice of ½ lemon
1 garlic clove, crushed
1 small bunch mint, finely chopped
1 small bunch dill, finely chopped

1. *Make the meatloaf:* Preheat the oven to 400°F (200°C). Line a baking sheet with parchment paper.
2. Place the beef, lamb, oats, onion, parsley, paprika, salt, allspice, oregano, coriander, nutmeg, pepper, and sumac in a large bowl. Use your hands to thoroughly mix the ingredients until everything is well distributed (you may need to mix for a little longer than you think is necessary to make sure it's all even).
3. Form the mixture into an 8 × 4-inch (20 × 10 cm) loaf on the baking sheet.
4. Mix the harissa and honey in a small bowl and then spoon the mixture on top of the meatloaf.
5. Bake for 35 to 40 minutes, until the meat is cooked through, browned on the outside, and crisping around the edges. It should reach an internal temperature of 160°F (71°C).
6. *Meanwhile, make the tzatziki:* Grate the cucumber into a strainer set over a large bowl, sprinkle it lightly with salt, and mix. Let sit for 10 minutes to allow the salt to draw the liquid out of the cucumber.
7. Squeeze the cucumber well between your hands to remove as much of the remaining liquid as you can. Transfer the cucumber to a small bowl and add the yogurt, lemon zest and juice, garlic, mint, and dill. Mix and taste, then add additional salt if needed.
8. Remove the meatloaf from the oven and let rest for 5 minutes. Slice and serve in pita bread with dollops of the tzatziki!

SUNDAY ROAST CHICKEN

SERVES 6

Rest: 45 minutes
Prep: 15 minutes
Cook: 1 hour, 50 minutes

Dairy Free
Follicular Phase
Gluten Free
Luteal Phase

Perhaps it's my English roots, but I think roast chicken is essential. Roasting is such a simple and effective cooking method—max flavor with very little input—plus you can pick the leftover meat off the bones to use in a second meal (soup, tacos, pasta—literally anything) and then boil the bones for broth (see page 159)! It's one of my favorite ways to hack food prep for the week. While the oven's on, throw in some Crispy Smashed Taters (page 129) or Gochujang and Honey-Glazed Carrots (page 133), whip up the gravy (see Fig and Sage Gravy; page 202), and Bob's your uncle—a Sunday roast!

One 3-to-4-pound (1.4 to 1.8 kg) chicken, thawed if frozen

RUB

1 tablespoon brown sugar
1 tablespoon sea salt
2 teaspoons onion powder
1 teaspoon garlic powder
1 teaspoon smoked paprika
1 teaspoon black pepper
1 teaspoon mustard powder (optional)
1 teaspoon dried thyme or other herbs (optional)

FOR ROASTING

4 large or 5 small carrots, roughly chopped
1 large yellow onion, roughly chopped
Sea salt and black pepper, to taste
⅓ cup (80 ml) avocado oil, divided, plus more for greasing and drizzling
2 or 3 fresh sage, rosemary, thyme, tarragon, or parsley sprigs
1 small lemon, washed

1. Bring the chicken to room temperature by leaving it out of the fridge, wrapped in its packaging, for 30 minutes to 1 hour. Remove any giblets from the center cavity. You can save these in the freezer for broth or roast with the chicken for gravy.
2. Meanwhile, preheat the oven to 475°F (245°C).
3. *Make the rub:* Combine the brown sugar, salt, onion powder, garlic powder, paprika, and pepper, and the mustard powder and thyme (if using) in a small bowl. Gently mix.
4. *Roast the chicken:* Place the carrots and three-fourths of the onion in a large roasting pan and sprinkle with salt and pepper. Drizzle in a little avocado oil, and toss gently.
5. Place the chicken, breast-side up, on top of the vegetables. Shove the remaining one-fourth of the onion and your herb(s) of choice into the center cavity. Prick the lemon all over with a knife, and place it into the cavity as well—it will probably stick out a little, but that's cute.
6. Drizzle half of the avocado oil over the chicken, using your hands to spread it evenly over the surface. Sprinkle half of the rub on the chicken, rubbing it all over.
7. Flip the chicken breast-side down and rub the underside with the remaining spices and oil. Keep the chicken upside down.
8. Reduce the oven temperature to 375°F (190°C) and immediately place the chicken in the oven. Roast for 1 hour and 45 minutes, or until a thermometer reads 165°F (75°C) when inserted into the thickest part of the thigh or a leg pulls off easily.
9. Check the chicken halfway through cooking, scooping up some of the drippings to baste it if it's looking a little dry. You can use a basting brush or just spoon it over.
10. Remove the pan from the oven and use tongs to carefully flip the chicken so it's breast-side up. Baste the chicken with some of the juices and then broil in the oven for 5 to 7 minutes, until the skin is crispy.
11. Transfer the chicken to a cutting board to rest for 15 minutes. Scoop out the carrots to serve (they are so good), and use the drippings for gravy (page 202) if desired.

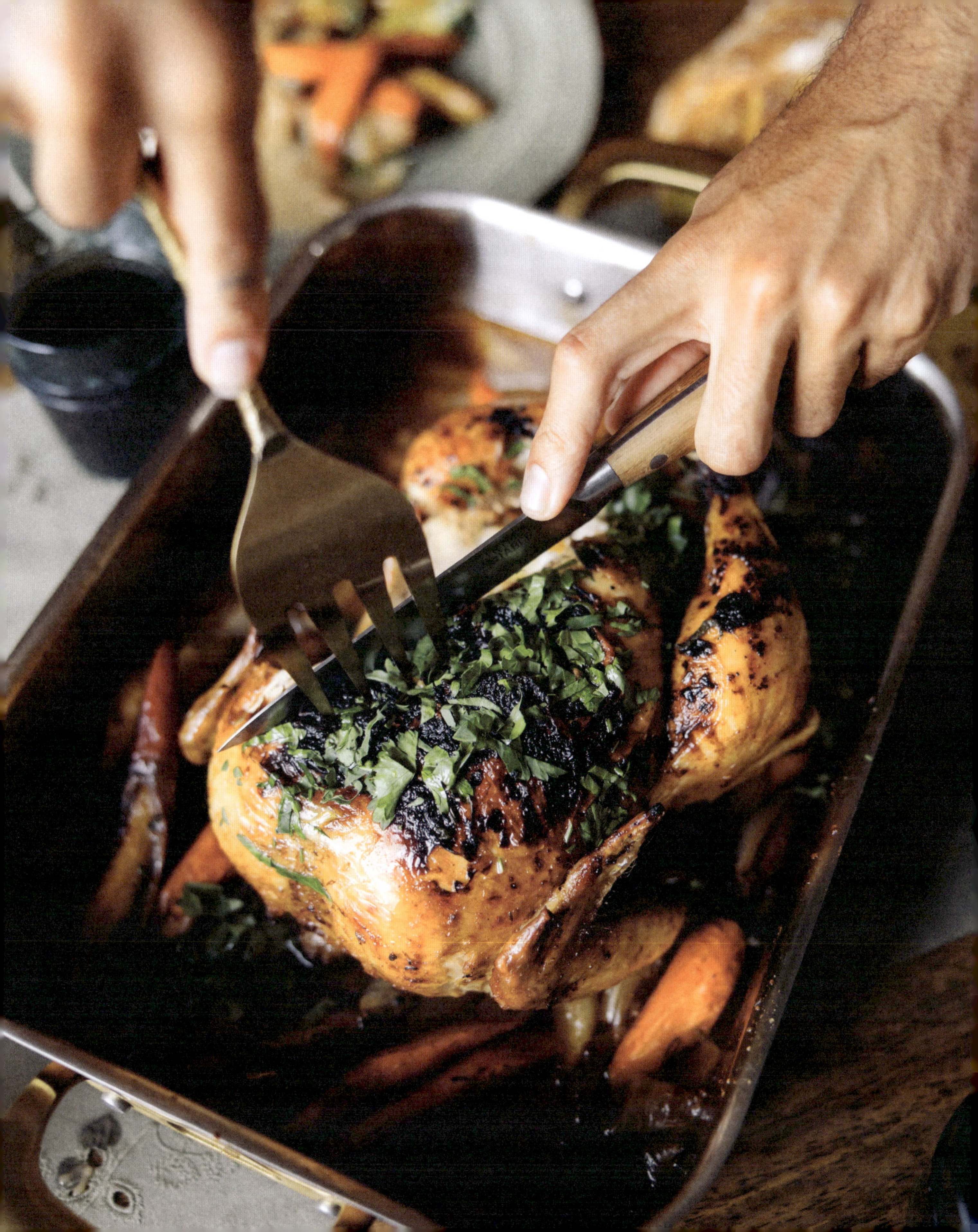

FIG AND SAGE GRAVY

MAKES 4 CUPS (960 ML)

Cook: 20 minutes

Follicular Phase

Gravy can make or break a meal, and if you can learn the secrets of gravy making, you can whip one up from almost anything! With the right flavors, you don't even need actual meat drippings or bouillon. You just need a fat source (drippings, butter, or oil), umami flavor (caramelized onion, meat juices, Worcestershire sauce, or miso), thickener (flour or cornstarch), acid (vinegar, lemon, or alcohol), liquid (meat juices, broth, or water), and a hint of sweetness, saltiness, and aromatics. Yes, gravy does also offer health benefits! Fats are essential for metabolizing nutrients, so it's really in your favor to eat veggies and lean meats with them. And butter or meat drippings are about as good as it gets!

¼ cup (57 g) butter or meat drippings and/or fat (see Tip 1)

½ medium white or yellow onion, finely chopped

Sea salt and black pepper, to taste

¼ cup (30 g) all-purpose flour

3 to 4 cups (720 to 960 ml) roast chicken juices or chicken Bone Broth (page 159), divided

1 tablespoon fig jam or 2 teaspoons brown sugar

1 teaspoon white wine vinegar

1 teaspoon Worcestershire sauce

2 fresh sage sprigs or ¾ teaspoon ground sage

½ cup (120 ml) heavy cream or whole milk (optional)

1. Melt the butter in a large pan over medium heat.
2. Add the onion to the pan with a little sprinkling of salt. Sauté over low heat until the onions soften and brown, 5 to 7 minutes (see Tip 2).
3. Add the flour to create a roux. Whisk until the flour soaks up all the fat and makes a thick paste. Spread this paste across the pan and allow it to cook, stirring occasionally, until the floury smell is replaced with a slightly nutty fragrance and the roux is a light brown, 1 or 2 minutes.
4. Add ½ cup (120 ml) of the meat juices and quickly whisk into the roux. It will thicken up fast. Continue to add the liquid, about 1 cup (240 ml) at a time, whisking to combine fully before adding more. As the liquid content increases, the roux will take a little longer to thicken. Increase the heat to medium and keep an eye on it as it thickens, adding liquid until you reach your desired thickness (my sweet spot is around 3½ cups/840 ml of liquid; see Tip 3).
5. Add the jam, vinegar, Worcestershire sauce, sage, salt, and pepper. Taste and adjust the seasonings as you go, especially if you added extra liquid to bulk out the gravy. Allow a few minutes for the flavors to meld before panic-adding anything!
6. Voilà! The gravy can very gently simmer while the rest of dinner cooks, but keep an eye on it so it doesn't evaporate too much or begin to stick on the bottom.
7. Let the gravy cool slightly before adding the cream (or leave it out to keep this dairy-free). Remove the sage just before serving. The gravy will thicken as it cools, but it should come back to the same consistency when reheated, or you can always add a splash more liquid. The leftovers are great in soup!

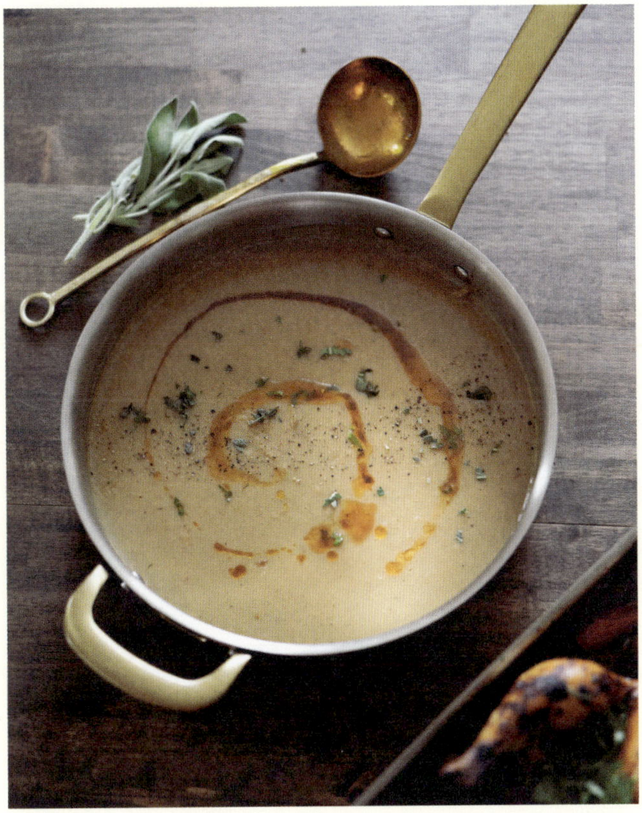

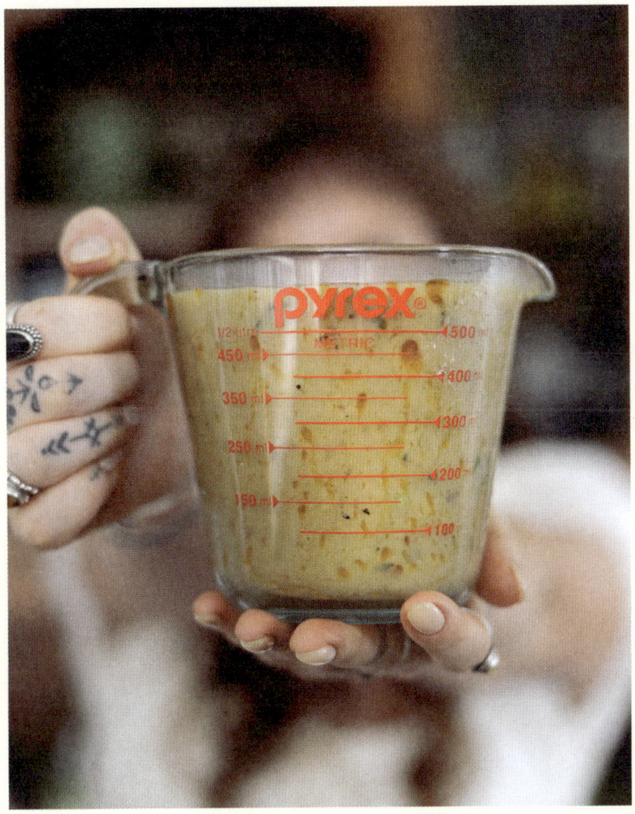

TIPS

1. If you have just roasted chicken in a roasting pan, you can put this pan directly onto the stovetop, deglaze with a couple tablespoons of vinegar, then add the flour and whisk it quickly to make a thin roux. Most likely there won't be enough meat juices in the pan to also account for the broth, so you should be able to just proceed with the recipe as normal, but if it was a very juicy chicken, scoop out most of the juices first, leaving just about 1/2 cup (120 ml) drippings in the pan, make the roux, and then proceed.

2. If you want to add any other aromatics or flavors to your gravy, add them right after step 2. Garlic, mushrooms, peppers, and dried herbs are good options. If using fresh herbs like rosemary, sage, or bay leaves, add whole sprigs after the liquid is incorporated in step 5, then simmer over very low heat before removing the sprigs when the gravy is done cooking.

3. If the gravy is too thin, mix together 1 tablespoon flour with 1/4 cup (60 ml) of the warm gravy in a small bowl to make a thick slurry and then add that to the pan. Gently simmer for 1 or 2 minutes and then turn the heat down a little to see how thick it gets. Repeat until you have your desired thickness!

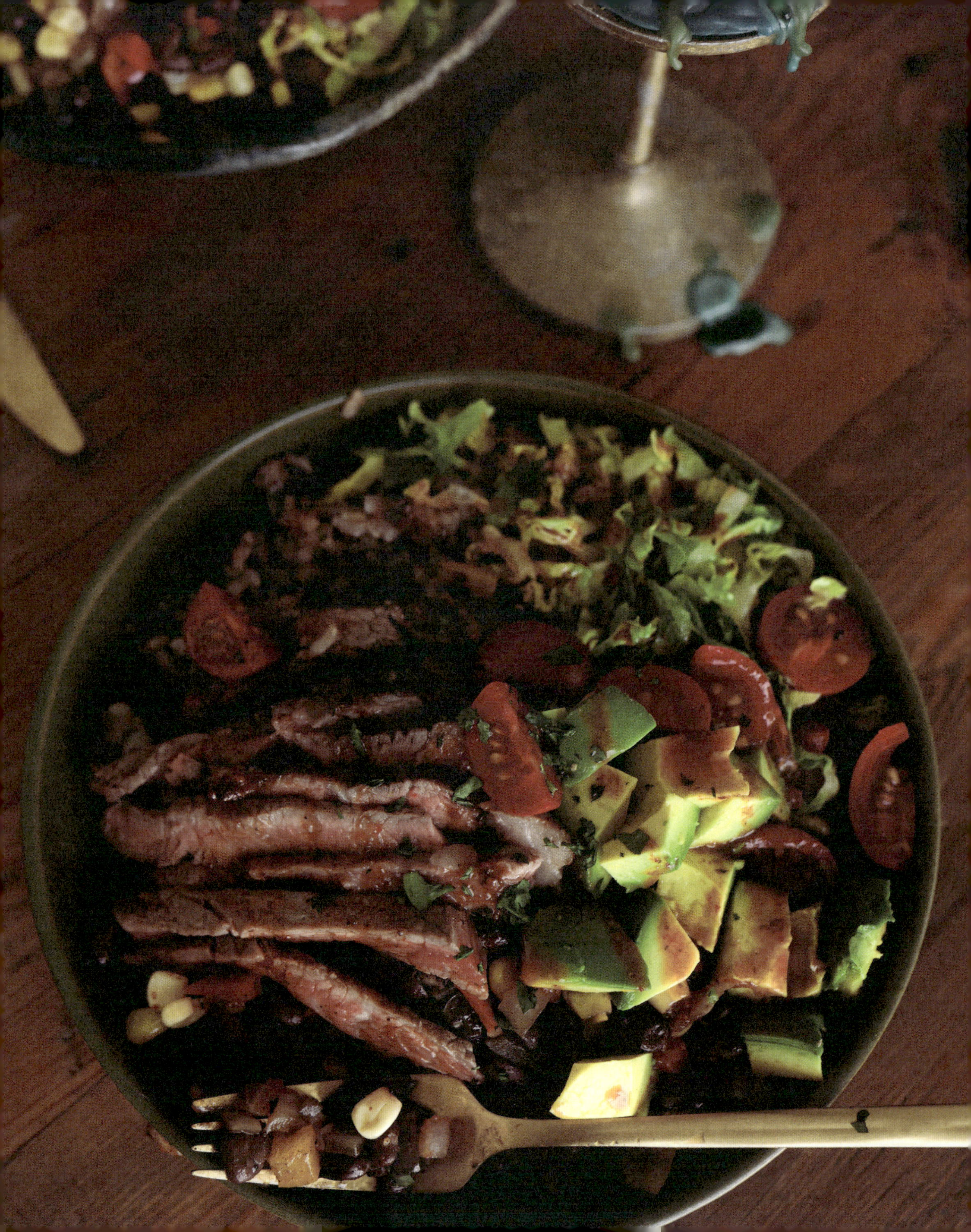

CHIPOTLE STEAK BOWLS

SERVES 4

***Prep:* 50 minutes**
***Cook:* 25 minutes**

Gluten Free
Luteal Phase
Menstrual Phase

I used to say I wasn't really a steak person—I blame immature taste buds and weird ideas about healthy foods—but now I will happily eat steak as often as I can afford to! It's easy to cook and a great source of easily bioavailable heme iron and protein. Plus, if you are able to source local, grass-fed, and grass-finished beef, you are actually supporting the positive environmental impact of small farmers and grazing animals. This one is great for meal prep!

Two 1-inch-thick (2.5 cm) ribeye steaks (about 1½ pounds/680 g)
1 batch Holy Chipotle Dressing (page 210)
4 tablespoons avocado oil, divided
¼ red or orange bell pepper, diced
½ small red onion, diced
1 teaspoon sea salt, divided, plus more for sprinkling
6 garlic cloves, 3 crushed and 3 whole, divided
1½ cups (258 g) cooked black beans
½ cup (80 g) fresh or frozen corn kernels
2 cups (330 g) wild rice, cooked
½ teaspoon ground cumin
½ teaspoon smoked paprika
Black pepper, to taste
1 small bunch cilantro, chopped, divided
2 tablespoons salted butter

FOR SERVING

Diced avocado
Chopped lettuce
Chopped tomatoes

1. Remove the steaks from the fridge. Place in a shallow dish, add ⅔ cup (160 ml) dressing, cover, and marinate while the steaks reach room temperature, about 45 minutes.
2. Meanwhile, heat a large skillet over medium heat and add 2 tablespoons avocado oil.
3. Throw in the bell pepper and onion, sprinkle with ½ teaspoon salt, and sauté, stirring occasionally, until softened, 4 to 5 minutes.
4. Make a space in the center of the pan and add the crushed garlic, stirring until fragrant, about 1 minute, then stir to combine.
5. Add the beans and corn and cook, stirring occasionally, until the veggies are slightly charred, 5 more minutes.
6. Add the rice, along with ½ teaspoon salt, the cumin, paprika, and black pepper, and half the cilantro and stir.
7. Reduce the heat to low and cover while you cook the steaks.
8. Heat another large skillet over medium-high heat and add the remaining 2 tablespoons avocado oil.
9. Completely dry the steaks with a clean cloth or paper towel, removing as much of the marinade as possible, then sprinkle liberally with salt and pepper. Discard the marinade.
10. Melt the butter in the pan and throw in the whole garlic cloves. Immediately add the steaks. You should hear a loud sizzling sound as soon as the steaks touch the pan; if not, the pan isn't hot enough.
11. Cook until both sides are seared and the inside is cooked to your desired doneness. For medium-rare steak, reduce the heat to medium and cook for 3 to 4 minutes per side; for medium steak, cook for 4 to 5 minutes per side; and for well-done steak, cook for 6 to 8 minutes per side.
12. Transfer the steaks to a cutting board to rest for 5 minutes. (This is so important! It allows the juices to settle into the meat, keeping it moist. Otherwise, they will run right out onto your cutting board and leave you with dry steak.)
13. Slice the steaks against the grain and serve on top of the rice and bean mixture. Garnish with the remaining cilantro and serve with avocado, lettuce, tomatoes, and of course a generous drizzle of the remaining Holy Chipotle Dressing.

CHAPTER EIGHT

DIPS & DRESSINGS

EAT WHAT YOU WANT—JUST MAKE IT YOURSELF,

is never more applicable than with dips and dressings. Store-bought dressings, like ranch, so often just add excess calories with little nutritional function, whereas a homemade ranch made with avocado oil mayo, kefir, and fresh herbs has so many nutritional benefits!

I take particular joy in dressings and have been dubbed "the sauce queen" by my loved ones, often called on when I was younger to make a fun dressing or sauce for an otherwise plain meal, so you could call me biased. But dressings are a great way to sneak in extra nutrients, to incorporate seeds for hormone health, and to elevate your food prep and make you actually want to eat raw carrots.

In fact, vegetables need to be eaten with fats so that your body can make the most of their micronutrients, so forcing yourself to down plain broccoli is not actually the "healthy" option you may think it is. Drizzling on a healthy fat like some olive oil or a fat-filled dressing like the Tahini Dressing (page 208) or Herbaceous Green Dressing (page 210) is actually ideal. Unfortunately, this book isn't called *Simple Saucy Magic*, so in this chapter I've limited myself to a few of my very favorites.

TAHINI DRESSING

MAKES 1 CUP (240 ML)

Prep: 5 minutes

Tahini is made of ground sesame seeds. That means it's full of estrogen-regulating lignans and zinc which together support immune health and progesterone production, along with protein, healthy fats, and tons of minerals. Sesame seeds are anti-inflammatory, too, which makes this dressing a great staple for those of us with chronic inflammatory conditions.

½ cup (120 ml) tahini (see Note)
Juice of 1 lemon, plus more to taste
1 garlic clove, crushed, plus more to taste
½ teaspoon sea salt, plus more to taste
½ cup (120 ml) ice water, plus more as needed

1. Place the tahini, lemon juice, garlic, and salt in a food processor or blender. You can also mix this with a whisk in a medium bowl.
2. While blending (or aggressively whisking), slowly pour in the ice water. This will make the tahini seize up (!) and thicken, but it will quickly become smoother, fluffier, and lighter in color. Add water until you reach your desired consistency.
3. Taste and adjust the lemon, garlic, and salt as needed. Store in a sealed jar in the fridge for up to 2 weeks. The dressing may thicken but you can loosen it up by mixing in a little water before serving.

NOTE

Try to get organic tahini paste made from 100 percent sesame seeds. It should be light in color and very smooth in texture. If it has a darker color or a strong, bitter odor or taste, it's rancid and should be discarded.

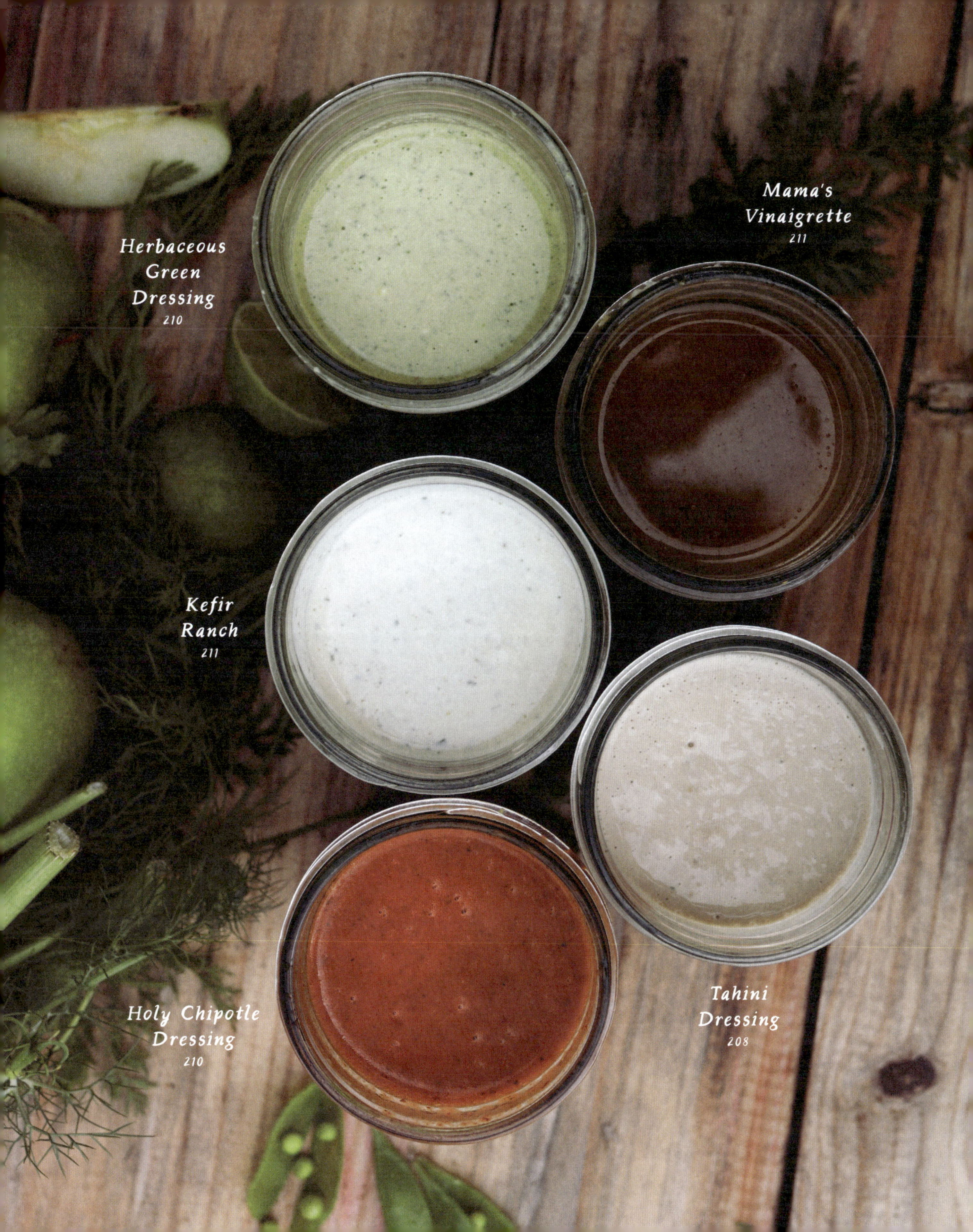
Herbaceous Green Dressing
210
Mama's Vinaigrette
211
Kefir Ranch
211
Tahini Dressing
208
Holy Chipotle Dressing
210

HERBACEOUS GREEN DRESSING

MAKES 2 CUPS (480 ML)

Prep: 5 minutes

This is a shortcut to getting tons of goodies in one fell swoop. It has fresh herbs for digestion, healthy fats for nutrient absorption, garlic for all the things (see page 272), egg yolk for choline, and hemp seeds for a protein and omega-3s! You can easily adjust this for your cycle by switching up the seeds (see page 230). Play with the herbs and seeds to create different flavor profiles!

1 cup (about 20 g) packed fresh herbs (some combination of parsley, cilantro, dill, or carrot tops)
⅓ cup (40 g) hemp seeds
1 tablespoon sunflower seeds or pumpkin seeds (see Headnote)
1 tablespoon sesame seeds or flaxseeds
½ cup (120 ml) plus 2 tablespoons extra virgin olive oil
3 tablespoons apple cider vinegar (with the mother)
Juice of 1 lemon, or more to taste
2 garlic cloves, or more to taste
1 egg yolk
1 teaspoon dried oregano or 1 small sprig fresh oregano
1 avocado
½ teaspoon sea salt, or more to taste
¼ teaspoon black pepper, or more to taste
Honey, to taste (optional)

1. Place the fresh herbs, seeds, olive oil, vinegar, lemon juice, garlic, egg yolk, oregano, avocado, salt, and pepper in a high-speed blender. Blend until completely smooth, 2 to 3 minutes.
2. Add more garlic, lemon juice, salt, and/or pepper, or even a drop of honey to taste. Store in a sealed jar in the fridge for up to 3 days.

HOLY CHIPOTLE DRESSING

MAKES 1½ CUPS (360 ML)

Prep: 5 minutes

I will eat anything with this stuff on it—it's sweet and smoky, with a tiny bit of heat. Inspired by the dressing I can't eat a Chipotle bowl without, it goes with anything and even makes a great meat marinade!

2 chipotles in adobo sauce, plus 1 teaspoon adobo sauce, or more to taste
¾ cup (180 ml) avocado oil
¼ cup (60 ml) red wine vinegar
¼ cup (60 ml) honey
2 tablespoons apple cider vinegar (with the mother)
1½ teaspoons sea salt
½ teaspoon dried oregano
¼ teaspoon ground cumin
¼ teaspoon smoked paprika
Black pepper, to taste

1. Blend the ingredients in a high-speed blender on high until smooth, about 30 seconds. Alternatively, place the ingredients in a 16-ounce (480 ml) mason jar and use an immersion blender to combine.
2. Store in a sealed jar in the fridge for up to 1 month.

MAMA'S VINAIGRETTE

MAKES ABOUT 1½ CUPS (380 ML)

Prep: 5 minutes

This is my mom's classic everyday salad dressing. It's perfectly zingy and fresh, bringing even the simplest salad to the next level. For different flavor profiles, add herbs like oregano, parsley, or mint; use orange instead of lemon; or add spices like cardamom, cumin, or coriander.

1 cup (240 ml) extra virgin olive oil, plus more to taste
⅓ cup (80 ml) apple cider vinegar (with the mother)
¼ cup (60 ml) balsamic vinegar
2 garlic cloves, crushed or finely grated, plus more to taste
1 tablespoon honey
1 tablespoon brown or Dijon mustard, plus more to taste
1 teaspoon lemon juice
1 teaspoon sea salt

1. Combine the ingredients in a 16-ounce (480 ml) mason jar. Shake the jar super hard until the dressing emulsifies and comes together.
2. If the dressing is too sharp or salty, add some oil; if you want stronger flavors, add extra mustard or garlic.
3. Seal the jar and store at room temperature for a few weeks or in the fridge almost indefinitely (it will solidify in the fridge and need to come to room temperature before use).

KEFIR RANCH

MAKES 2 CUPS (480 ML)

Prep: 5 minutes

This long-perfected recipe tastes just like the classic dressing, except this version contains homemade mayo and kefir, so it's packed with probiotics and healthy fats and is anti-inflammatory. Serve with roasted veggies for a super nourishing and easy-to-digest snack that adds a massive flavor boost to the traditional crudité tray.

1 cup (240 ml) Avocado Oil Mayo (page 212)
1 cup (240 ml) Kefir (page 69)
1 or 2 garlic cloves, crushed, plus more to taste
2 teaspoons lemon juice, plus more to taste
1 teaspoon honey
1 teaspoon onion powder
½ teaspoon dried dill or 1 teaspoon finely chopped fresh dill
½ teaspoon mustard powder or Dijon mustard
½ teaspoon parsley flakes or 1 teaspoon finely chopped fresh parsley
½ teaspoon sea salt, plus more to taste
¼ teaspoon black pepper

1. Add the ingredients to a 16-ounce (480 ml) wide-mouth mason jar, whisking with a fork as you go.
2. Adjust the garlic, lemon juice, and salt to taste.
3. Cover the mason jar and store in the fridge for up to 1 week.

AVOCADO OIL MAYO

MAKES $1^1/_4$ CUPS (300 ML)

Prep: 5 minutes

Mayo isn't intrinsically bad for you, but the oil choice makes a big difference. Using avocado oil instead of canola, sunflower, or vegetable oil turns mayo from an inflammatory fat into a healthy fat. Plus, using great-quality eggs increases those good fatty acids, vitamins, and minerals. The most important thing is that the egg and oil get properly emulsified. I recommend an immersion blender for this, although it can also be made in an upright blender if you drizzle in the oil slowly.

1 large egg
1 egg yolk
1 cup (240 ml) avocado oil
1 teaspoon sea salt
2 teaspoons lemon juice
1 teaspoon white vinegar
1 teaspoon granulated sugar (optional)

1. Add the egg and egg yolk to a wide-mouth 16-ounce (480 ml) mason jar. Gently add the avocado oil and salt on top of the eggs, trying not to disturb them too much.
2. Add the lemon juice, vinegar, and sugar (if using) on top and then gently insert an immersion blender all the way to the bottom of the jar.
3. Blend, without moving the blender, until the mixture thickens on the bottom and draws in oil from the top. Slowly move the blender around, gradually moving your way up the jar until the mixture is thickened and emulsified (see Tip).
4. Pump the blender from top to bottom a couple of times to ensure everything is combined.

KETCHUP

MAKES 2 HEAPING CUPS (ABOUT 520 ML)

Prep: 5 minutes
Cook: 20 minutes

We have a ketchup-obsessed toddler and have spent a few too many dollars on organic, sugar-free ketchup... we've also run out of ketchup a lot, and hence, homemade ketchup has become somewhat of a necessity. You can make it by cooking down fresh tomatoes, but I've never had time for that, so this whips up quickly using tomato paste as the base!

Two 6-ounce (170 g) cans tomato paste
½ cup (120 ml) apple cider vinegar (with the mother)
⅔ cup (160 ml) water
½ cup (120 ml) honey
½ teaspoon onion powder
¾ teaspoon sea salt
¼ teaspoon curry powder
¼ teaspoon garlic powder

1. Whisk the ingredients in a medium saucepan.
2. Bring the mixture to a boil, reduce the heat to low, and cover partially with a lid to keep it from splattering and allow the steam to escape. Simmer for 20 to 30 minutes, until the mixture thickens to a scoopable consistency and reduces by half.
3. Remove from the heat and cool, then decant into a jar or squeeze bottle.
4. Keep in the fridge for . . . as long as you would keep store-bought ketchup!

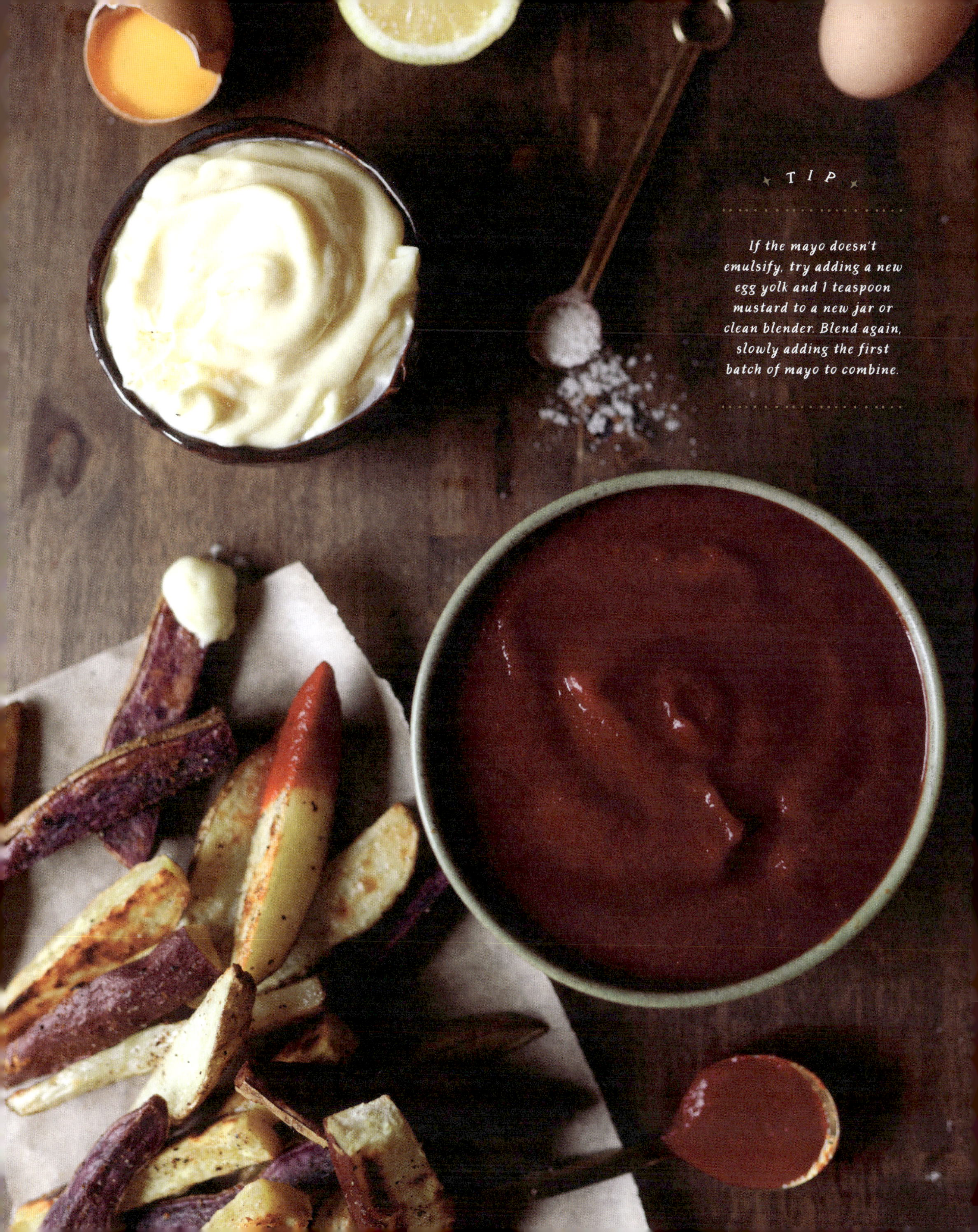

TIP

If the mayo doesn't emulsify, try adding a new egg yolk and 1 teaspoon mustard to a new jar or clean blender. Blend again, slowly adding the first batch of mayo to combine.

SPROUTED HUMMUS

MAKES 3 CUPS (720 G)

Rest: 8 to 48 hours
Prep: 15 minutes
Cook: 45 minutes

"Why on earth would I want to sprout my hummus?" you may ask. Good question! Chickpeas, while they are a great source of protein, fiber, and micronutrients, are legumes and can be pretty rough on the stomach for a lot of people. Allowing them to soak in water until they sprout releases some of that hard-to-digest phytic acid, making them much easier for your body to process. Alternatively, you can just soak them overnight, which will still help with digestion and make them cook more quickly.

5 to 6 cups (1.2 to 1.4 L) filtered water
1 cup (165 g) dried chickpeas (see Note 1)
½ teaspoon baking soda
1½ teaspoons sea salt, divided, plus more to taste
½ to ⅔ cup (120 to 160 g) tahini (see Note 2)
1 or 2 garlic cloves, plus more to taste
2 tablespoons lemon juice, plus more to taste
¼ to ½ cup (60 to 120 ml) ice water

FOR SERVING (OPTIONAL)

Olive oil
Za'atar
Lemon zest
Sautéed peppers
Roasted garlic
Baked chickpeas

1. Place the chickpeas in a large bowl with the filtered water. Cover with a plate and let sit at least overnight or, if sprouting, for 36 to 48 hours (until you see little sprouts poking out). Drain the water and rinse the chickpeas.
2. Transfer the chickpeas to a medium pan and cover them with about ½ inch (1 cm) water. Add the baking soda, bring to a boil, and skim off any scum that comes to the surface. Reduce the heat to low, cover, and let simmer for about 20 minutes. Then, add 1 teaspoon of salt.
3. Cover and simmer until the chickpeas are soft and easily smashable, 20 to 25 minutes. When the chickpeas are almost done, you'll notice little skins starting to float to the surface. Agitate the chickpeas with a slotted spoon, knocking off as many of these skins as possible, and use the spoon to remove them when they come to the surface—this will create a smoother texture.
4. Save about ¼ cup (60 ml) of the chickpea water and drain the rest.
5. Transfer the chickpeas to a food processor or blender along with 2 tablespoons of the reserved chickpea water, the remaining ½ teaspoon salt, and the tahini, garlic, and lemon juice. Blend until smooth, then slowly drizzle in the ice water, 1 tablespoon at a time, as you blend, until you reach your desired consistency. This will make the hummus super creamy and fluffy.
6. Taste the hummus and add more salt, garlic, or lemon to your preference.
7. Spread the hummus on a plate or scoop into a bowl, top with a swirl of olive oil, a sprinkle of za'atar, some lemon zest, sautéed peppers, roasted garlic, and/or baked chickpeas. Store, covered with a thin layer of olive oil, in the fridge for up to 1 week.

VARIATIONS

BEET HUMMUS

- Roast 1 to 3 beets (about 1 cup/135 g) according to page 141.
- Add the beets to the food processor before adding the chickpeas in step 5.

GREEN GODDESS HUMMUS

- Add a large handful of herbs (any combination of parsley, dill, tarragon, cilantro, or chives) to the food processor before adding the chickpeas in step 5.
- Serve topped with 1 or 2 tablespoons chopped herbs.

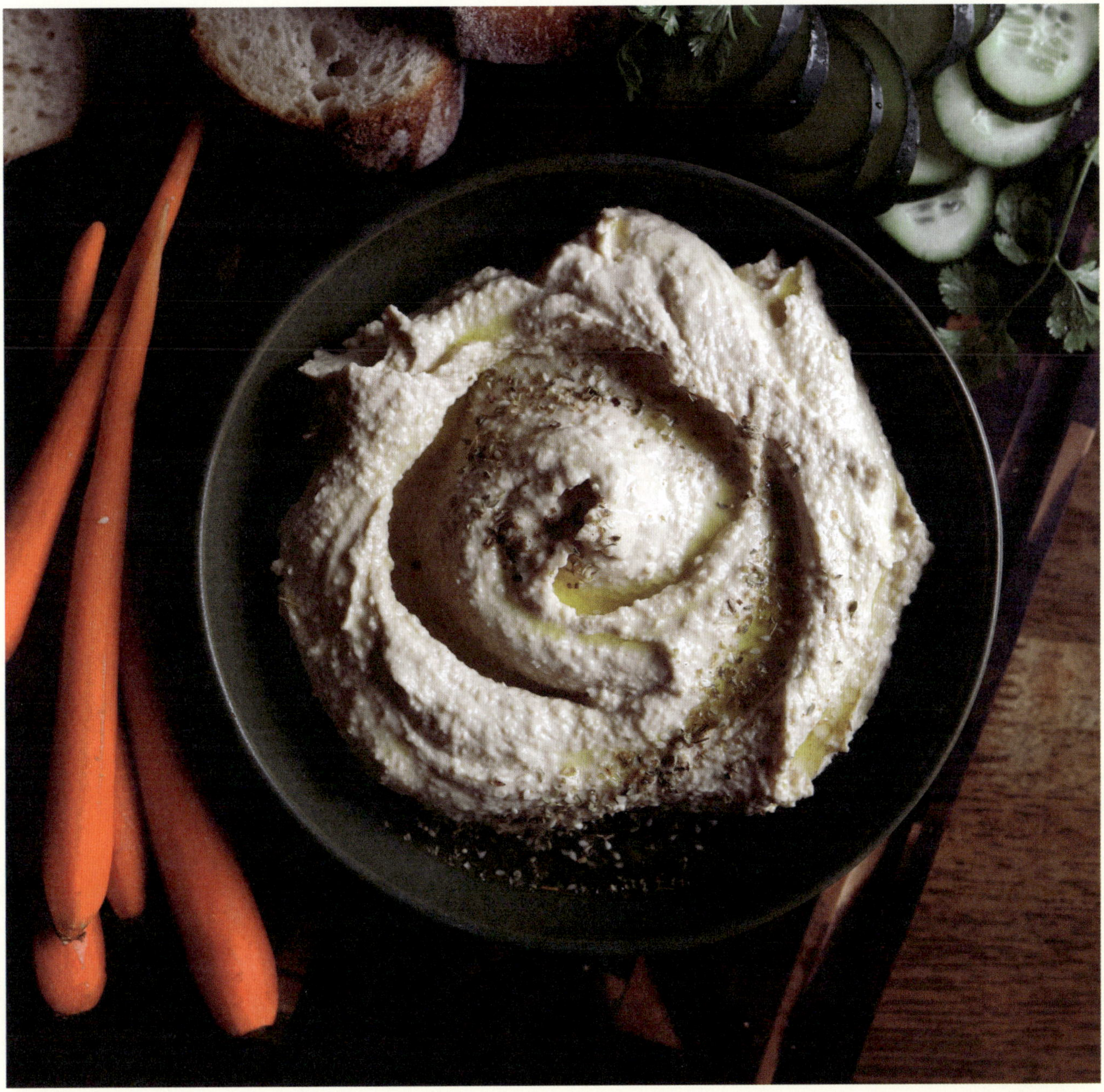

CHOCOLATE HUMMUS

- Substitute peanut butter for the tahini in step 5, if desired. Instead of the salt, garlic, and lemon juice, add ¼ to ½ cup (60 to 120 ml) maple syrup, honey, or agave; ¼ cup (21 g) cacao or cocoa powder, 2 teaspoons vanilla extract, and a pinch of salt.
- Serve topped with mini chocolate chips, a drizzle of maple syrup, and/or coconut cream. Serve with fruit, pretzels, or bread, or just eat it by the spoonful!

✦ NOTES ✦

1. In a pinch, you can also use two 15-ounce (400 g) cans of chickpeas. Drain and rinse them, then skip to step 3 and cook for 15 minutes instead of 20.

2. To make seed cycling hummus for the menstrual or follicular phases, replace the tahini with pumpkin seed butter. Make this by blending roasted pumpkin seeds with a little sea salt in a food processor until they form a butter, adding a little drizzle of oil if necessary.

CHAPTER NINE

NUTRIENT-DENSE TREATS

EVERYONE NEEDS TREATS— AND I MEAN REAL TREATS.

I refuse to believe that it's sustainable for anyone to commit to never having sugar or chocolate or other sweet things. The key is to plan for them and make treats that serve your body as well as your soul.

You can do this simply by making them yourself. Even the most traditional white-sugar-and-flour homemade goods will be one thousand percent better for you than store-bought items. To take it a step further, choose unrefined sugar sources, add extra fiber, and use targeted ingredients to serve your needs and turn your creations into actually healthy goodies.

We used to tease my mom a lot for always trying to make treats healthy. "I'm making a cake!" she would announce, and then proceed to use whole-wheat flour, significantly less sugar, and extra raisins. Needless to say, there were some flops, but over the years she's perfected the art of a healthier homemade treat. Those are the kind of treats I've included here. I have no problem making a white-sugar-white-flour cake dripping with buttercream, but you can find those recipes everywhere. These are the recipes I've developed that genuinely serve a purpose in your body without sacrificing flavor and while satisfying that sweet tooth. The Power Muffins (page 234) are inspired by my mom's go-to carrot muffins with just a little extra pizazz, and they're a favorite food prep item of mine. I love to whip up the Berry Crumble (page 227) on a weeknight, and my Gluten-Free Oatmeal Chocolate Chip Cookies (page 219) may be gluten free, but they are actually my favorite cookie recipe ever. Most importantly, these are recipes that I want you to enjoy totally guilt-free, even the ones that have *actual sugar* in them!

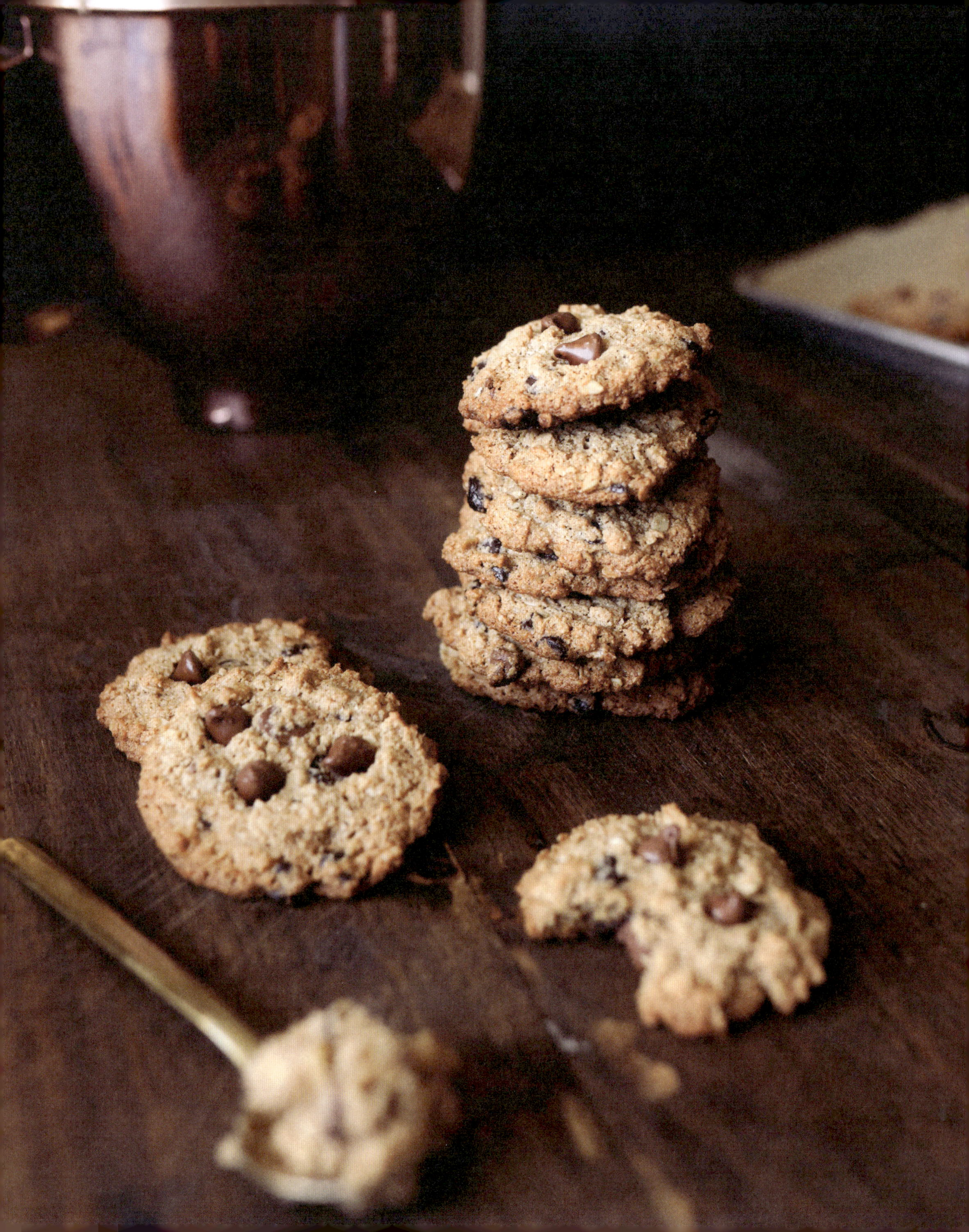

GLUTEN-FREE OATMEAL CHOCOLATE CHIP COOKIES

MAKES 24 COOKIES

Prep: 10 minutes
Cook: 10 minutes

Follicular Phase
Gluten Free
Ovulation Phase

A good chocolate chip cookie feels like home to me—and there's no reason cookies can't serve your body, too! These cookies are gluten free, full of fiber, and low in sugar (compared to most cookies). If you are gluten intolerant, be sure to check that your oats are in fact gluten free and, as always, try to get organic, glyphosate-free oats. If you choose to use dark chocolate or sugar-free chocolate chips, these cookies can be even lower in sugar, and you can enjoy all the great antioxidant benefits of chocolate!

1 cup (226 g) salted butter, softened
1 cup (220 g) brown sugar
2 large eggs
2 teaspoons vanilla extract
3 cups (300 g) almond flour
1 cup (80 g) quick oats
1 cup (80 g) rolled oats
1½ teaspoons ground cinnamon
1 teaspoon baking powder
½ teaspoon baking soda
1½ cups (255 g) semisweet chocolate chips

1. Preheat the oven to 350°F (175°C). Line two baking sheets with parchment paper.
2. Cream the butter (with either elbow grease or an electric mixer) in a medium bowl. Add the brown sugar and mix until well incorporated and fluffy. Add the eggs and vanilla extract and whisk again to combine.
3. Add the almond flour, quick and rolled oats, cinnamon, baking powder, and baking soda, stirring together with a spoon or spatula. Mix in the chocolate chips.
4. Scoop generous tablespoon-sized balls of cookie dough onto the baking sheets, placing them 1 to 2 inches (2.5 to 5 cm) apart (you should be able to fit up to 8 dough balls on one sheet). Flatten the balls a little with your hands or the back of a spoon.
5. Bake for 10 (softer/chewier) to 12 minutes (crispier), depending on the texture you like!

TIP

I love to bake up half the mixture (about 12 cookies) and then roll up the extra dough into a log shape, wrap it in parchment paper, and freeze it for later use. Freeze for up to 1 month, and bring to room temperature before slicing and baking.

BANANA BLENDER MUFFINS

MAKES
12 MUFFINS

Prep: **15 minutes**
Cook: **25 minutes**

Dairy Free
Follicular Phase
Gluten Free
Luteal Phase

These muffins are very delicate and soft by nature, so they will sink a little as they bake! If they are a bit undercooked, they will sink more. If they are overcooked, they will be a little dry. Other than that, they are very forgiving and can be made with just one banana or one egg instead of two. You can also add chocolate chips or flaxseeds—feel free to mix it up!

Avocado or coconut oil, for greasing the pan
2 medium ripe bananas
2 large eggs
½ cup (130 g) natural peanut or almond butter
½ cup (40 g) rolled oats
¼ cup (60 ml) honey or maple syrup
1 tablespoon apple cider vinegar
1 teaspoon baking soda
1 teaspoon vanilla extract
½ teaspoon ground cinnamon

1. Preheat the oven to 350°F (175°C).
2. Grease a muffin pan with avocado oil. (I prefer not to use liners, as the muffins tend to stick to them.)
3. Place the bananas, eggs, peanut butter, oats, honey, vinegar, baking soda, vanilla, and cinnamon in a blender or food processor and—yup—blend 'em up!
4. Pour the mixture into the muffin cups, leaving a ¼-inch (6 mm) space for rising at the top of each cup.
5. Bake for 20 to 25 minutes, until the muffins puff up, darken in color, and are dry to the touch in the center.
6. Remove from the oven, let the muffins cool for a few minutes in the pan, and then turn them out! If need be, run a knife around the edge of each muffin before tipping the pan upside down and lightly banging to get them out.
7. Store in the fridge for up to a week, although they are best eaten immediately (and very often disappear quickly).

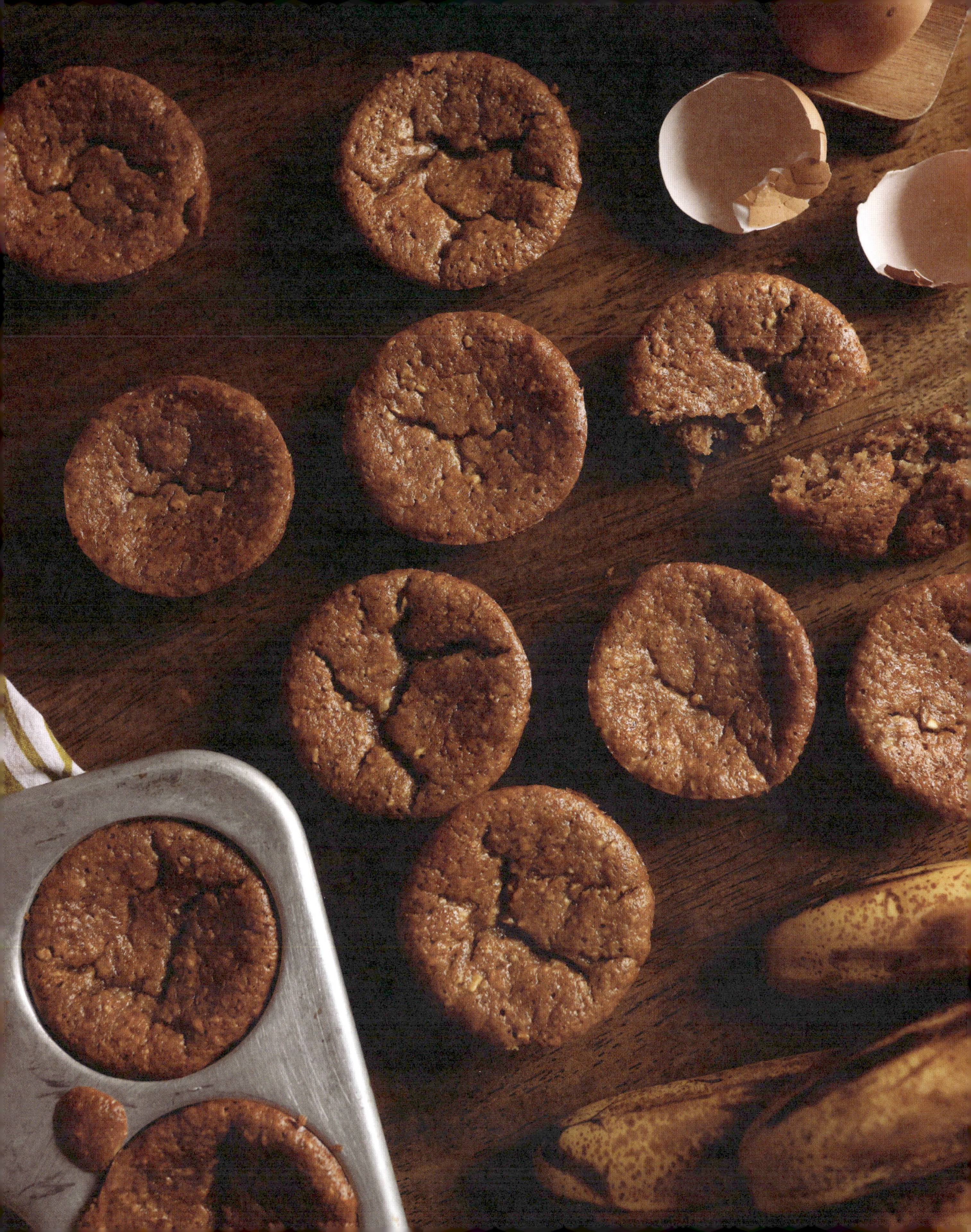

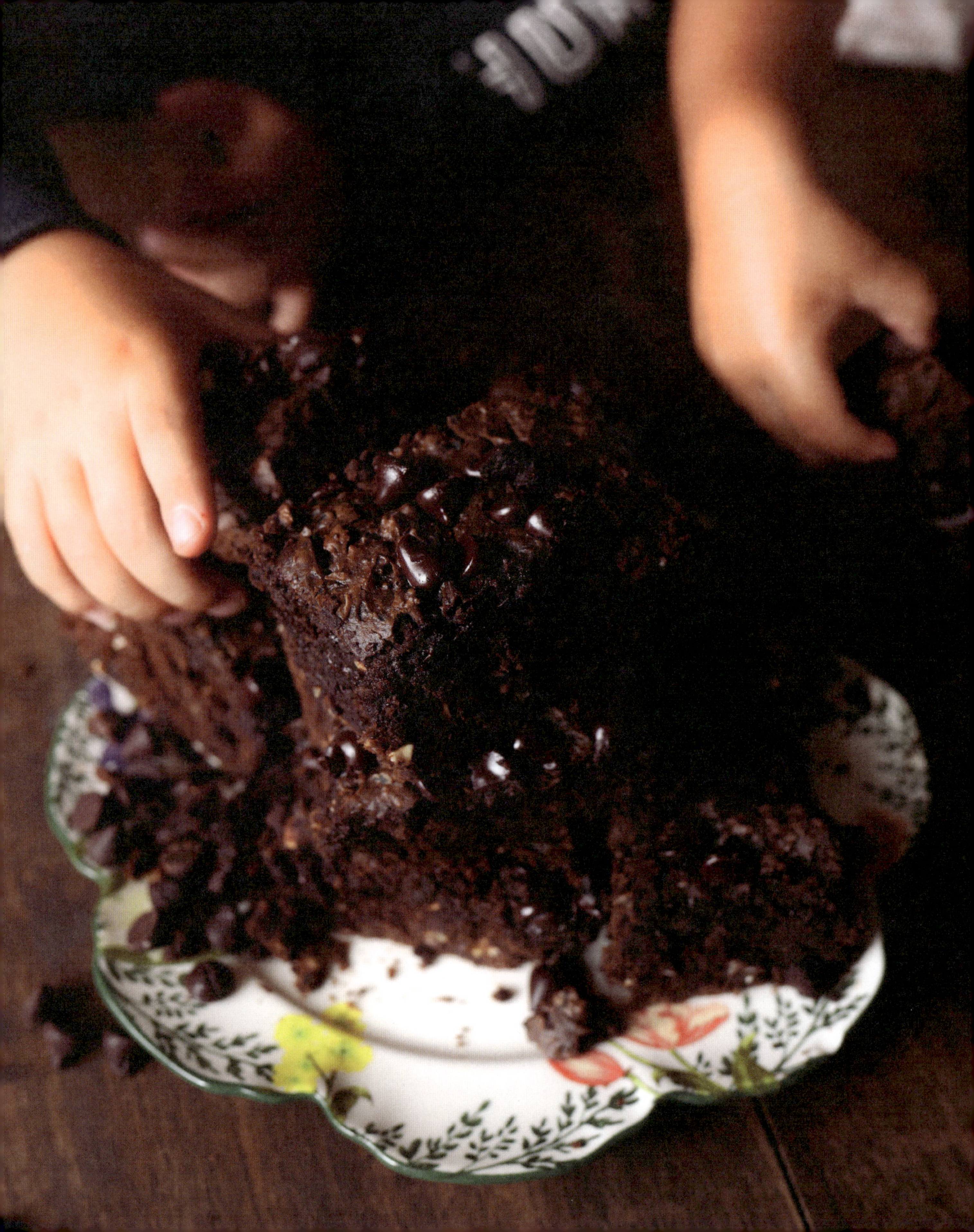

BLACK BEAN BROWNIES

MAKES 12 BROWNIES

***Prep:* 10 minutes**
***Cook:* 30 minutes**

Dairy Free
Gluten Free
Menstrual Phase

You wouldn't believe the number of incredulous looks I receive when I announce that the brownies I just served are "bean brownies" after everyone and their mom, plus all the pickiest kids, have just devoured them. They're rich, fluffy, and just sweet enough, with zero flour and a good amount of protein. The chocolate chips are essential here, but you can use a sugar-free or stevia-sweetened option if you really want to make these a no-nonsense treat!

Avocado or coconut oil, for greasing the pan
Two 15.5-ounce (439 g) cans black beans, drained and rinsed
2 large eggs
1 cup (260 g) creamy natural peanut butter
½ cup (40 g) oats, quick or rolled
⅓ cup (80 ml) maple syrup or honey
¼ cup plus 2 tablespoons (32 g) cocoa powder
3 teaspoons vanilla extract
1 teaspoon baking powder
1 teaspoon ground cinnamon
1 cup (170 g) dark chocolate chips, divided

1. Preheat the oven to 350°F (175°C). Lightly oil a 9-inch (23 cm) square baking dish.
2. Place the beans, eggs, peanut butter, oats, maple syrup, cocoa powder, vanilla extract, baking powder, and cinnamon in a food processor. Blend on high until smooth.
3. Remove the blade from the food processor and stir in ⅔ cup (115 g) chocolate chips.
4. Scoop the batter into the baking dish and smooth into an even layer, then sprinkle liberally with the remaining ⅓ cup (55 g) chocolate chips.
5. Bake for 30 minutes, or until the brownies are firm to the touch and a knife or toothpick comes out clean.
6. Store the leftovers (if you manage to save any!) in an airtight container in the fridge for up to 1 week.

BAKED APPLE CRUMBLES

MAKES 5 APPLES

Prep: 15 minutes
Cook: 55 minutes

Blood Sugar Balancing
Dairy Free
Gluten Free
Luteal Phase

Baked apples were one of those childhood staple desserts my mom made. I may have zhuzhed up the recipe a little, and now it is a major fave. It hits the sweet spots while being great for blood sugar and easily adaptable to different flavors and phases of the cycle. And the soft-cooked apples are so rich in prebiotic pectin, which feeds your healthy gut bacteria! I've added a whipped coconut cream topping, but you can totally use regular heavy whipping cream or even Greek yogurt with a drop of vanilla extract and a bit of honey to sweeten.

5 Granny Smith apples
6 large dates, chopped
1 cup (120 g) chopped walnuts
½ cup (50 g) almond flour
½ cup (40 g) rolled oats
Zest of 1 orange (about 2 tablespoons)
3 tablespoons coconut oil
2 tablespoons brown sugar
1 teaspoon ground cinnamon
½ teaspoon ground ginger
½ cup (45 g) unsweetened shredded coconut (optional)
1 cup (240 ml) warm water

TOPPING

One 13.5-ounce (400 ml) can coconut cream, chilled in the fridge for 24 hours
½ teaspoon vanilla extract
1 tablespoon maple syrup (optional)

1. Preheat the oven to 375°F (190°C).
2. Cut a thin section off the top of each apple, exposing the flesh and core. Cut around the core with a sharp knife, then scoop out the core along with about ¼ inch (6 mm) of extra flesh around it, but don't scoop any extra flesh underneath it—be sure to leave a good 1 inch (2.5 cm) of apple at the bottom. Set the apples in an 8-inch (20 cm) square baking pan.
3. Place the dates, walnuts, almond flour, oats, orange zest, coconut oil, brown sugar, cinnamon, ginger, and coconut (if using) in a medium bowl. Combine with your hands, rubbing everything through your fingers to distribute the oil. The mixture should be crumbly but stick together when squeezed.
4. Fill each apple with the mixture, adding a good amount to the top and pressing gently to create a little mound of crumble.
5. Add the water to the pan and bake in the oven for 30 minutes, or until the apples begin to soften.
6. Carefully remove the pan from the oven and gently cover with a sheet of foil. Return to the oven and bake for 20 to 25 more minutes, until the apples reach your desired softness and the crumble topping is a deep brown. Let cool slightly.
7. *Meanwhile, make the topping:* Remove the chilled coconut cream from the fridge. Scoop the cream into a medium bowl, leaving any clear coconut water behind.
8. Using a hand mixer, whisk until fluffy, gently circulating the mixer around the bowl until soft peaks form, 3 to 5 minutes. Add the vanilla extract and maple syrup (if using) and whisk again briefly.
9. Once the apples are cool enough to eat, serve with dollops of coconut cream on top!

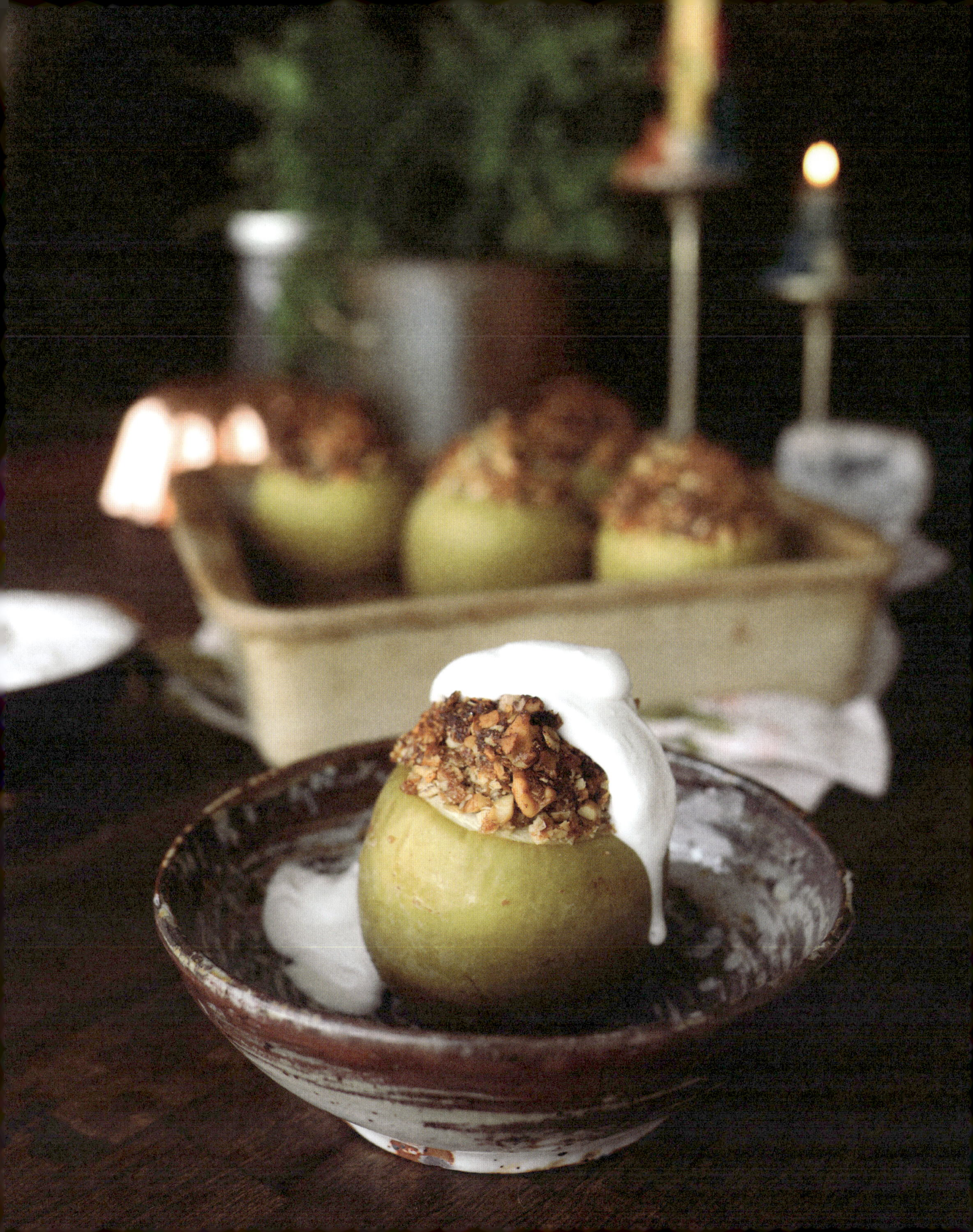

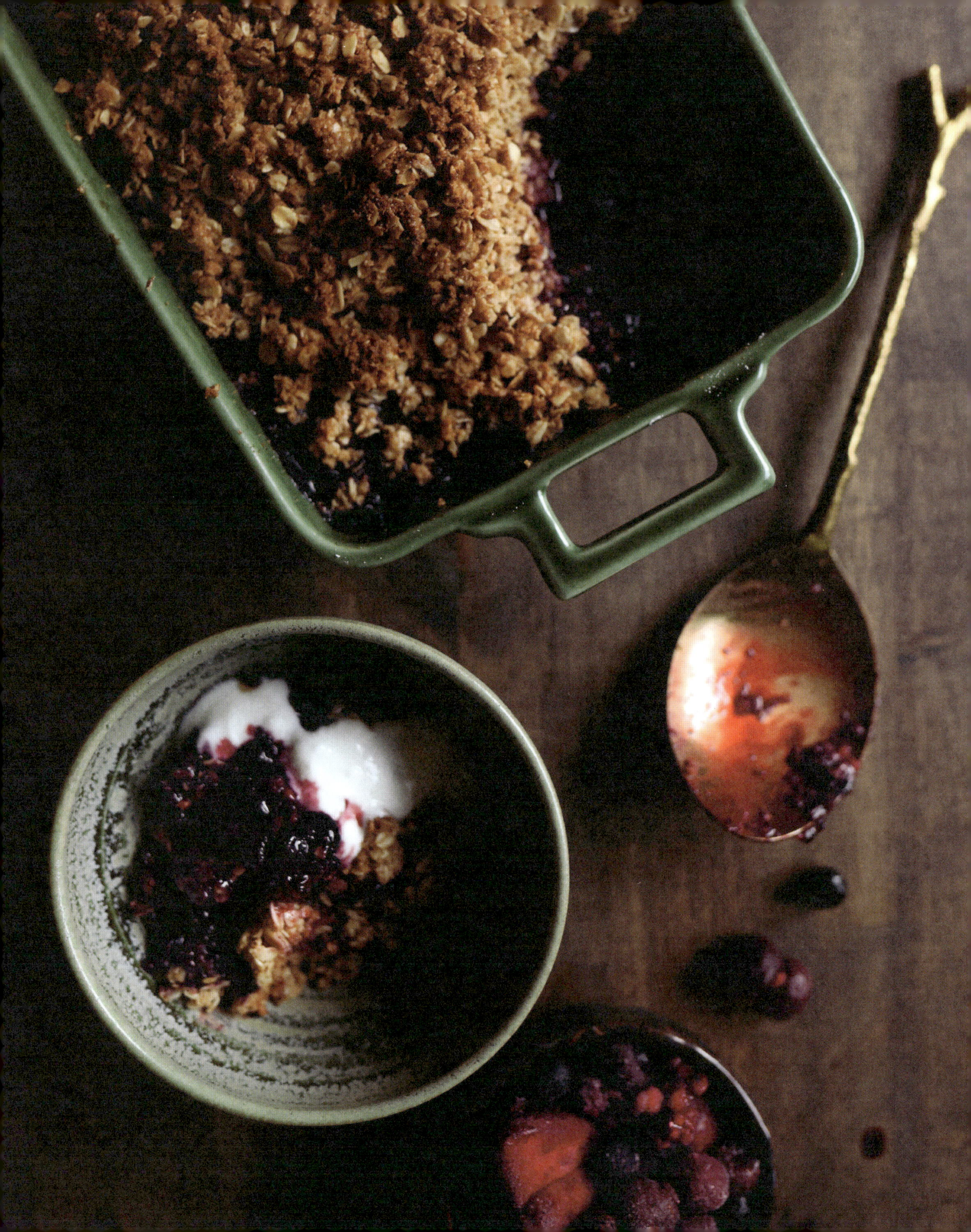

BERRY CRUMBLE

A dessert made completely out of pantry staples ? Talk dirty to me. Really, though, if you count frozen berries as a staple (which I absolutely do), you can whip this up anytime. Healthy ? Perhaps. Definitely full of antioxidants, fiber, and flavor.

SERVES 6

***Prep:** 15 minutes*
***Cook:** 1 hour*

Gluten Free
Ovulation Phase
Menstrual Phase

½ cup (113 g) butter, at room temperature
1 cup (80 g) rolled oats
1 cup (80 g) quick oats
¾ cup (75 g) almond flour
½ cup (110 g) plus ¼ cup (55 g) brown sugar or coconut sugar, divided
1 teaspoon ground cinnamon
1 teaspoon ground ginger, divided
6 cups (900 g) frozen berries
¼ cup (30 g) cornstarch
Zest of 1 orange (about 2 tablespoons)
Zest of 1 lemon (about 1 tablespoon)
Whipped cream, coconut cream, or yogurt, mixed with honey and vanilla extract to taste, for serving (optional)

1. Preheat the oven to 350°F (175°C).
2. Combine the butter, rolled and quick oats, almond flour, ½ cup (110 g) brown sugar, the cinnamon, and ½ teaspoon ginger in a medium bowl. Mix well with your hands, rubbing the ingredients together until everything is incorporated and clumps together easily. Set aside.
3. Pile the berries into a 9-inch (23 cm) square baking dish. If it looks like a lot, don't worry—they will reduce a ton once cooked.
4. Sprinkle thoroughly with the remaining ¼ cup (55 g) brown sugar, ½ teaspoon ginger, the cornstarch, orange zest, and lemon zest. Rifle the mixture around as best you can to spread the ingredients throughout (you can do this in a separate bowl, but I just prefer to save the mess).
5. Evenly distribute the crumble on top of the berry mixture, leaving the crumble in little chunks so it can crisp up.
6. Bake for 1 hour, or until cooked through, bubbling, and deeply browned on top.
7. Serve with whipped cream, coconut cream, or yogurt mixed with a little honey and a dash of vanilla, if desired.

WATERMELON MINT SORBET

SERVES 4 TO 6

Prep: 5 minutes

Dairy Free
Gluten Free
Menstrual Phase

This is one of the most refreshing things I have ever consumed. Watermelon is mostly water, as we know, but it does contain a nice little serving of minerals, and with the addition of lime juice and sea salt, it becomes a little electrolyte slushie. This recipe is the perfect way to avoid wasting the other half of a giant watermelon in the summertime! Adding fresh ginger provides an extra zing that I absolutely love.

Small handful of mint leaves, plus more for serving
4 cups (600 g) frozen watermelon chunks (see Note 1)
Juice of 2 limes, or more if needed
2 tablespoons honey
¼ teaspoon sea salt
1 teaspoon grated fresh ginger (optional)
¼ cup (60 ml) water (optional)
Flaky salt, for serving (optional)

1. Place the mint leaves in a blender (putting them in first ensures they blend well), followed by the watermelon, lime juice, honey, salt, and ginger, if using.
2. Blend until smooth, 2 to 3 minutes, scraping down the sides regularly.
3. Add extra lime juice if more liquid is needed. If you prefer not to add extra sourness, a little water will do, but only add a tiny bit at a time, just barely enough to get it blended (see Note 2).
4. Garnish with a mint leaf and flaky salt if you please, and serve immediately.

NOTES

1. To freeze watermelon, remove the rind and cut into 1- to 2-inch (2.5 to 5 cm) chunks. Place in a freezer-safe ziplock or reusable silicone bag and freeze for at least 12 hours.

2. A powerful blender should be able to blend this into a thick, smooth texture with very little liquid, but otherwise you'll need a little water to encourage it to blend! Just go slowly, a tablespoon or so at a time.

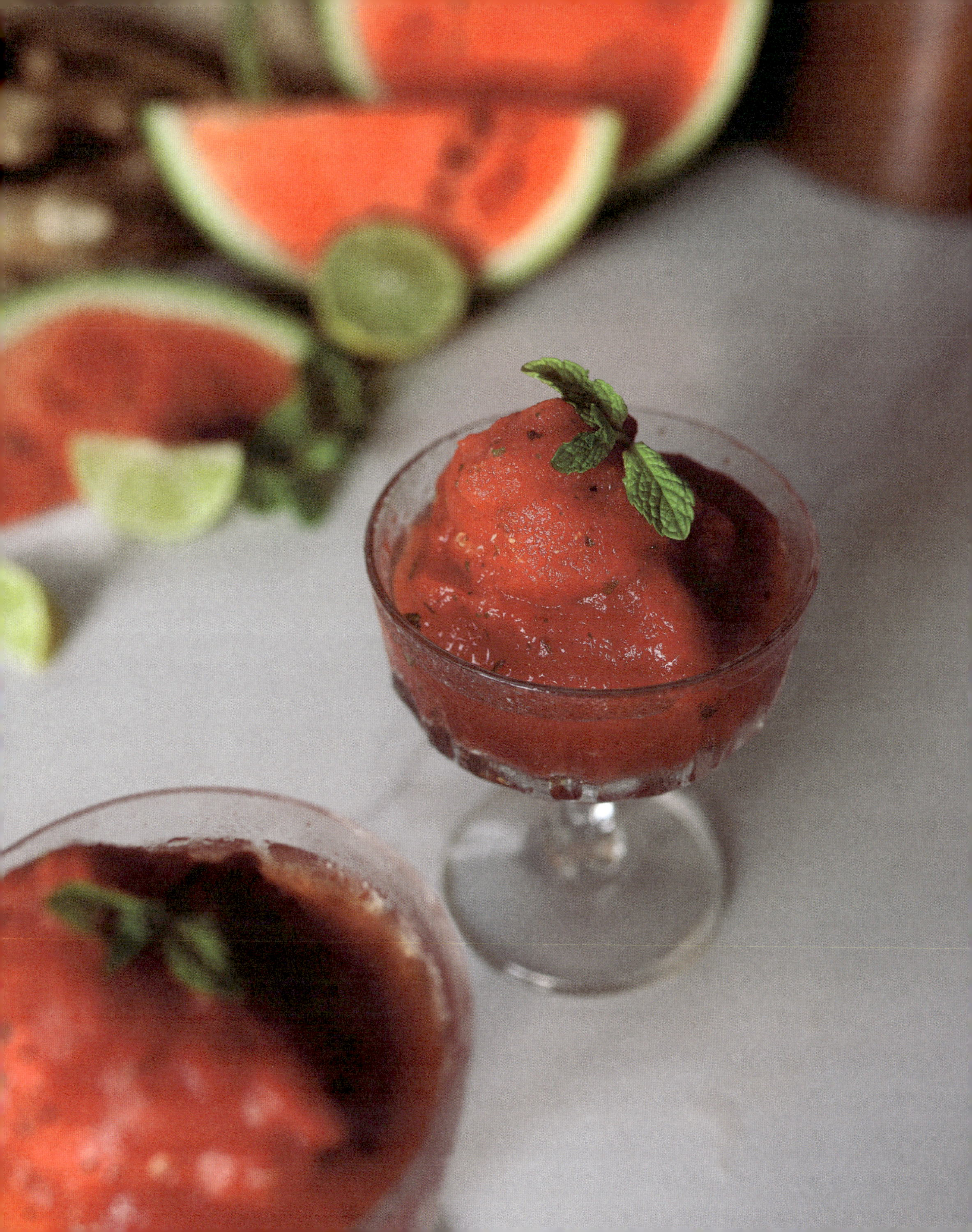

SEED CYCLING

One of the simplest ways you can leverage nutrition to support your hormones is through seed cycling. This is, quite literally, eating different seeds at different phases of your cycle, with each seed offering targeted benefits for your hormonal needs. It sounds laughably simple, but seed cycling has been studied for women with PCOS, and it shows significant positive results that support hormone balance for all women. Here's how it works.

Menstrual and Follicular Phases

PUMPKIN SEEDS AND GROUND FLAXSEEDS

1 to 2 tablespoons of each daily

These seeds primarily support estrogen balance. The large amounts of lignans (phytoestrogens that help balance estrogen) in pumpkin seeds and especially in flaxseeds help prevent excess estrogen as levels rise. Pumpkin seeds offer zinc to support testosterone and rising progesterone for the next phase. They're also a source of tryptophan, which supports sleep (many women note better sleep quality within a couple of weeks of seed cycling).

Be sure to buy raw (unroasted) seeds, as they will have the most nutritional benefit, and buy organic if possible. If buying in bulk, store in an airtight jar or in the freezer if it will take you a very long time to use them!

Ovulation and Luteal Phases

SUNFLOWER SEEDS AND GROUND SESAME SEEDS

1 to 2 tablespoons of each daily

These seeds primarily support progesterone production, a priority in this phase, as both seeds contain large amounts of vitamin E and zinc. The small amount of lignans in sesame seeds continues to offer estrogen-balancing support. Sesame seeds also help lower inflammation and support cholesterol metabolism, which are directly linked to hormone health.

These seeds can be added to smoothies, dressings, and baked goods, as you will see throughout the recipes in this book, notably the Herbaceous Green Dressing (page 210), Cycle Syncing Buckwheat Granola (page 233), Seed Cycling Bliss Balls (page 237), and Power Muffins (page 234). For optimal metabolism, the smaller seeds—flaxseeds and sesame—should be ground (you could also grind the pumpkin and sunflower seeds, but it isn't as essential).

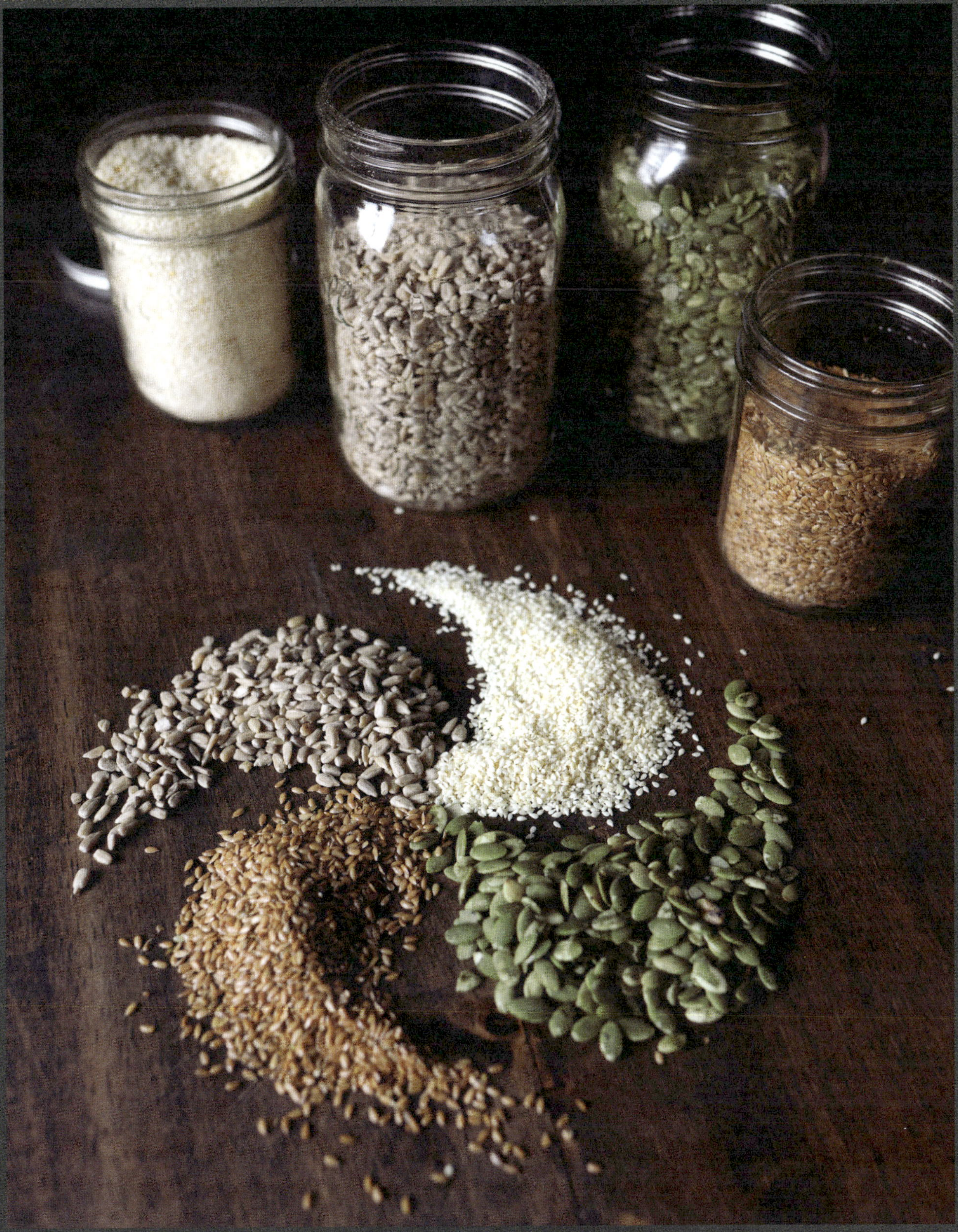

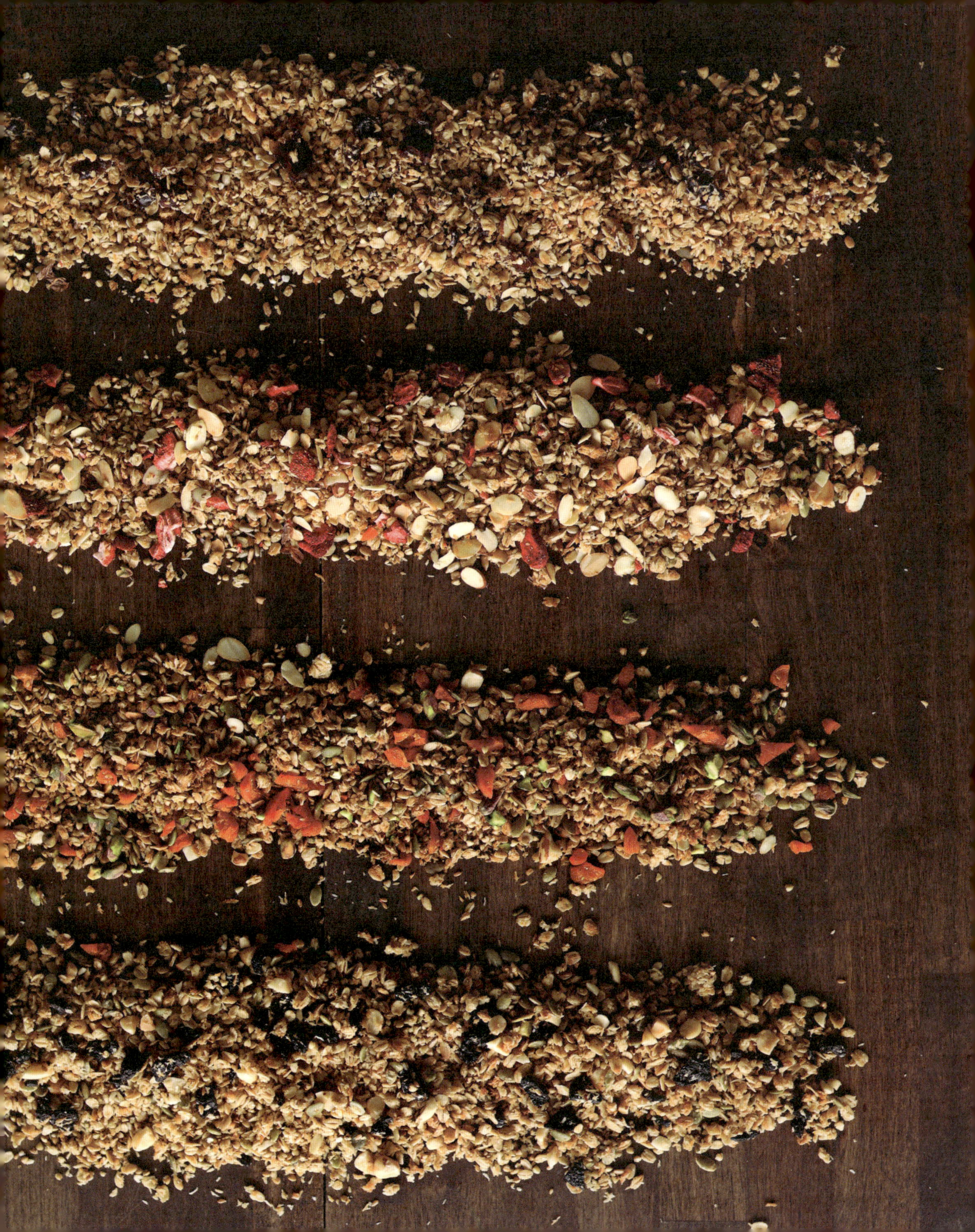

CYCLE SYNCING BUCKWHEAT GRANOLA

MAKES 8 CUPS (780 G)

***Prep:* 10 minutes**
***Cook:* 30 minutes**

Dairy Free
Gluten Free

Homemade granola is so easy to make and so much better than anything you can buy! Once you learn the basics, you can switch it up so easily, making this a great recipe for cycle syncing and seed cycling. You can add whatever nuts and seeds you like into the mix, so I've left that up to you. But if you want to eat with your menstrual cycle, I've provided some specific options below that are particularly supportive for each phase.

½ cup (120 ml) coconut oil
⅓ cup (80 ml) maple syrup
3 tablespoons water
1 tablespoon orange zest
1 teaspoon vanilla extract
Pinch of sea salt
2 tablespoons brown sugar (optional)
2 cups (160 g) rolled oats
1 cup (165 g) buckwheat groats
1 cup (85 g) coconut chips
½ cup (about 65 g) raw cashews, roughly chopped
½ cup (about 65 g) other raw nuts of choice (see phase recipes)
1 cup (160 g) raisins or other dried fruit of choice (see phase recipes)
1 cup (about 130 g) seeds of choice (see phase recipes)

MENSTRUAL PHASE

½ cup (70 g) chopped Brazil nuts
1 cup (70 g) dried cherries
½ cup (75 g) pumpkin seeds
½ cup (85 g) flaxseeds

FOLLICULAR PHASE

½ cup (65 g) shelled pistachios
1 cup (95 g) chopped apricots
½ cup (75 g) pumpkin seeds
½ cup (85 g) flaxseeds

OVULATION PHASE

½ cup (75 g) almonds, roughly chopped
1 cup (40 g) freeze-dried raspberries
½ cup (65 g) sesame seeds
½ cup (65 g) sunflower seeds

LUTEAL PHASE

1 cup (120 g) chopped walnuts
1 cup (85 g) chopped dates
½ cup (65 g) sesame seeds
½ cup (65 g) sunflower seeds

1. Preheat the oven to 325°F (160°C).
2. Place the coconut oil, maple syrup, water, orange zest, vanilla, salt, and brown sugar (if using) in a small pot and gently melt together over medium-low heat, 3 to 4 minutes.
3. Combine the oats, buckwheat, coconut chips, cashews, and nuts of choice in a large bowl.
4. Whisk the liquid mixture in the pot and immediately pour over the dry mixture, stirring to coat completely. Transfer the granola to a large baking sheet, spreading it into an even layer.
5. Bake for 20 minutes, or until golden at the edges, then rotate the pan 180° and bake for 7 to 10 more minutes, until darker brown around the edges (see Tip).
6. Remove from the oven and sprinkle the dried fruit and seeds of choice over the top. Let cool.
7. Stir the granola, breaking up any chunks if necessary, and then store in an airtight container at room temperature for up to 1 month.

TIP

If you prefer chunky granola, don't stir your mixture during baking or right after. Instead, break it up once it has cooled. If you prefer loose granola, remove the pan from the oven a couple of times while baking to stir the mixture.

POWER MUFFINS

MAKES 20 MUFFINS

***Prep:* 15 minutes**
***Cook:* 20 minutes**

Dairy Free
Follicular Phase
Menstrual Phase

These are called Power Muffins because they will charge you up—they're not your coffee shop chocolate chip muffins (which are essentially icing-less cupcakes). These muffins are designed to fuel you quickly and efficiently while also tasting divine. They're great for kids and good for freezer prep; I love to defrost them under the broiler so they get a li'l toasty and then slather one in a good blob of grass-fed butter.

½ cup (120 ml) coconut oil
⅓ cup (80 ml) maple syrup
¼ teaspoon sea salt
1 cup (120 g) all-purpose flour
1 cup (90 g) oat flour (see Note)
½ cup (110 g) packed light brown sugar or coconut sugar
¼ cup (25 g) flaxseed meal
1 teaspoon baking powder
1 teaspoon baking soda
1 teaspoon ground cinnamon
½ teaspoon ground ginger
¼ teaspoon ground nutmeg
2 large eggs
½ cup (120 ml) coconut milk
⅓ cup (80 ml) water
2 cups (220 g) shredded carrots
1 cup (90 g) shredded coconut
½ cup (80 g) raisins or other dried fruit
½ cup (60 g) chopped walnuts or other nuts
⅓ cup (45 g) pumpkin seeds (or flax, sesame, or sunflower seeds; see page 230)
Butter, for serving, optional

1. Preheat the oven to 350°F (175°C). Line two muffin pans with liners.
2. Heat the coconut oil, maple syrup, and salt in a small saucepan over low heat until the oil liquefies, about 5 minutes.
3. Meanwhile, combine the all-purpose flour, oat flour, light brown sugar, flaxseed meal, baking powder, baking soda, cinnamon, ginger, and nutmeg in a large bowl.
4. Make a well in the center of the dry ingredients. Add the eggs, coconut milk, water, and the melted oil and maple syrup. Stir until just combined; don't overmix. Fold in the carrots, coconut, raisins, and walnuts.
5. Fill each liner about three-quarters of the way with batter (use about ¼ cup/50 g in each). Sprinkle with the pumpkin seeds.
6. Bake for 20 minutes, or until a toothpick comes out clean but not dry.
7. Try a muffin hot and fresh with butter, if desired, and freeze any extras in an airtight container for up to 1 month.

NOTE

I just throw oats, any type, in a blender to make oat flour at home.

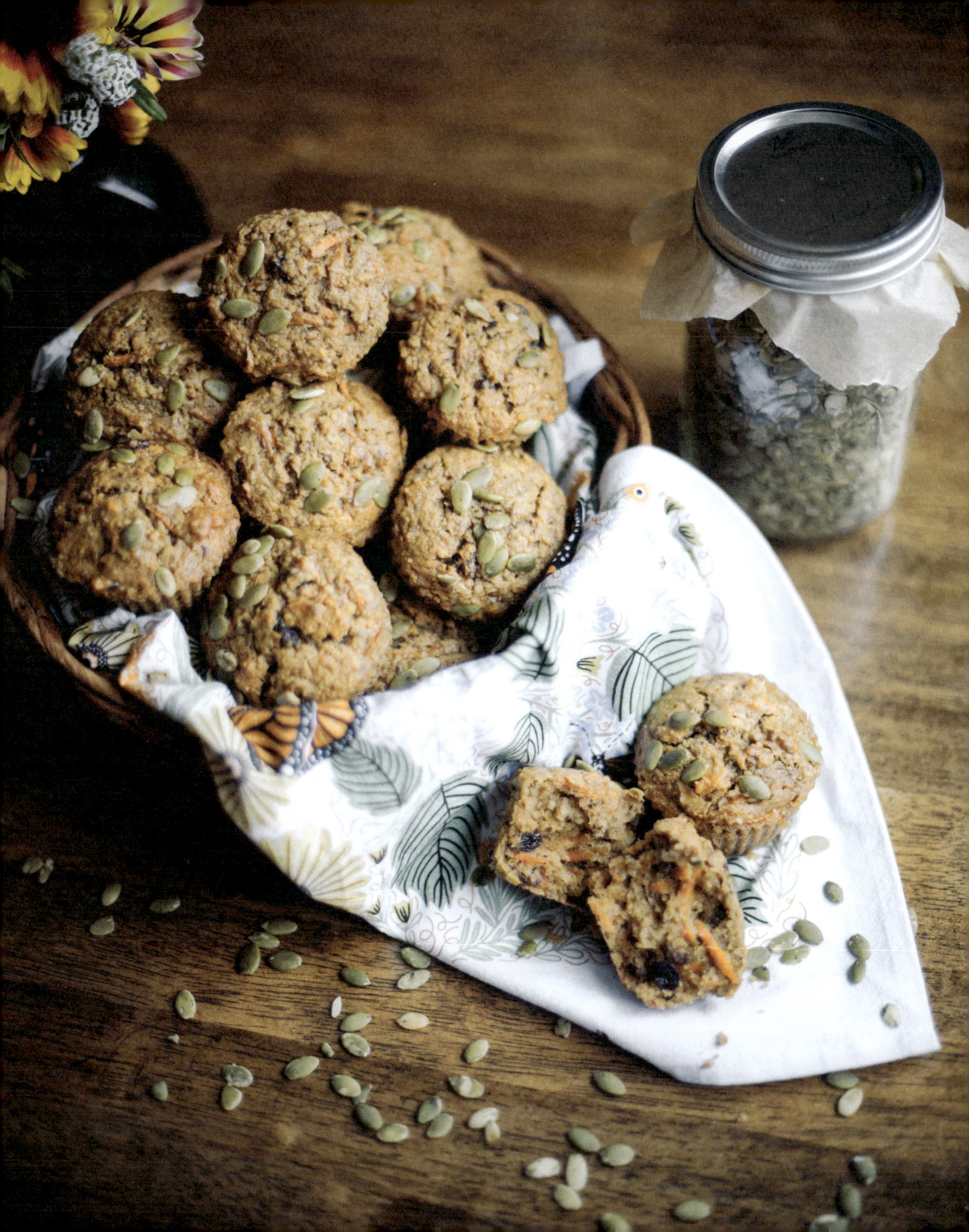

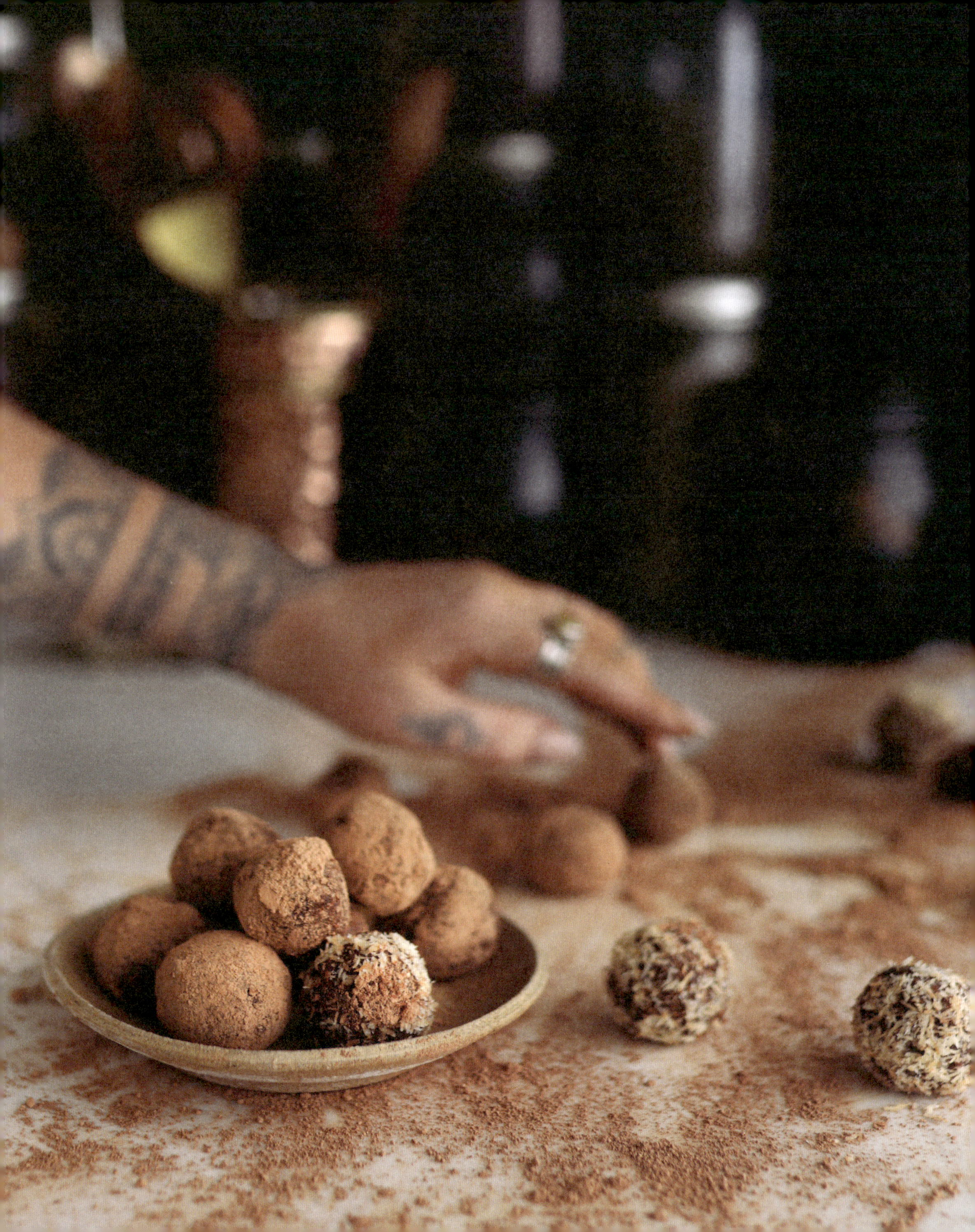

SEED CYCLING BLISS BALLS

MAKES ABOUT 16 BALLS

Prep: 35 minutes

All Phases
Dairy Free
Gluten Free

This is a food prep secret weapon: yummy little bites that pack a whole ton of goodness but are still super delicious. If you are seed cycling for your hormones, this is a great way to make sure you get that daily dose of blended seeds. Just switch them up depending on the phase of your cycle and you're good to go. These bliss balls tend to be a pretty big hit with toddlers, too, which is always a plus.

1 cup (130 g) cashews
¼ cup (35 g) sunflower seeds or (28 g) ground flaxseeds
¼ cup (40 g) sesame seeds or pumpkin seeds
10 Medjool dates, pitted, plus more as needed
⅓ cup (30 g) rolled oats, plus more as needed
3 tablespoons cocoa powder
Pinch of sea salt

FOR COATING (OPTIONAL)

Unsweetened shredded coconut, as needed
Cocoa powder, as needed
Chopped nuts or seeds, as needed

1. Soak the cashews, sunflower seeds (if using flaxseeds, leave them out), and sesame seeds or pumpkin seeds in hot water for 30 minutes. Drain and set aside.
2. If your dates are dry and not soft and sticky, soak them in hot water also, for about 5 minutes or until softened, then drain.
3. Transfer the soaked cashews and seeds to a food processor and pulse briefly, then scrape down the sides and add the dates, oats, cocoa, and salt. Blend until smooth, scraping down the sides as necessary. The mixture should be soft and a little sticky, but easily moldable. If it's too sticky and mushy, add more oats and blend again. If it's too dry, add a few more soaked dates and blend again.
4. *If you like, coat the bliss balls:* Sprinkle your coating of choice on a small plate.
5. Use a tablespoon to scoop out portions of the mixture, then gently roll each portion into a ball between your palms. Roll in the coating of your choice.
6. Store in the fridge for up to 1 month.

COCONUT "CARAMEL" COOKIES

MAKES 12 COOKIES

Prep: 20 minutes
Cook: 25 minutes
Rest: 30 minutes

Blood Sugar Balancing

Dairy Free

Gluten Free

Ovulation Phase

I used to love Samoas, the classic Girl Scout cookie, but when I steered away from sugar I was inspired to figure out a simple, whole-food, unprocessed version for myself. It took a lot of trial and error to get there, but folks... I think we did it. In fact, now I don't even enjoy the "real" thing; these are so much better! I leaned on the magic of dates—although they are super sweet, they have a balancing effect on blood sugar due to their high fiber content. They feed good gut bacteria and fight inflammation, too!

10 Medjool dates, pitted
1½ cups (135 g) unsweetened shredded coconut
¼ cup plus 1 tablespoon (75 ml) coconut oil, divided
1 teaspoon vanilla extract
1¾ cups (190 g) extra-fine-ground almond flour
Pinch of sea salt
9 ounces (255 g) dark chocolate chips

1. Preheat the oven to 325°F (160°C). Line a baking sheet with parchment paper.
2. Soak the dates in a bowl of hot water for about 10 minutes to get them really soft. Pour out the water and place them in the fridge to cool.
3. Evenly spread the coconut on the baking sheet and toast in the oven for about 5 minutes. Remove from the oven, stir and re-spread with a spatula, and then bake for another 5 minutes, or until completely golden. (Keep an eye out; the coconut can burn super fast!)
4. Place the dates in a food processor and blend on high until mostly chopped, 20 to 30 seconds. Add ¼ cup (60 ml) coconut oil and the vanilla extract and blend until smooth, about 1 minute.
5. Scoop the date-and-coconut-oil mixture into a large bowl and then add the toasted coconut, almond flour, and salt. Stir until combined—the dough should be sticky enough to hold its shape.
6. On the lined baking sheet, form the dough into twelve rounds and use your finger or a chopstick to make holes in the centers, smushing them back together if they crack.
7. Bake for 20 to 25 minutes, until slightly crisped on the outside but still soft on the inside.
8. Melt the chocolate chips by bringing about 2 inches (5 cm) of water to a boil in a medium, heavy-bottomed pot. Place the chips and 1 tablespoon coconut oil in a glass or metal bowl that is big enough to rest on the rim of the pot without the bottom of the bowl touching the water. Place the bowl on top of the pot and allow the chips and coconut oil to melt most of the way. Quickly stir to combine and then remove from the heat.
9. Stab one cookie at a time with a fork, dunk its little bottom into the chocolate, and then place chocolate side up on a cooling rack. Once all the cookies have been dunked and the chocolate is ever so slightly hardening, flip the cookies and use a fork or spoon to drizzle chocolate across the tops.
10. Refrigerate or freeze the cookies until the chocolate hardens completely, about 30 minutes in the fridge or 15 minutes in the freezer. Enjoy.
11. If you have any left, store them in an airtight container in the refrigerator for up to 1 week.

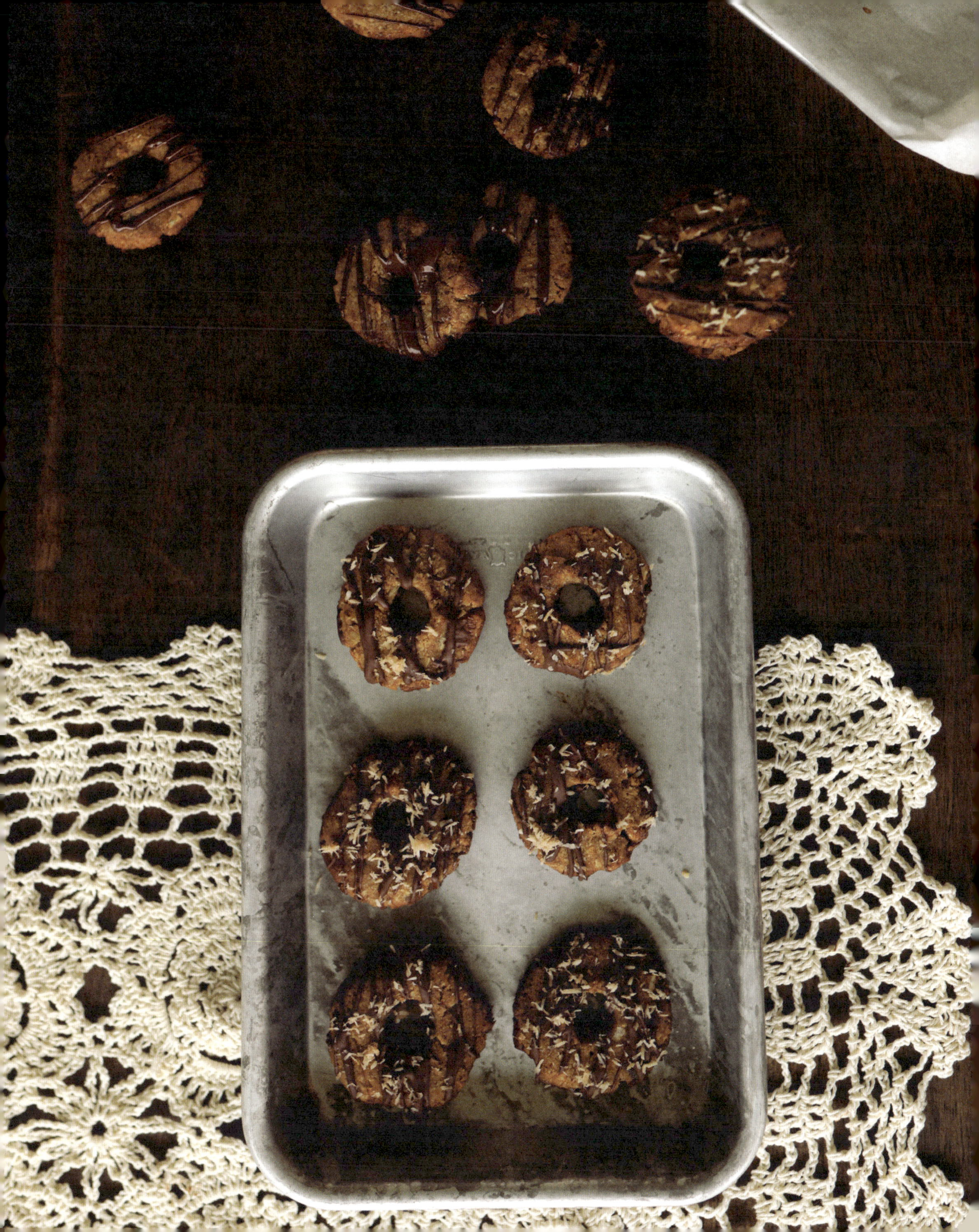

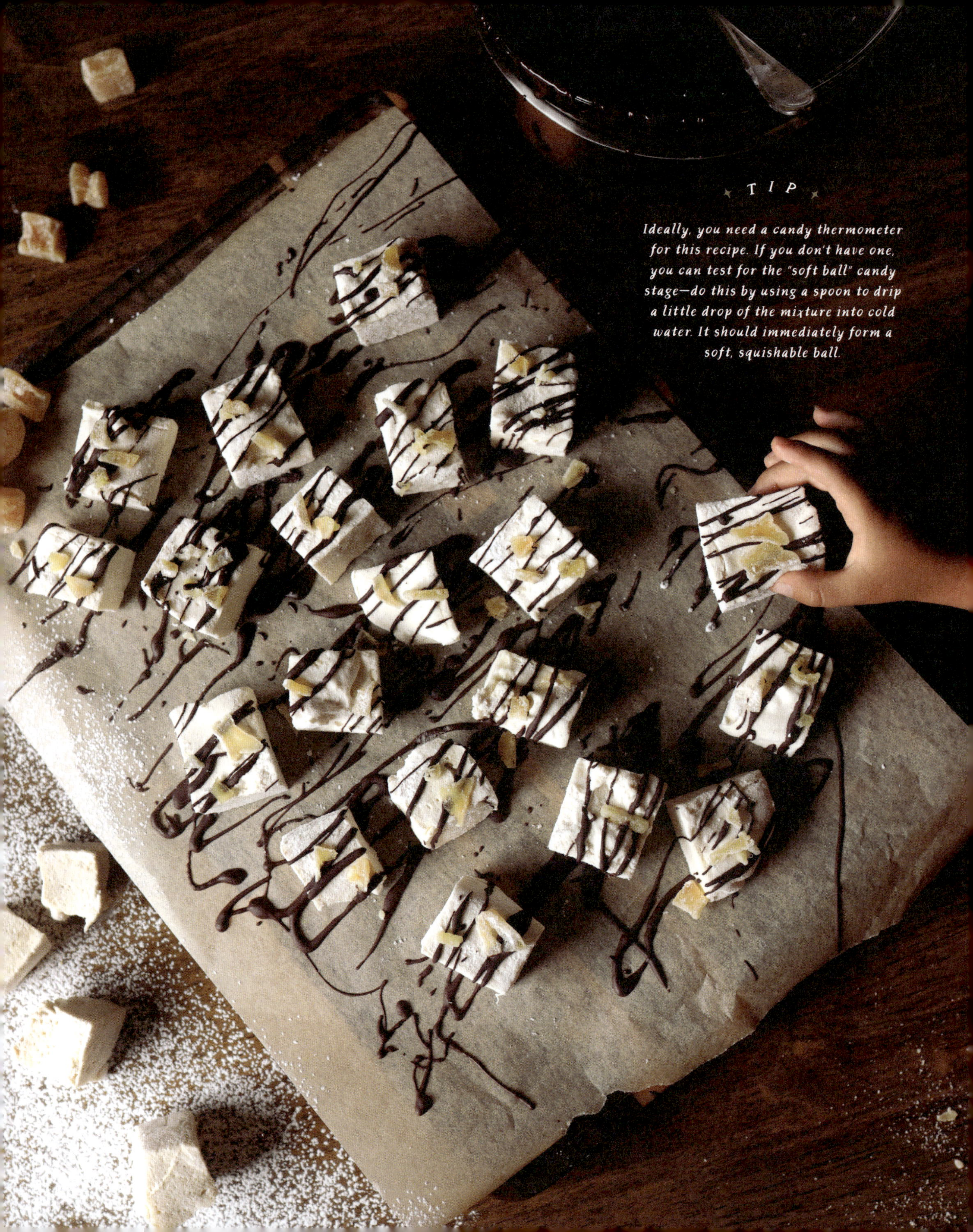

TIP

Ideally, you need a candy thermometer for this recipe. If you don't have one, you can test for the "soft ball" candy stage—do this by using a spoon to drip a little drop of the mixture into cold water. It should immediately form a soft, squishable ball.

MEDICINAL MARSHMALLOWS

MAKES 20 MARSHMALLOWS

Prep: 25 minutes
Rest: 11 hours
Cook: 20 minutes

Dairy Free
Gluten Free
Luteal Phase
Ovulation Phase

Marshmallow root is super beneficial for the body's mucus membranes due to its mucilaginous nature. This makes it soothing for the throat, protective for the gut, and calming for inflammation. Combining it with beef gelatin and ginger for more gut-and-throat-soothing benefits makes this recipe a pretty Mary Poppins–esque way to take your medicine.

2 cups (480 ml) water
1 inch (2.5 cm) fresh ginger, grated
¼ cup (15 g) shredded or chopped dried marshmallow root
2 tablespoons plus 1 teaspoon grass-fed beef gelatin
1 cup (240 ml) maple syrup
Pinch of sea salt
¾ cup (48 g) arrowroot powder, divided
¼ cup (40 g) crystallized ginger, finely chopped, for garnish (optional)
Melted chocolate (see step 8 on page 238), for drizzling

1. The night before marshmallow making, combine the water and fresh ginger in a small pot over medium heat. Bring to a gentle boil and then cover, reduce the heat to low, and simmer for at least 10 minutes. Remove from the heat and let cool.
2. Pour the infusion into a medium jar and add the marshmallow root. Put the lid on and give it a little shake to combine. Let rest for at least 8 hours or overnight, until the liquid becomes thick and slimy.
3. When you're ready to make the marshmallows, strain the infusion to remove the chunks of ginger and marshmallow root.
4. Place the gelatin in a large bowl or the bowl of a stand mixer with ½ cup (120 ml) of the marshmallow infusion. Stir and then let rest for the gelatin to "bloom," meaning it has soaked up some liquid and become a slightly granular, wobbly mass, 5 to 10 minutes.
5. Meanwhile, add another ½ cup (120 ml) of the infusion to a medium pot along with the maple syrup and salt. (If you have a little leftover infusion, you can save it to drink.) Stir well, and then don't stir again.
6. Bring to a boil and cook on medium-high heat, 10 to 14 minutes. It will get super frothy and bubble up a few times during boiling. Once the temperature reaches 230 to 240°F (110 to 116°C) or is at the "soft ball" candy stage (see Tip), remove from the heat.
7. Immediately and slowly pour the hot candy mixture into the bowl with the gelatin, mixing constantly on medium-high speed (I don't recommend attempting this by hand, but you can use a handheld mixer).
8. Mix continuously for a long time—7 to 10 minutes—until the mixture becomes frothy and white and holds soft peaks, like whipped cream or marshmallow fluff.
9. Line a 9-inch (23 cm) square baking dish with parchment paper and use a sieve to coat the pan with ¼ cup (16 g) of the arrowroot powder.
10. Scoop all the marshmallow mixture into the pan and use a spatula to spread it out evenly. Sprinkle the top with the crystallized ginger (if using) and leave the marshmallows on the counter to harden, 2 to 3 hours.
11. Use the parchment paper to lift the marshmallows from the pan and slice them into roughly 2-inch (5 cm) squares with a warm, sharp knife.
12. Add the remaining arrowroot powder to a plate and dip each cut side of the marshmallows in it to prevent them from sticking to each other.
13. Drizzle with melted chocolate. Store in an airtight container at room temperature for up to 1 week.

CHAPTER TEN

POTIONS & BEVVIES

THIS CHAPTER IS THE BRIDGE BETWEEN FOOD AND MEDICINE.

For the home healer, the kitchen is so much more than a fridge and an oven—it's the center for countertop consultations, the apothecary, the alchemist's studio. I am deeply thankful for modern medicine—it is absolutely necessary in so many instances—but it is so empowering to have the tools to heal yourself and your loved ones when need be. Rather than leaning on over-the-counter drugs at the first sign of illness, we can turn to the plant world, which has supported our wellness for thousands of years and has so much to offer! And in uncertain times, when many folks don't have consistent medical access, knowledge really is power. As a girlie raised in England, it's been ingrained in me since birth that there is almost nothing a good cuppa tea can't fix. As I've progressed along my herbal learning journey, I've come to see just how true that really is. I am a bevvy babe, a libation lass. If you come to my house, beware. I will likely ask how you're feeling, dive into my herb hutch, brew up something mildly weird, and shove a series of tincture droppers at you.

In this chapter, you will find all my favorite liquid concoctions, plus a few more remedies: the everyday beverages, like Adrenal Cocktails (page 244) for stress support, and the specialty refreshments like the sunny Saffron Cordial (page 253) that will lift your mood. There's a deep dive into teas, of course, because there is so much to unpack there, along with a resource list you can use to choose your brew. Then we move into true medicines—from traditional, hardworking kitchen remedies in the Allium Alchemy section (page 272) to a crash course on making your own tinctures (page 262).

It is worth noting that, with most natural remedies, the key is consistency. Eating one garlic clove or brewing one cup of tea is not going to fix you. These remedies are most effective when applied at the onset of symptoms and continued regularly, multiple times a day, until you are completely clear. Many of them will not mask symptoms in the same way an over-the-counter drug will, but will instead work with your body to address the underlying causes, while also providing symptom relief. There is a depth and wealth of wisdom that can be used to craft a cure that is tailored to each individual, taking into account their unique attributes and the complexity of each herb. However, the remedies laid out here are simple, safe, and a great starting point for anyone.

Note: If in doubt, always do your own research, check for contraindications for your particular situation, and consult a professional when needed.

ADRENAL COCKTAILS

If you haven't yet heard of the adrenal cocktail, let me introduce you to some true kitchen magic. The concept is simple, but the effects are powerful. An adrenal cocktail is basically like a homemade electrolyte drink with no added junk, specifically targeted to support physical and mental stress. It does this by supplying the specific nutrients your adrenal glands need to help balance cortisol production in a readily bioavailable, quickly metabolized form.

THE KEY MAGICAL COMPONENTS ARE:

375 mg potassium
460 mg sodium
60 mg whole-food vitamin C

Here's how it works: When you are under stress—physical stress from sleepless nights, long workdays, or poor nutrition, or mental stress from colicky babies, work calls, or constant worry—your body perceives a threat. This sends you into fight-or-flight mode, and your adrenal glands (your stress regulation centers) start releasing the hormones adrenaline and cortisol. Those hormones use up tons of vitamin C, which quickly gets depleted when you are consistently stressed. That isn't the only thing that gets depleted, though: Minerals like potassium and sodium are often particularly lacking in depleted and stressed-out bodies. This stresses your body even more, as it searches for the fuel it needs to perform necessary functions. And when it doesn't have what it needs, the body shuts down lots of "unnecessary" functioning and switches on its "battery saver" mode. This can affect everything from digestion to sleep, and it inevitably has a negative effect on your hormone function, as your endocrine system gets imbalanced trying to overcompensate for the lacking nutrients and the overworked adrenals.

In chronically stressed folks (which many of us are), this creates a vicious cycle that leaves our adrenal glands constantly overworked, our cortisol so overused that we have none left when we need it (like to wake up in the morning), and our body in a constant mineral deficit. When you supply your stressed body with these essential nutrients, it signals that you are safe and have what you need to function, and it can begin to return to a "rest-and-digest" mode, with your parasympathetic nervous system in charge. This is a healthy, relaxed body that can digest food well and sleep well, doesn't have brain fog, and has healthy hormone function.

Can you get all these nutrients from food? Yes, ideally. But many of us are busy, so it's normal to have some gaps. Plus, the fact that this drink contains very little fiber means all those nutrients get into your system far faster than if you had to digest food to extract them. This helps tired, poorly functioning systems get a quick and easy lift.

Anyone can drink an adrenal cocktail. In times of major stress and adrenal fatigue, drink one in the morning and one in the afternoon, between meals. When you need a little support, have one whenever you think of it, always on an empty stomach.

When you first begin drinking them, if you are chronically stressed, your body may react to getting what it needs by entering deep rest, making you feel sleepy and low in energy. But if you stick with it, you will quickly see a change. For most, however, there is an almost immediate difference. Adrenal cocktails can become a pick-me-up that replaces your afternoon coffee and prevents that midday slump.

Once you get the hang of it, you can mix and match your ingredients, add things, use different juices—just make sure you are hitting the milligram amounts listed on page 244 (and that you don't exceed 375 mg of potassium).

And don't be concerned about the sugars in the orange juice. It's such a small amount, and those carbs do a job, too: They provide a nice little hit of energy and help to fuel your nervous system. If you are diabetic, check out my Hibiscus Adrenal Cocktail (page 246) for a sugar-free alternative.

If you want more sustained energy, you can add a fat like coconut cream (2 to 3 tablespoons) and/or protein in the form of collagen powder (1 to 3 tablespoons). Both will help to slow the release of sugars into your system. The fats give you another energy source, and the amino acids in collagen help your body more effectively metabolize the vitamins and minerals in the drink. This is because amino acids are the building blocks for the hormones and enzymes that facilitate nutrient absorption and cellular communication.

The adrenal cocktail is truly magical. Turn the page for a few of my favorite variations. It's best to drink them at room temperature so they can assimilate into your system more quickly, but you can chill them if you like.

A note on ingredients

ORANGE JUICE

Fresh-squeezed is ideal (and also usually the cheapest), but in a pinch you can use bottled juice. Just use the best-quality juice you can find, ideally in glass bottles and with pulp.

SEA SALT

This should be good-quality, raw salt from the ocean (not iodized or kosher salt). Some good brands are Eden, Redmond, and Celtic—or if you feel ambitious, you can harvest your own!

CREAM OF TARTAR

This is easily found in the spice section of most stores, but quality does matter. I like Frontier Co-op brand!

COCONUT WATER

Be sure to get a brand without added sugar (you would be surprised at how many are not actually pure coconut water!).

EACH RECIPE SERVES 1

Prep: 5 minutes

Classic Adrenal Cocktail

This is the cheapest and simplest version. It contains fresh-squeezed OJ for whole-food vitamin C, sea salt for trace minerals, and cream of tartar for potassium.

Juice of 2 large oranges (about ½ cup/120 ml)
¼ teaspoon sea salt
¼ teaspoon cream of tartar

1. Add the ingredients to a tall glass and stir to combine. Drink as is or top with water to dilute to taste.

Coconut Water Adrenal Cocktail

This is the most popular version. The coconut water makes it sweeter and lends additional minerals and potassium, so there's no need for cream of tartar.

Juice of 2 large oranges (about ½ cup/120 ml)
¼ teaspoon sea salt
1 cup (240 ml) pure coconut water

1. Add the ingredients to a tall glass and stir to combine. Drink as is or top with water to dilute to taste.

Hibiscus Adrenal Cocktail

This is a sugar-free version for those who have to watch their blood sugar. Hibiscus contains less vitamin C and potassium than orange juice, so we use a full 12 ounces (360 ml) of tea and add cream of tartar to make up for it.

1½ cups (360 ml) strong hibiscus tea
¼ heaping teaspoon cream of tartar
¼ teaspoon sea salt

1. Add the ingredients to a tall glass and stir to combine. Drink as is or top with water to dilute to taste.

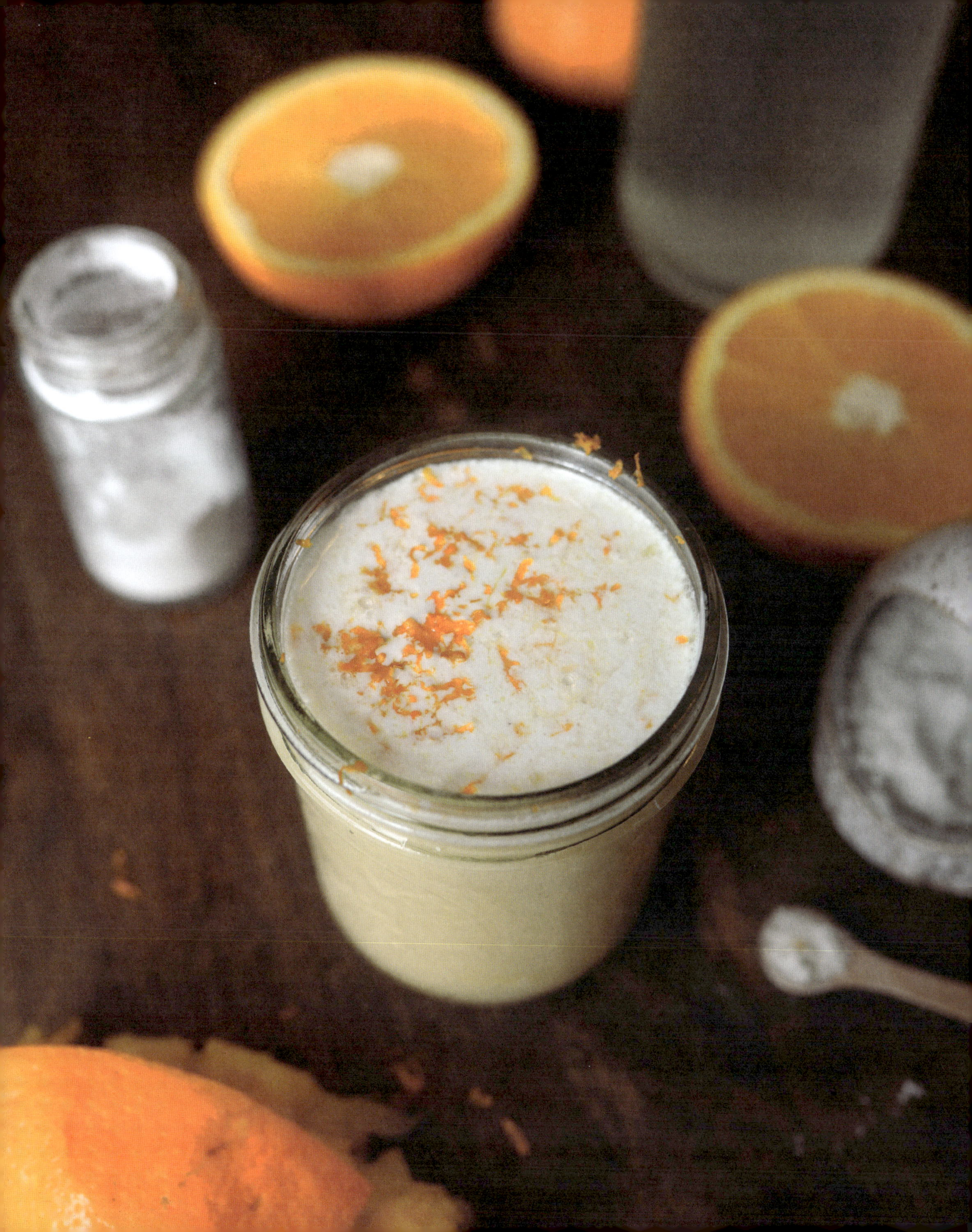

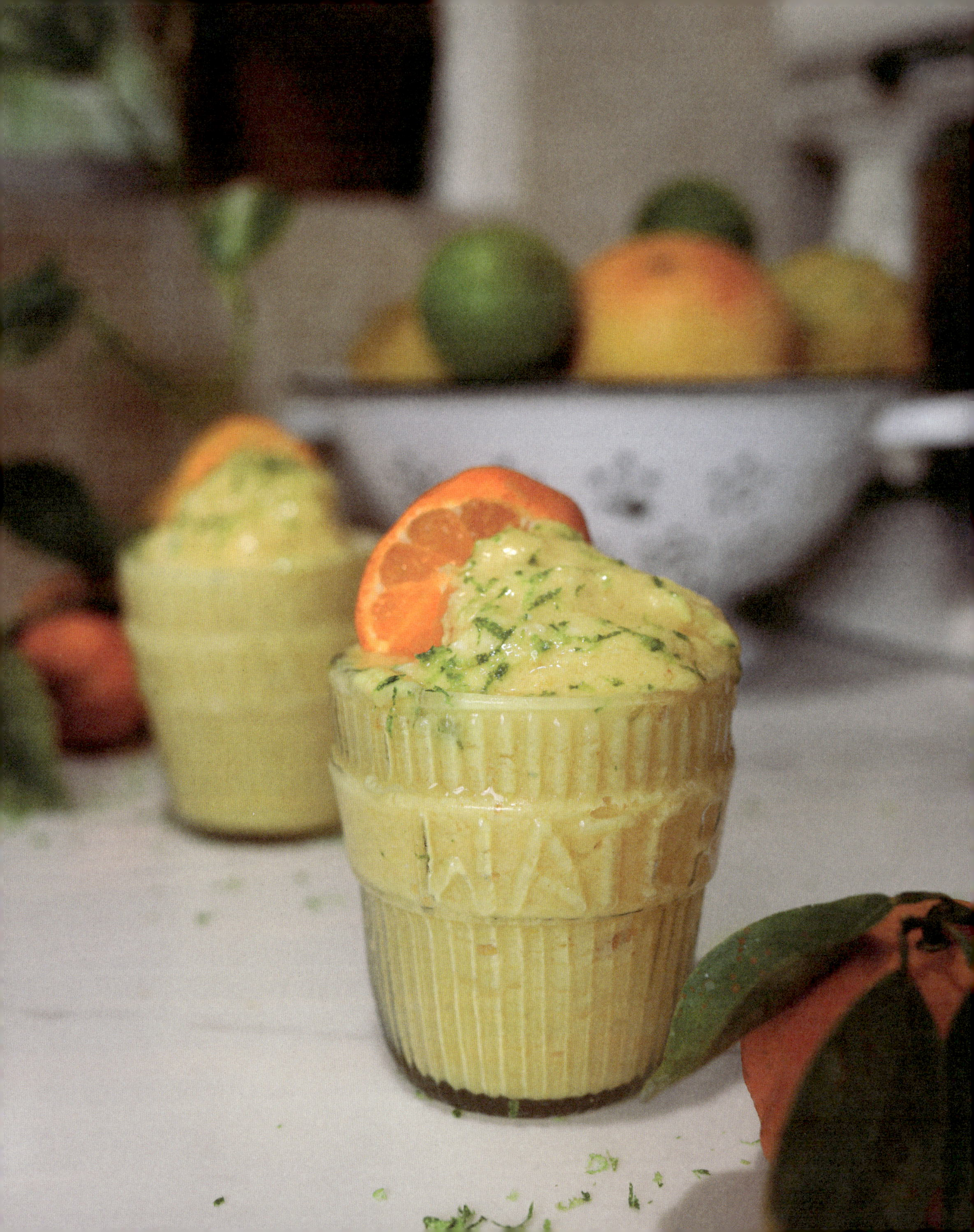

BOOSTED ORANGE SLUSHIE

MAKES 6 CUPS (1.4 L)

Prep: 5 minutes
Rest: 8 hours

If an adrenal cocktail and an Orange Julius had a baby who went to the islands and found a little spice, it would be this slushie. It's so refreshing—sour with a little sweetness—with probiotic goodness from the yogurt, anti-inflammatory benefits from the turmeric (don't skip the pinch of black pepper that helps to activate the powerful curcumin in the turmeric!), and minerals from the salt and cream of tartar. What's not to love? You can play with the flavors; I like to add a little lime zest, but you could even throw in some vanilla extract or a dash of cinnamon.

6 medium navel oranges, divided
1 cup (250 g) plain full-fat yogurt
½ cup (120 ml) coconut water
¼ cup (60 ml) maple syrup, plus more to taste
2 inches (5 cm) fresh turmeric or 2 teaspoons ground turmeric
Zest of 1 lime (about 2 teaspoons; optional)
½ teaspoon cream of tartar
¼ teaspoon sea salt
Pinch of black pepper

1. Line a baking sheet with parchment paper. Peel five of the oranges, leaving a good amount of the white pith on them, then break the segments apart. Place on the sheet pan and freeze in a single layer until firm, then transfer to a freezer-safe container and freeze overnight (or for at least 8 hours).
2. When ready to make the slushie, juice and zest the remaining orange.
3. Place the orange segments in a blender with the orange juice, orange zest, yogurt, coconut water, maple syrup, turmeric, lime zest (if using), cream of tartar, salt, and pepper.
4. Blend on high until completely smooth, about 30 seconds. Add more maple syrup for extra sweetness if necessary, but let the sour flavor shine! Serve immediately.

SWEET DREAMS MOCKTAIL

SERVES 1

Prep: 5 minutes

This mildly sweet and slightly sour mocktail combines all the heavy-hitting sleep aids to help you drift off. The amino acid glycine in collagen lowers your core body temperature, which naturally triggers sleep. It also increases serotonin (the precursor to melatonin) and has a calming effect on brain activity. Chamomile is a sedative known to calm anxiety, and tart cherry juice is loaded with melatonin and tryptophan, which are both major sleep inducers! This drink is safe during pregnancy and breastfeeding and can be made without honey for a very low-sugar option.

3 tablespoons dried chamomile flowers or 2 chamomile tea bags
1 cup (240 ml) boiling water
2 tablespoons collagen powder
1 tablespoon honey
2 tablespoons Tart Cherry Reduction

1. Place the chamomile and boiling water in a jar or French press. Cover and steep for 5 minutes, or chill and save for later.
2. Spoon the collagen and honey into your favorite mug. Add 2 tablespoons of the chamomile tea to help the mixture dissolve, then mix with a spoon or small frother.
3. Pour the remaining tea into the mug with the honey and collagen.
4. Drizzle in the Tart Cherry Reduction, stir, and enjoy a good night's sleep!

Tart Cherry Reduction

MAKES $1\frac{1}{2}$ CUPS (360 ML)

Cook: 45 minutes

This method can be used to turn any juice into a refined, no-sugar-added syrup. By gently reducing the juice, you not only strengthen the flavors but also double down on the benefits. This reduction contains vitamins A and C; potassium, copper, magnesium, iron, and antioxidants; and melatonin and tryptophan to promote relaxation.

3 cups (720 ml) pure tart cherry juice

1. Pour the juice into a medium saucepan (ideally not nonstick).
2. Bring almost to a boil and then reduce to a gentle simmer over low heat until the mixture reduces by more than half, stirring occasionally, 45 minutes to an hour. The bubbles should become larger and slower, and the mixture should coat the back of a spoon. Remove from the heat immediately and let cool.
3. Store in a sealed jar in the fridge for up to 2 weeks.

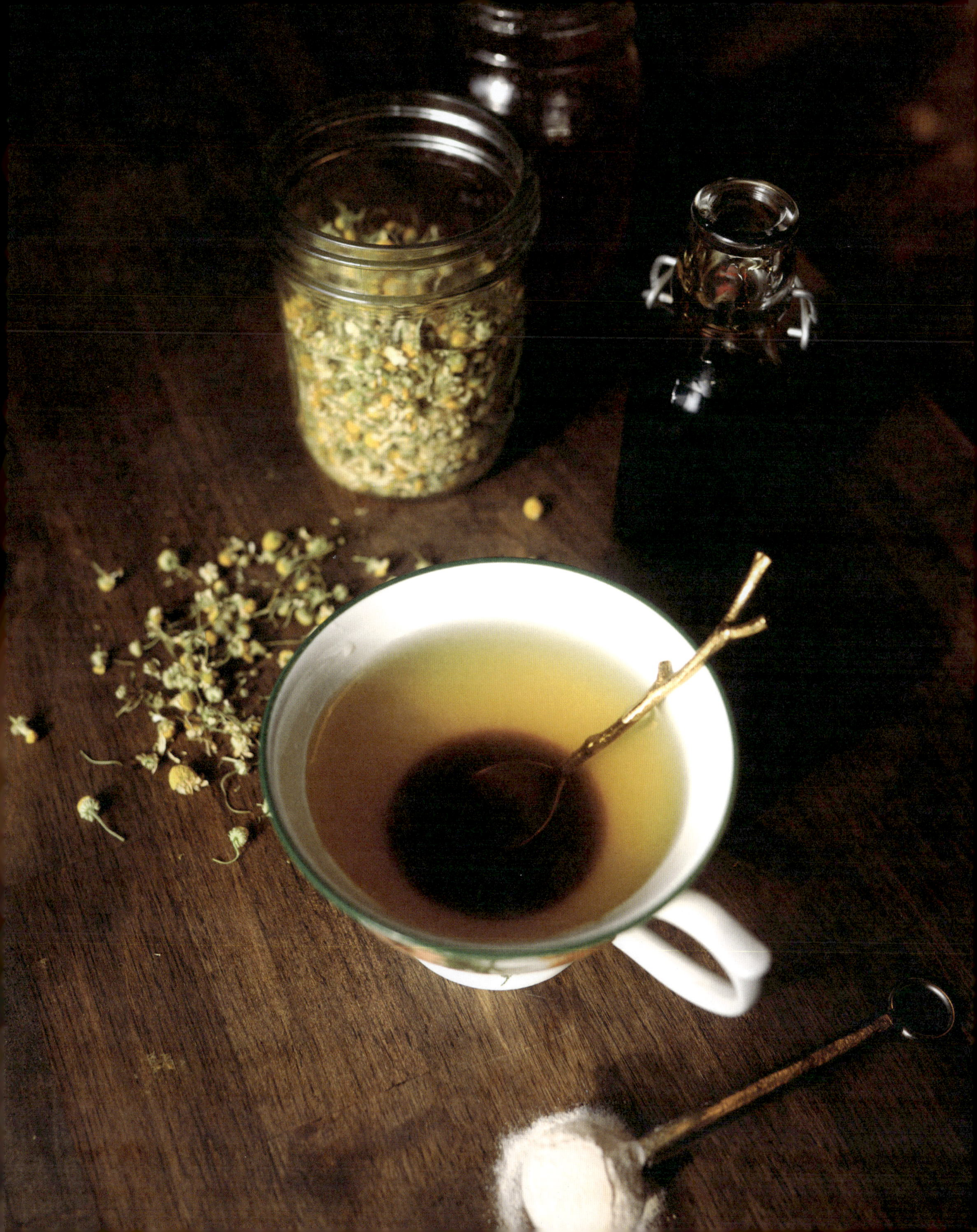

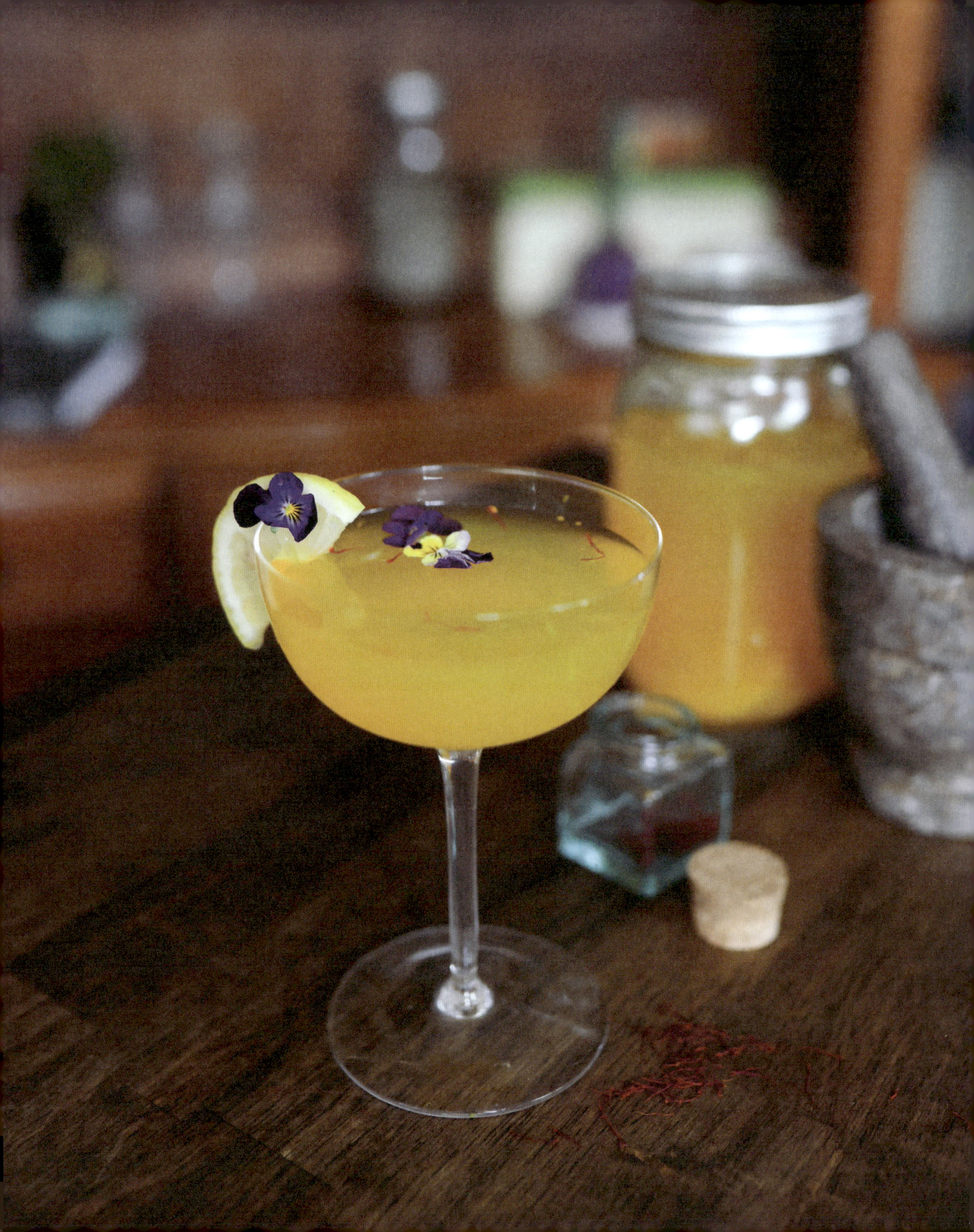

SAFFRON CORDIAL

SERVES 4

Prep: 10 minutes
Cook: 5 minutes
Cooling: 1 hour

This cordial originates in Persia, where it is known as safran şerbeti. Saffron is associated with sunshine, happiness, and wealth and has been used for centuries for well-being. Its benefits include increasing serotonin signaling (similar to a gentle SSRI medication), supporting dopamine pathways, regulating stress response by reducing cortisol, and having mild anxiolytic effects! For this cordial, I add turmeric for extra anti-inflammatory benefits, which makes the color even more vibrant.

15 to 20 strands saffron (about ¼ teaspoon)
2 teaspoons cane sugar
4½ cups (about 1 L) water
1 teaspoon grated ginger
1 lemon, washed and thinly sliced, plus extra slices for serving
¼ teaspoon ground turmeric
Pinch of black pepper
¼ cup (60 ml) raw honey, or more to taste

1. With a mortar and pestle or coffee grinder, grind the saffron and sugar until finely ground.
2. Place the water, ginger, and lemon slices in a small pot. Cover and bring to a boil for a few minutes, until fragrant. Remove from the heat.
3. Stir in the saffron sugar, turmeric, and pepper and let steep until cool enough to touch, then remove the lemon slices.
4. Stir in the honey, tasting for your desired level of sweetness and adding more if need be.
5. Pour into a large jar and chill for a few hours before serving over ice with a lemon slice. Store in the fridge for up to 1 week.

BONE BROTH HOT COCOA

MAKES 2 CUPS (480 ML)

Prep: 5 minutes
Cook: 10 minutes

Calm down—don't turn the page on me yet. Yes, I said "bone broth" and "cocoa" in the same sentence, and yes, it might sound vile, but if you follow this recipe, I promise it will change your mind. The key is to use unsalted, unflavored bone broth. This is, admittedly, hard to find in the store, so this recipe is definitely best with homemade broth! When I make bone broth, I often don't season or add extra ingredients for this very reason. Combining the gut-soothing, mineral-rich, anti-inflammatory benefits of broth with the mood-boosting antioxidants of cacao and some well-chosen spices makes this not only a super delicious treat but also a much more functional way to enjoy chocolate! Top with Medicinal Marshmallows (page 241) for extra goodness.

1 cup (240 ml) unseasoned Bone Broth (page 159)
1 cup (240 ml) whole milk
2 cardamom pods, lightly smashed
⅛ teaspoon Ceylon cinnamon powder
Dash of chili powder
Pinch of black pepper
¼ cup (25 g) cacao powder or plain cocoa powder (see Note)
¼ cup (60 ml) maple syrup, or to taste
2 tablespoons heavy cream, divided

1. Combine the Bone Broth, milk, cardamom, cinnamon, chili powder, and pepper in a small saucepan and gently warm over medium heat until fragrant, 3 to 5 minutes.
2. Add the cacao powder and maple syrup and whisk to combine.
3. Continue to heat until just before the mixture boils, whisking regularly, about 4 minutes.
4. Remove from the heat, taste, and add more maple syrup to adjust the sweetness if necessary.
5. Remove the cardamom pods, pour into mugs, and stir 1 tablespoon heavy cream into each. (Optionally, whip or froth the cream a little first and then add on top!)

NOTE

CACAO VS COCOA: If you're using chocolate for its magical benefits (aren't we all?), cacao is the way to go. It's made from raw, unroasted, cold-pressed cocoa beans, so all of the minerals and vitamins are preserved in the powder. Cocoa powder has a less bitter flavor, but it's roasted at high temperatures, which greatly reduces the nutritional benefits.

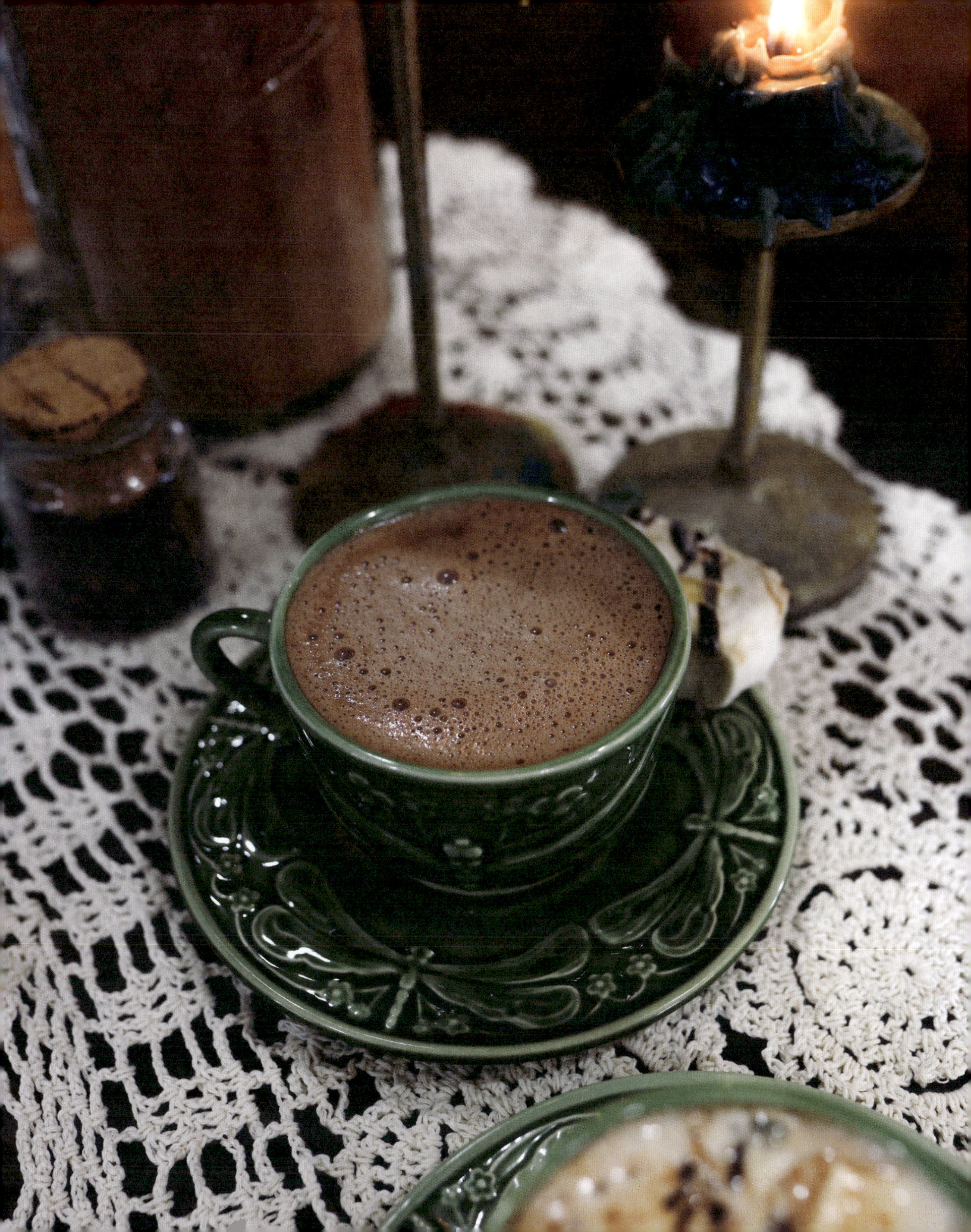

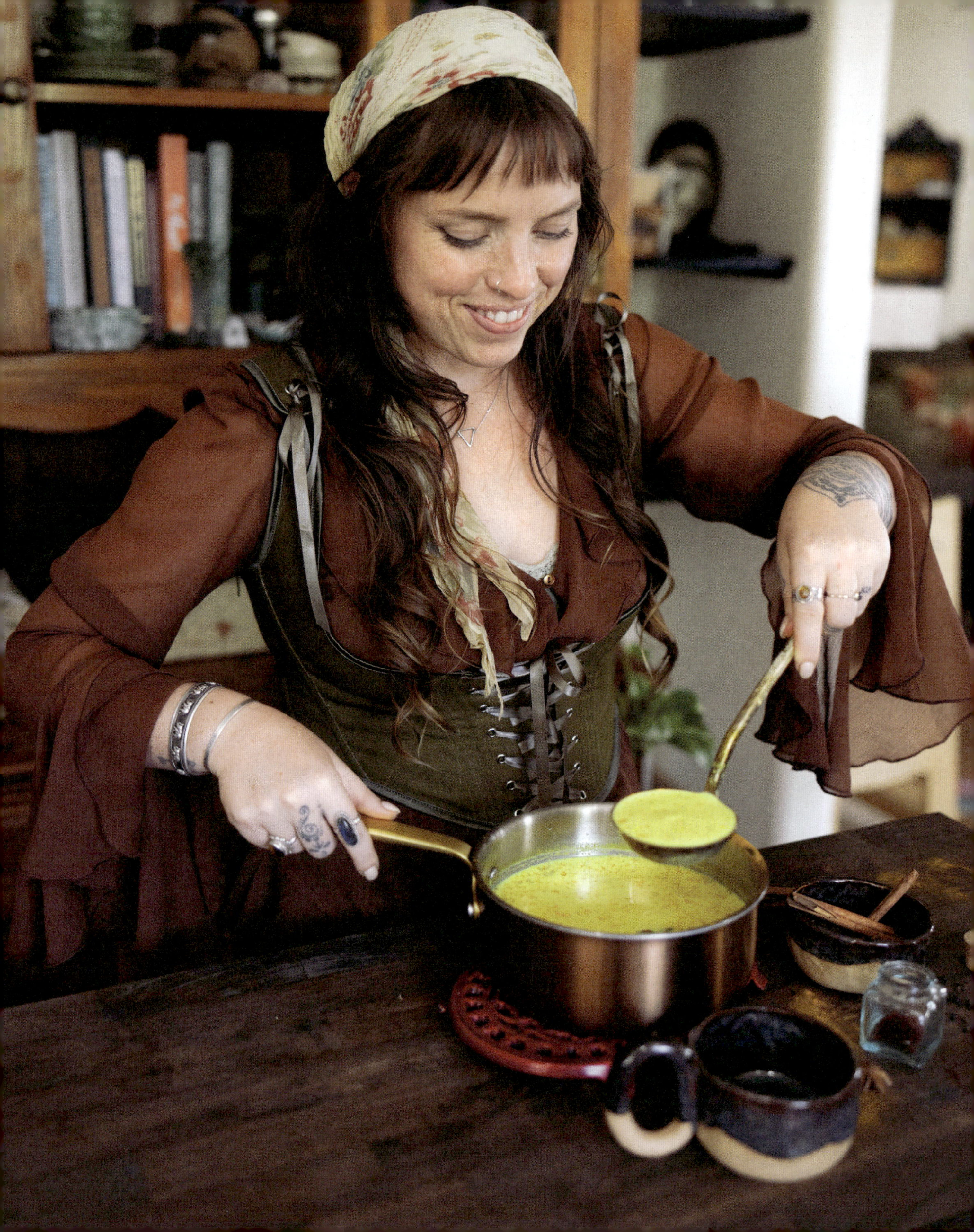

CHAI-SPICED GOLDEN MILK

MAKES 2 CUPS (480 ML)

Prep: 5 minutes
Cook: 15 minutes

Golden milk is like hot chocolate's cool herbal auntie. I love to drink it at night to get all the warming, relaxing goodness without a sugar hit before bedtime. This powerfully healing elixir harnesses the anti-inflammatory power of curcumin from the turmeric—along with the digestive benefits of ginger and pepper and the antimicrobial and immune-boosting properties of all those other spices—by utilizing the butterfat of milk and ghee to extract the fat-soluble compounds of those ingredients. The saffron helps calm nerves and promote a sunny mood. Many of the ingredients are optional, except for the milk, peppercorns, turmeric, and (in my opinion) sweetener—so make it your own!

¾ cup (180 ml) water
2 cups (480 ml) whole milk or coconut milk
6 to 8 whole black peppercorns
6 to 8 strands saffron
2 whole cloves
1 or 2 star anise pods
1 cardamom pod, lightly smashed
1 cinnamon stick or ⅛ teaspoon ground Ceylon cinnamon
1 inch (2.5 cm) fresh ginger, chopped, or ½ teaspoon ground ginger
1½ teaspoons ground turmeric
½ teaspoon vanilla extract
Pinch of sea salt
1 tablespoon maple syrup or honey, or to taste
1 teaspoon ghee or coconut oil, or to taste

1. Warm the water and milk in a small saucepan over medium-high heat. Add the peppercorns, saffron, cloves, star anise, cardamom, cinnamon, ginger, turmeric, vanilla, and salt.
2. Stir occasionally for 3 to 5 minutes, then turn the heat down to low as soon as the mixture begins to bubble (to avoid boiling the milk).
3. Let stew for 5 to 10 more minutes, ensuring that the turmeric is fully incorporated and the spices are infused. Remove from the heat.
4. Stir in the maple syrup and ghee. Strain into mugs, add more maple syrup and ghee to taste, and enjoy!

FUN FACT

Curcumin is most bioavailable when consumed with piperine, a compound found in black pepper, so to get the benefits of turmeric, always add even a tiny pinch of pepper. Additionally, both curcumin and piperine are fat-soluble, so they're always best consumed with a healthy fat source (like the whole milk and ghee in this recipe!).

Teas & Tinctures

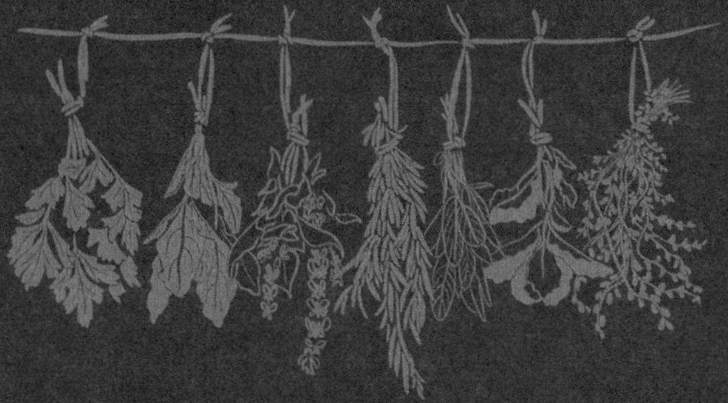

It's impossible to talk about kitchen magic without delving into the world of teas and tinctures. They are the absolute gateway into herbalism and some of the oldest and simplest ways to extract the beneficial (magical) properties of herbs and spices.

Teas are a great quick and easy way of getting herbal goodness along with lots of hydration and mineral support. They are emotionally soothing and warming, making them irreplaceable for wellness and recovery as well as daily enjoyment.

Tinctures are far more concentrated. They are fast-acting and potent, more suited to acute needs or for practical daily use (think of them like the homemade equivalent of vitamin pills, but with far more varied benefits, as each plant contains such numerous compounds and applications). They are ideal for convenience and long-term storage.

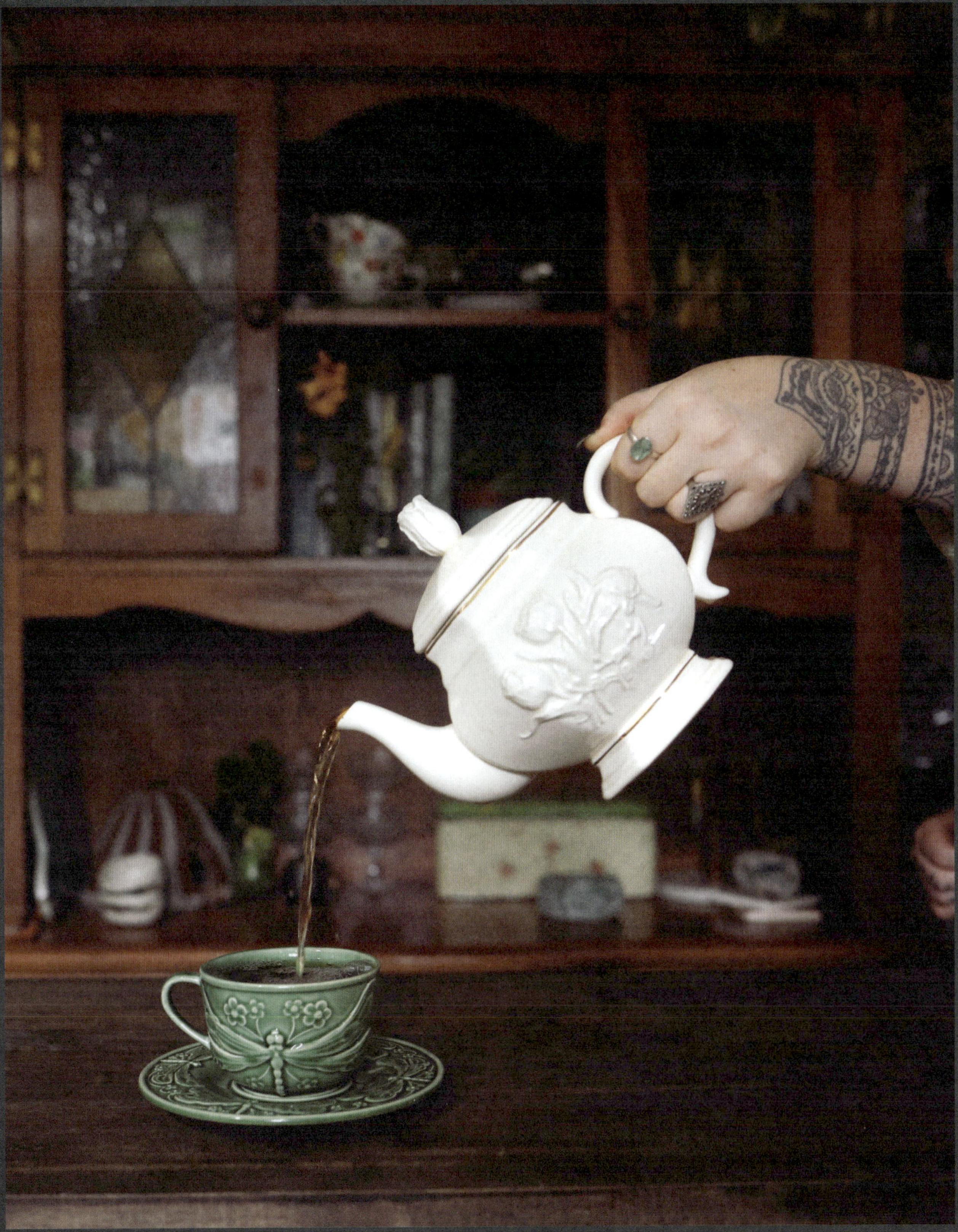

BREWS

Teas are one of the oldest, simplest, and most effective medicines we have. Making tea is the quickest way to extract the goodness from plants—and a powerful form of food magic that anyone can harness. Energetically, teas offer comfort and a chance to slow down, rest, and receive. When I was growing up in England, drinking tea was a daily occurrence for me, offered everywhere I went. But if you weren't raised on tea, there are a few things you should know—and if you're new to tea as medicine, this may be helpful, too.

Medicinal plant brews fall into two basic categories: *infusions* and *decoctions.*

FUN FACT: Herbal teas aren't actually "tea"; they're herbal infusions. "Tea" is technically just the name for an infusion of leaves from the Camellia sinensis (tea) plant (this refers to black, green, or white tea, among others).

How to Brew Herbs

SELECTING YOUR HERBS

Use the herb list on page 38 to find herbs that serve your particular needs. You can blend multiple herbs together for their health benefits or for taste! In fact, I recommend experimenting with making your own blends to serve different needs and tastebuds. It's so fun.

Most herbs you can measure with your heart. A traditional serving size for a strong medicinal cup is a "palmful" of dried or a "handful" of fresh herbs. Spices and very aromatic herbs like thyme should be used in smaller amounts, or they will overpower the brew. Very powerful sedatives or potent medicinal herbs should be used even more sparingly.

MAKING AN INFUSION

Infusions are made using the soft leaves or flowers of plants and can be brewed hot or cold. A strong infusion should brew for up to 4 hours, but a few minutes will do at the very least.

To make a hot infusion:

1. Use 3 teaspoons dried or 3 tablespoons fresh herbs (for a single serving).

2. Bring 12 ounces (1½ cups) of clean, filtered water to a full rolling boil.

3. Leave the water to cool slightly for 2 to 3 minutes. (Different herbs may require different brewing temperatures—delicate herbs or those with stronger flavors can become bitter at high temperatures, while others don't brew well at lower ones—but this is a good general rule.)

4. Place the herbs in a 16-ounce (480 ml) jar or French press and pour the hot water over them, stirring to submerge.

5. Steep for 5 to 20 minutes, depending on your herbs. The longer the infusion steeps, the stronger the flavor and medicinal properties will be, although some herbs can become bitter if brewed for too long.

6. Cover the tea while it steeps, particularly if it has lots of volatile oils (oils that can escape through steam). Herbs with volatile oils include mint, chamomile, lavender, rosemary, and other teas with strong scents.

7. If using a jar, strain the tea into a mug before serving, or depress the French press lid and pour to serve.

COLD INFUSIONS are often preferred for large batches, particularly for aromatic herbs with volatile oils that are more likely to go bitter when brewed too long at higher temperatures. This gentle method allows for a long infusion while preventing extraction of the bitter compounds.

To make a cold infusion:

1. Use about 8 teaspoons of dried herbs or 8 tablespoons of fresh herbs.

2. Pour 4 cups (960 ml) of filtered, room-temperature water into a large jar.

3. Place the herbs in a mesh or muslin cloth, tied loosely enough to allow the herbs to move around. Dip them in the water to wet them slightly before submerging fully.

4. Keep the bundle of herbs suspended by trailing the end of the cloth over the lip of the jar and loosely screwing the lid over it to hold it in place. (You can also brew this with loose herbs and strain the infusion through a sieve before serving.)

5. Set the jar on the countertop, place it in the fridge, or set it outside in a sunny spot to make sun tea!

6. Cold infusions usually take 12 to 24 hours, depending on where you place them, but the timing isn't an exact science. You can taste the infusion and see if you think it's ready to drink!

MAKING A DECOCTION

Decoctions are made from the harder parts of plants: the roots, bark, berries, or seeds.* A strong decoction should brew for up to 24 hours, but an hour will do at the very least.

To make a decoction:

1. Use 8 teaspoons of dried or 8 tablespoons of fresh herbs.

2. Place the herbs in a medium pot and add about 1 quart (1 L) of cold water, then bring to a simmer over medium heat.

3. Cover with a lid and simmer for around 30 minutes, then remove from the heat and steep for 15 to 30 more minutes, adding more delicate leafy or floral herbs to steep at this point if desired.

4. Strain before serving.

**The exceptions are marshmallow root and burdock root: Both prefer a long, cold infusion so as not to harm the beneficial constituents.*

While there is an art to brewing and blending herbs, and particular ways to craft a perfect potion, these basics will get you a long way. Most plants are very forgiving and intuitive to use once you start experimenting with them, so don't worry too much, and get to brewing!

TINCTURES

If you want to delve a little deeper into the medicinal side of herbs, it's good to know how to make a basic tincture. Tinctures pull all the goodness out of herbs and spices and make them super easy to use in liquid form. There are some herbs whose compounds extract just fine with water (an infusion or tea; see page 260), but you will get more goodness from certain herbs with a longer extraction, most commonly by using clear alcohol or vinegar. You can also use oil, honey, wine, or glycerin; different methods work better for different plants. You can get very specific with tincture making, using precise measurements and methods to get the utmost out of each herb. But you can also get a long way with the old-school, heart-measured folk medicine method. This will work perfectly for most herbs.

You can use a tincture any time you might otherwise use a tea, and the herbal applications are generally the same (see the list on page 38 for herbs and their uses), but tinctures are far more concentrated and fast-acting. They are best for acute issues or convenient daily use and long-term storage.

Dried herbs are easier to measure and control, and they have a lower moisture content, which makes them more stable than fresh herbs. You can use fresh herbs, but you'll need higher-proof alcohol (at least 95 percent alcohol by volume/ABV) or glycerin to account for the higher moisture content. The water content in the final product can still be too high to make it safe for long-term storage. A quick sun-dry of the fresh herbs before tincturing is the ideal solution!

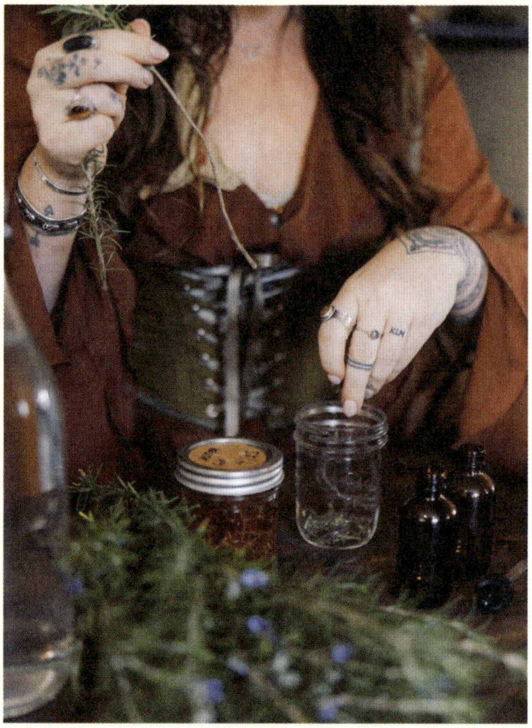

"Tinctures pull all the goodness out of herbs and spices and make them super easy to use in liquid form."

Sourcing Herbs

When making herbal remedies, quality really matters. You want to find either organic bulk herbs or clean, wild-gathered herbs from pollution-free areas.

To gather your own herbs, the most important thing is identification. Many basic medicinal herbs like nettle, raspberry leaf, chamomile, and dandelion are very clearly identifiable, but some are not, so be mindful. When gathering in the wild, never do so directly beside a busy road or in a polluted area, and always stay on public land. Never take all that you find, and always clean and dry your herbs thoroughly. You can also grow many herbs easily at home where you can control the environment!

To buy herbs, look for bulk spices and tea sections in local health-food stores, or shop online for well-sourced, high-quality organic herbs at good prices.

To begin building your herbal apothecary, start with common, gentle, nutritive herbs that have multiple applications. Some favorites are:

NETTLE · PEPPERMINT · RASPBERRY LEAF · CHAMOMILE · LEMON BALM · ECHINACEA

To make a tincture:

YOU WILL NEED:

- A clean 16-ounce (480 ml) mason jar
- Herbs, ideally dried, finely chopped
- High-proof, clear alcohol (vodka or gin; 40 to 60 percent ABV for leaves and flowers, 90 to 95 percent ABV for resin, roots, and barks)
- Jar labels
- A muslin cloth or fine-mesh strainer
- Amber or dark glass tincture bottles with dropper lids

1. Thoroughly wash the jar and your hands (no need to sterilize).

2. Fill the jar halfway with the herbs. Don't pack the herbs, but give the jar a gentle shake to make sure they are settled in.

3. Cover the herbs completely with alcohol, leaving about ½ inch (1 cm) of headspace. Screw the lid on tightly and give it a gentle shake.

4. Label the jar with the date, the name of the herb, and the type and proof of the alcohol.

5. Store the jar in a cool, dry place for 4 to 6 weeks (or more). Gently shake the jar every day, or as often as you think of it.

6. When ready to use, strain the mixture through a muslin cloth or fine-mesh strainer into a glass bowl or jug, making sure to squeeze all the liquid out of the herbs.

7. Be sure all the plant matter is removed, then pour into tincture bottles, label once again, and store in a cool, dark place until needed. You can store a properly made tincture pretty much indefinitely, just as you would alcohol.

8. Most common tinctures are recommended in doses of ½ to 1 teaspoon (2.5 to 5 ml), two to three times daily.

I HAVE A TEA FOR THAT

And, actually, I also have a tincture for that. The following herbs have generally the same properties *either* brewed into a tea or extracted into a tincture. It's up to you how you want to use them—whether you need a quick, comforting remedy (tea) or want a strong, long-lasting, convenient cure (tincture). Gather your jars and start collecting herbs, and soon enough you, too, will have a tea for that.

You can use the following herbs alone or in blends; there are very few occasions where you wouldn't want to blend two particular herbs. While I have described basic applications, if you have very particular health needs or are on certain medications, it's never a bad idea to do a quick search for contraindications of a particular herb, which will tell you if it's safe for your use.

The safest across the board are nutritive herbs that are also used as food—nettle, mint, chamomile, dandelion, hibiscus, rosehip, raspberry leaf, and many other commonly known herbs fall into this category and can be used very freely. Herbs that should be used with a little more caution or sparingly are marked with an asterisk. Herbs that have common contraindications are marked with two asterisks.

For instructions on how to use these herbs and in what amounts, turn to page 260 for brewing teas and page 262 for making tinctures.

Digestive Health

- **CONSTIPATION:** ginger, licorice**, peppermint, slippery elm
- **DIGESTION:** cardamom, cinnamon, clove, dandelion root, ginger
- **FOOD POISONING:** cinnamon, ginger, mulberry leaf, sage
- **IBS:** aloe vera, calendula*, cardamom, licorice**, valerian**
- **NAUSEA:** chamomile, ginger, marshmallow root

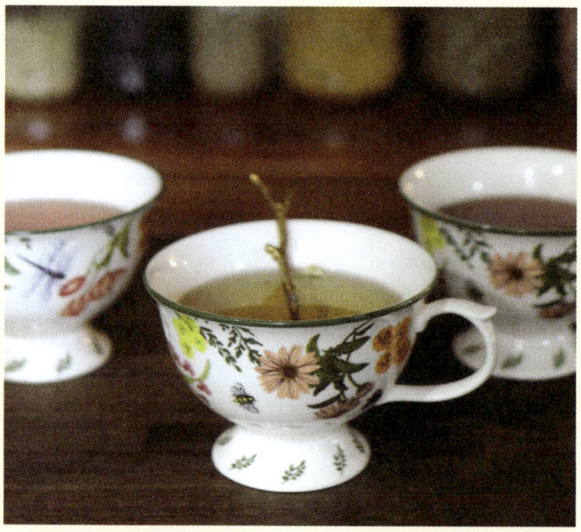

Hormone Health

- **FOLLICULAR PHASE:** holy basil, red clover, schisandra
- **OVULATION PHASE:** astragalus*, cinnamon bark, maca, red clover
- **LUTEAL PHASE AND PMS:** burdock, chamomile, ginger, saffron
- **MENSTRUAL PHASE:**

  Heavy Bleeding: ashwagandha, nettle, raspberry leaf, yarrow

  Cramps: chamomile, cramp bark, passionflower, thyme

  Menopause: black cohosh**, ginseng, sage, St. John's wort**

  Period Regularity: chasteberry*, dandelion, sage, shatavari

  PCOS and Hormone Balance: chasteberry, spearmint
- **BLOOD SUGAR BALANCE AND TYPE 2 DIABETES:** cinnamon, dandelion root, holy basil
- **INSULIN RESISTANCE:** cinnamon, fenugreek, licorice**, spearmint

Illness

- **ASTHMA:** lavender, mullein, nettle, thyme
- **COUGH:** clove, mullein, sage, thyme
- **DETOXIFICATION:** celery seed, fennel, milk thistle
- **FEVER:** black pepper, ginger, holy basil
- **HEADACHE:** feverfew**, ginger, peppermint
- **IMMUNE SYSTEM:** astragalus*, echinacea, elderberry, garlic, ginger, thyme

Mental Health

- **ADRENAL HEALTH:** holy basil, licorice**, rosemary
- **ANXIETY:** lemon balm, oat straw, St. John's wort**, valerian**
- **DEPRESSION:** saffron, rhodiola*, rosemary, St. John's wort**
- **MENTAL CLARITY:** ashwagandha*, rhodiola*, rosemary, sage
- **PHYSICAL EXHAUSTION:** angelica*, ginseng, maca
- **SLEEP:** lavender, nutmeg, passionflower*, valerian**
- **STRESS:** holy basil, rosemary, valerian**

Pregnancy

- **FIRST TRIMESTER:** lemon balm, oats, oat straw
- **SECOND TRIMESTER:** nettle, raspberry leaf
- **THIRD TRIMESTER:** alfalfa, peppermint, raspberry leaf, valerian**
- **LABOR:** clove, raspberry leaf
- **POSTPARTUM:** dandelion root, fennel, nettle

**Use sparingly or check for contraindications.*
***Use sparingly, has common contraindications.*

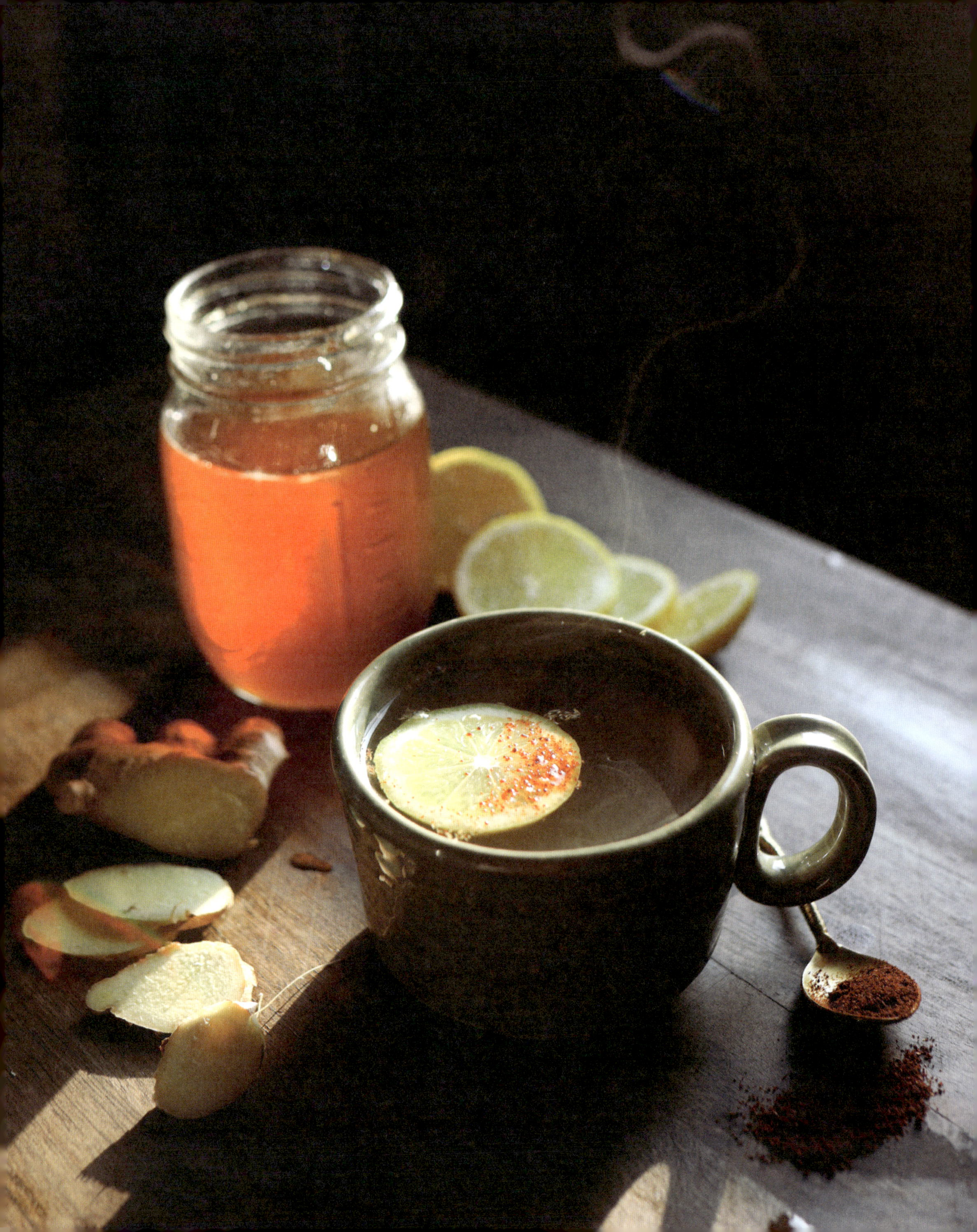

THE FLU BOMB

MAKES 1 CUP (240 ML)

Prep: *5 minutes*

This warm drink is adapted from the great old-school herbalist Barbara O'Neill's famous recipe, which she claims can get rid of a cold or flu in three days, and honestly, I might agree. It's basically just a single-serving cauldron of all the most heavy-hitting antibacterial, antiviral, anti-inflammatory, anti-everything kitchen ingredients, and if you can chug this three or four times a day when you come down with the lurgy, it should significantly shorten your sickness. Barbara's recipe includes a single drop of eucalyptus or tea tree oil, which is no longer recommended. Instead, I use oil of oregano (not oregano essential oil), which is well known to be one of nature's most powerful antibacterial, antifungal, and antiviral medicines. Follow the dosage instructions on your own bottle if using, but generally 1 to 3 drops, 2 to 3 times per day (depending on how much you can handle) is recommended. You can leave it out if it's contraindicated for you (see Note). If you find the ingredients too strong, use as much of each one as you can tolerate.

2 tablespoons raw honey, or more to taste

Juice of 1 lemon

1 garlic clove, finely grated

1 teaspoon finely grated ginger

Pinch of cayenne pepper, or more to taste (as much as you can handle)

1 to 3 drops oil of oregano (optional)

1. Combine the ingredients in a mug and top up with warm water (but not boiling water, which will kill the benefits of the raw honey). Stir well and drink as quickly as you can.

NOTE

Oil of oregano is not recommended during pregnancy. It can also interact with diabetes medications and lithium. It has a blood-thinning effect, which can amplify the effects of blood thinners.

MORNING SICKNESS ELIXIR

MAKES 2 QUARTS (2 L)

Prep: 10 minutes
Cook: 10 minutes
Steep: 10 minutes

Morning sickness is the bane of every pregnant woman's existence. While there can be multiple causes, huge contributing factors are blood sugar fluctuations, sluggish digestion, and hormone and mineral imbalances. This elixir targets all of those things; it's sweetened with honey to keep your blood sugar up and contains ginger and spearmint to support easy digestion and quell nausea. Spearmint is also high in magnesium, which can be transformational for morning sickness, and sea salt adds extra electrolytes and minerals. Keep this elixir in the fridge and sip it throughout the day to keep blood sugar levels balanced and nausea low!

7 cups (1.7 L) filtered water
1 cup (30 g) dried spearmint
3 to 4 tablespoons grated fresh ginger
Zest of 1 lemon
½ cup (120 ml) lemon juice
1 cup (240 ml) honey
½ teaspoon sea salt

1. Bring the water to a boil in a medium saucepan.
2. Add the spearmint, ginger, and lemon zest. Stir, cover, reduce the heat to low, and simmer for 5 minutes.
3. Remove from the heat and let steep, covered, for 5 to 10 minutes.
4. Strain the mixture into a large jar using a cheesecloth or fine-mesh sieve, squeezing out all the liquid from the herbs, then discard or compost the herbs.
5. Let cool to a comfortable drinking temperature, then add the lemon juice, honey, and salt.
6. Stir well to combine, refrigerate, and drink within 1 week.

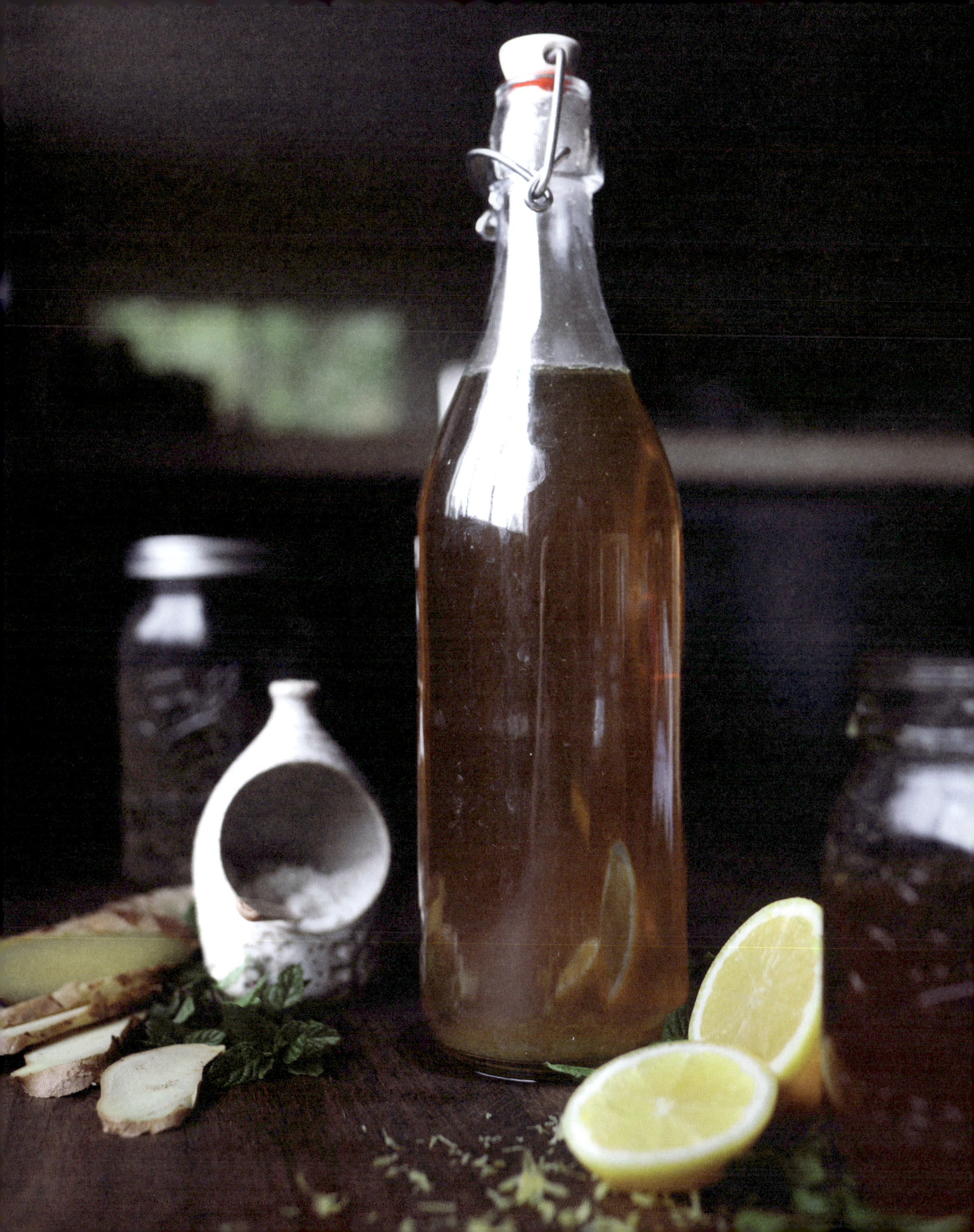

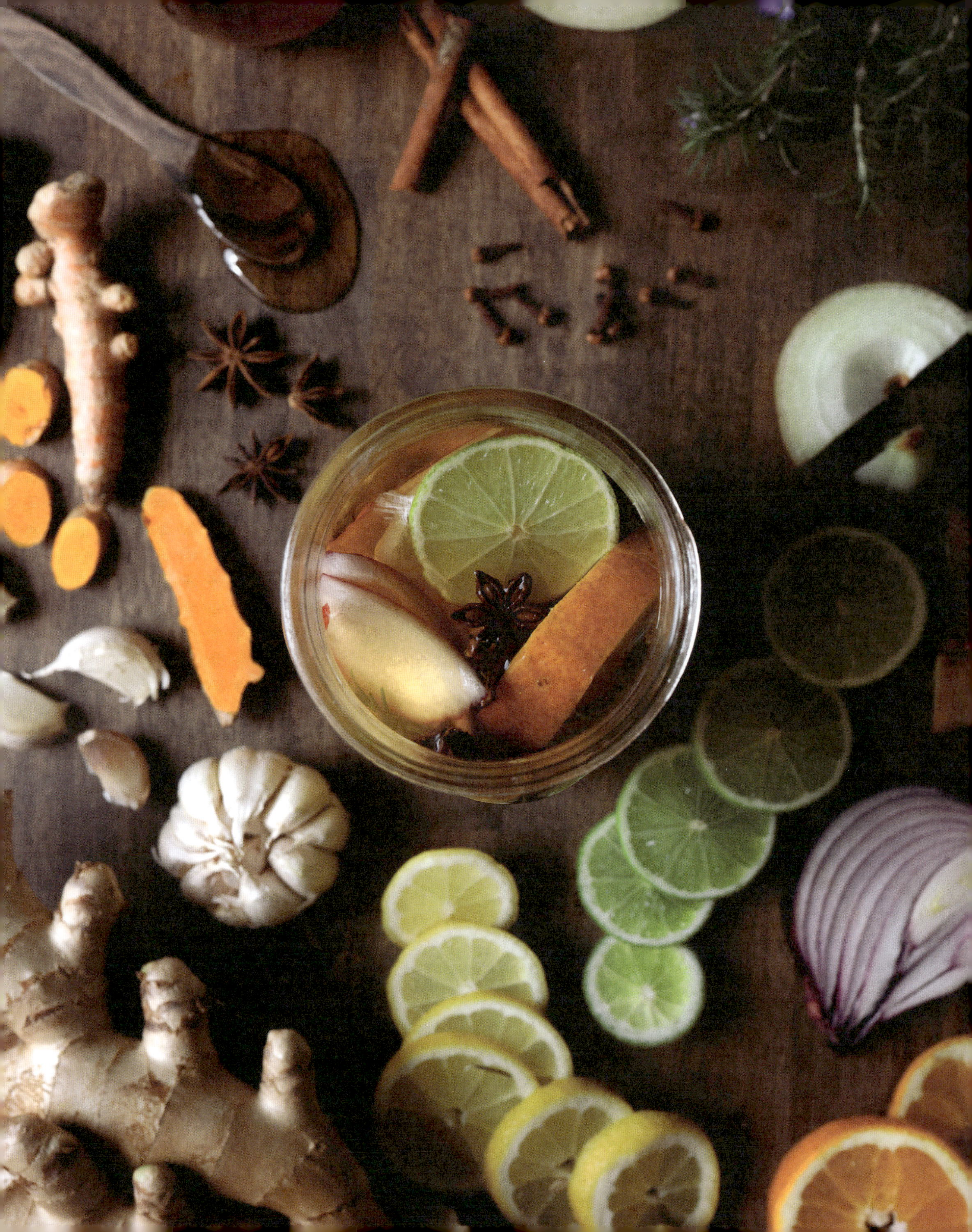

FIRE CIDER

MAKES 1¼ CUPS (300 ML)

Prep: 30 minutes
Fermenting: 4 to 6 weeks

Fire cider is an old faithful remedy that is easy to make, easy to use, and so widely applicable. Great for circulation, immune support, and gut health, it's the perfect entry-level potion to make in preparation for cold season! Fire cider is an oxymel, an infusion made with vinegar and sweetened with honey. Apple cider vinegar, the good, unfiltered kind with "the mother," is full of probiotic benefits and good bacteria, so it's great for your gut health. Because it's acidic, the vinegar also extracts beneficial properties from whatever you infuse it with. Fire cider is particularly potent, since it's infused with some of the most powerful cold- and flu-fighting ingredients, most notably horseradish and jalapeño peppers (hence the "fire"). Still, the beauty of it is that you can adjust the recipe according to whatever is available to you. Try to pack in as many of these ingredients as possible; a shot or two a day will help keep illness at bay. Fire cider can be made into tea by adding warm water, used as a salad dressing, or added to stews, soups, or veggies when cooking.

½ cup (65 g) grated fresh ginger
½ cup (65 g) grated fresh horseradish
½ cup (65 g) grated fresh turmeric
8 to 10 garlic cloves, roughly chopped
½ medium white onion, finely chopped
½ medium red onion, finely chopped
1 to 2 jalapeño peppers, with seeds, finely chopped
Peel of 1 lemon, thoroughly washed and chopped
Juice of 1 lemon
3 to 4 rosemary, oregano, sage, and/or thyme sprigs (whatever you have)
1 tablespoon black peppercorns
Raw, unfiltered apple cider vinegar (with the mother), as needed
¼ cup (60 ml) raw unfiltered honey, or more to taste

1. Layer the ginger, horseradish, turmeric, garlic, onions, jalapeño, lemon peel and juice, herb sprigs, and peppercorns in a 16-ounce (480 ml) wide-mouth mason jar.
2. Cover with apple cider vinegar by 1 to 2 inches (2.5 to 5 cm) and use a long knife or spoon to wiggle the ingredients around and ensure there are no air bubbles. Leave at least 1 inch (2.5 cm) of headspace at the top of the jar.
3. Seal the jar with a plastic lid or cover with a piece of parchment and seal with a metal lid (to prevent the vinegar from corroding the metal). Give it a good shake.
4. Store in a cool, dark place for 4 to 6 weeks. If you forget about it and it ferments longer, that's no big deal.
5. Strain the infused vinegar through a cheesecloth into a large jug or bowl. Squeeze the ingredients to get all the liquid gold out of them!
6. Add the raw honey and mix. Add more honey to taste if need be, but remember, it's fire cider—it should be fiery! If you're trying to add enough honey to cover up the fire . . . good luck. It should taste spicy, sour, and a little sweet.
7. Store in a clean jar in a cool, dry spot for up to a year. Take a shot of fire cider daily for immunity or to aid digestion after a big meal, or take a shot up to 3 times per day to ward off illness.

ALLIUM ALCHEMY

If you want hard evidence that food is medicine, look no further than the world of alliums. Garlic and onions, aside from being the foundation for good flavor in any meal, are healing powerhouses—and you can absolutely harness that healing. Most of their benefits come from the presence of sulfuric compounds: the things that make alliums pungent and eye-stinging, released when they are chopped or crushed.

Garlic is one of the most well-researched and widely accepted food medicines. Allicin is one of garlic's most iconic sulfuric compounds, proven to help lower cholesterol and blood pressure, fight free radicals and inflammation, and support cardiovascular and immune health. Interestingly, it is only present for a few minutes after cutting or crushing fresh garlic, and it loses potency once cooked. Garlic is packed with other beneficial compounds, though; it has powerful antiviral and antibacterial properties, which makes it effective against common colds and viruses like the flu but also many types of bacterial infections like E. coli, staph, strep, urinary tract infections, and even some antibiotic-resistant bacteria. It can even prevent the production of toxins, making it beneficial for treating food poisoning. To treat colds and flus, eating one or two fresh cloves per day is advised.

Onions are high in vitamin C, fiber, folic acid, and lots of minerals like potassium, making them great for immune function, iron absorption, metabolic health, nerve and cellular function, fluid balance, and muscle health, among other things. They are high in antioxidants that reduce the risk of age-related disease and support healthy aging by reducing inflammation and supporting liver health. Like garlic, they have antibacterial, antimicrobial, and antiviral properties, but their real magic for colds is due to their expectorant abilities. The sulfuric compounds and flavonoids in onions work to thin and loosen mucus and help your body expel gunk—these are the same compounds that form volatile gas and cause you to cry when cutting onions! There isn't a particular dosage, as onions are a very safe and gentle medicine that can be used as often as needed.

You can get lots of benefits just by cooking with alliums, but for all these powerful properties, you need to eat them freshly cut and raw. That can be . . . challenging, so here are some medicinal preparations that are worth keeping in your back pocket for when you feel a cold incoming.

All of the following preparations can be taken as is or incorporated into fresh (not heated) recipes. They add incredible depth of flavor to food while also offering their powerful medicine. Mix them into salad dressings or dips, or use them to garnish anything from eggs to pasta to avocado toast!

If you want hard evidence that food is medicine, look no further than the world of alliums.

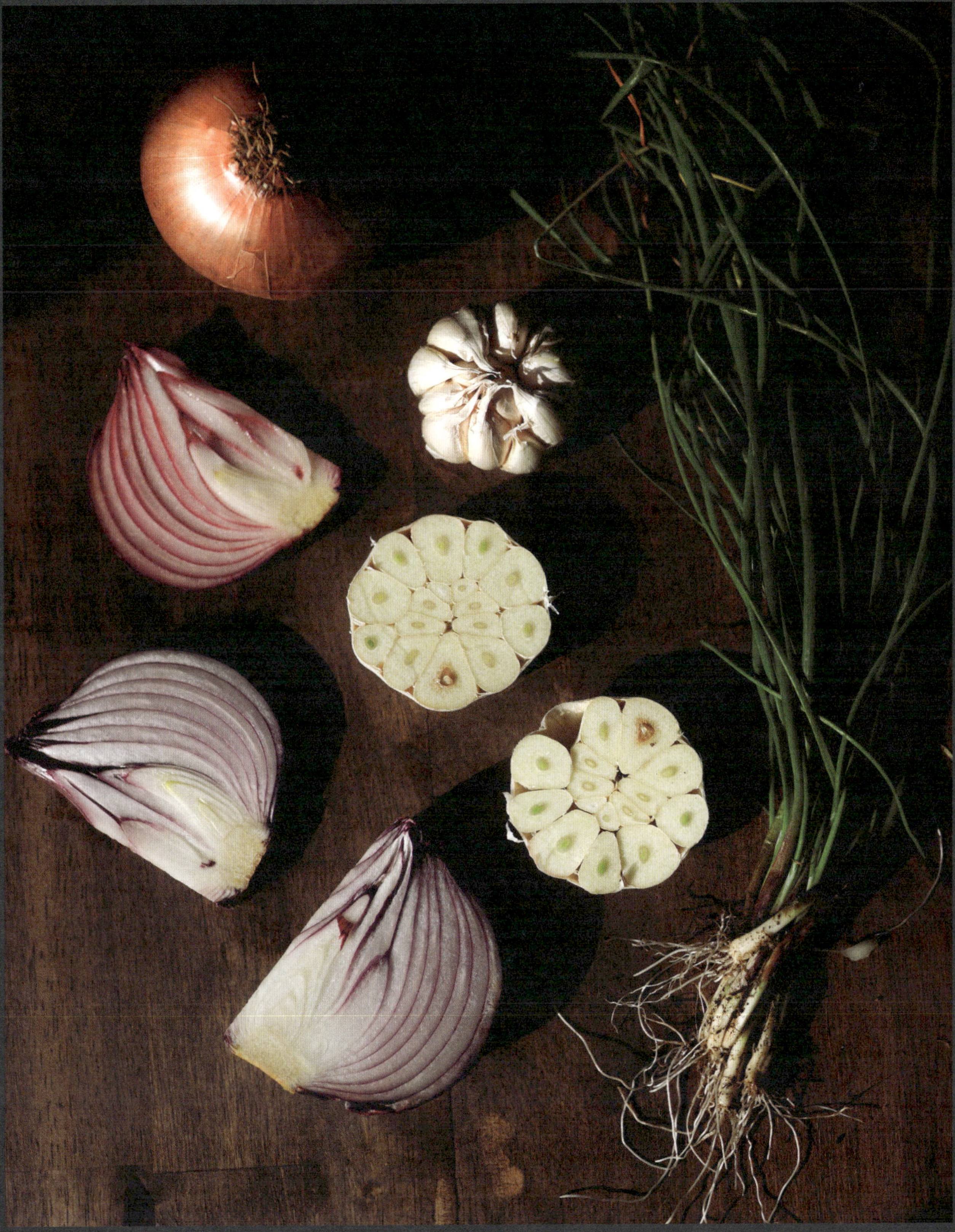

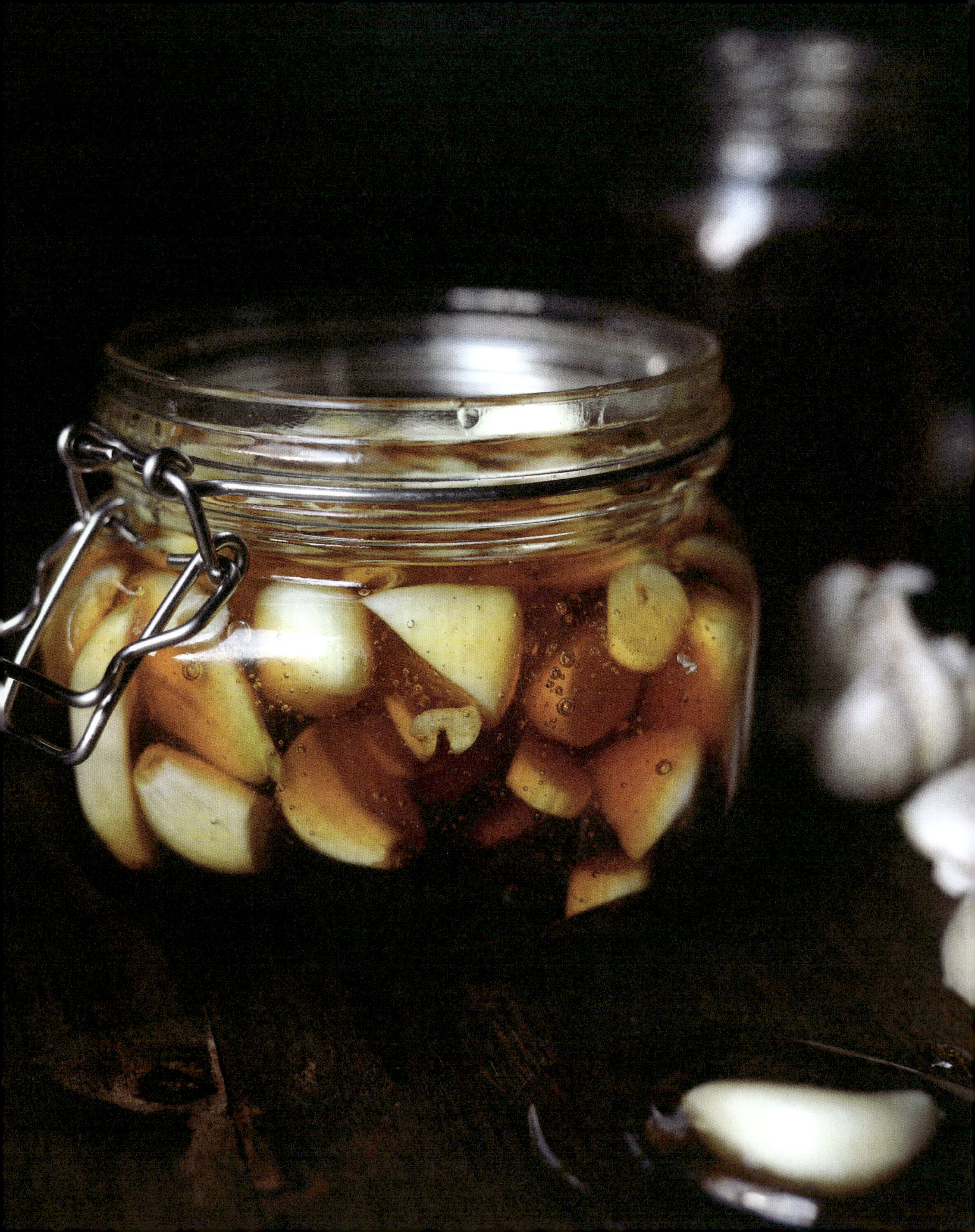

PICKLED GARLIC AND HONEY

MAKES 16 OUNCES (480 ML)

Prep: 15 minutes
Fermenting: 7 weeks

This mellow garlic concoction makes the medicine go down easy: You can eat a clove daily for long-term anti-inflammatory benefits or up to three a day for acute infections and colds.

5 to 6 garlic bulbs
Apple cider vinegar with "the mother," as needed
½ cup (120 ml) raw honey

1. Peel and lightly crush the garlic cloves. Let sit at room temperature to oxidize for 5 minutes.
2. Place them in a 16-ounce (480 ml) mason jar and cover completely with vinegar. If you have one, place a fermentation weight on top to keep the garlic below the surface of the vinegar.
3. Seal with a plastic lid or cover the mouth of the jar with parchment paper and seal with a metal lid. Leave in a cool, dark place for 3 to 4 weeks, until the garlic is pickled to taste.
4. Strain the garlic out and set aside. Transfer the vinegar to a small saucepan, add the honey, and gently warm over low heat until the honey dissolves, stirring to combine.
5. Return the garlic to the jar, then pour in the honey and vinegar mixture.
6. Seal tightly with a plastic lid or cover the mouth of the jar with parchment paper and seal with a metal lid. Return to a cool, dark place for another 3 weeks, until soft and sweet.
7. Store in the fridge for up to a year (or more). Eat one to three cloves daily as needed, using a clean spoon each time you remove the cloves.

NOTES

ON BOTULISM: Concern often arises with these fermented honey recipes, as honey itself is touted as a botulism risk. But it's safer than you think. For the bacteria that causes botulism to grow, it needs a low-oxygen and high-water environment, a pH over 4.6, and warm temperatures. Raw honey has very low water content and strong antimicrobial activity that combats the botulinum toxin. The fermentation lowers pH quickly below 4.6, and there's plenty of oxygen present. If you have concerns, the best thing to do is get pH strips and test regularly.

Don't give honey to children under the age of 1; it can contain spores that cause infant botulism.

QUICK GARLIC HONEY

MAKES ABOUT $^3/_4$ CUP (180 ML)

Prep: 10 minutes

This is a quick fix but has a stronger taste than pickled garlic. Take a teaspoon up to 3 times daily for coughs, colds and flu, urinary tract infections, and other infections.

1 garlic bulb
Raw honey, as needed
1 tablespoon apple cider vinegar with "the mother"

1. Peel and finely chop the garlic cloves. Let sit at room temperature to oxidize for 5 minutes. Transfer to an 8-ounce (240 ml) mason jar.
2. Add enough honey to cover the garlic by at least 1 inch (2.5 cm) and stir well. Add the apple cider vinegar and stir again.
3. Use immediately. Store in the fridge for up to 3 months.

GARLIC OIL

MAKES 2 CUPS (480 ML)

Cook: 5 minutes
Rest: 3 hours

This is a particularly gentle application for mild earaches (use 2 or 3 drops in the ear once or twice a day), occasional tooth pain (use an oil-soaked cotton ball on the area at whim), hair growth (massage it into your scalp a couple of times a week), or adding to fresh foods.

1 garlic bulb
2 cups (480 ml) extra virgin olive oil

1. Peel and gently crush the garlic cloves.
2. Place in a small pan, add the oil, and heat over medium-low heat until just uncomfortably warm to the touch, about 5 minutes. Remove from the heat and let sit for 2 to 3 hours.
3. Strain through a cheesecloth, pour the oil into a jar, and eat the cloves. Store in the fridge for up to 1 week.

ONION AND HONEY COUGH SYRUP

MAKES 8 OUNCES (240 ML)

Prep: 5 minutes
Chill: 8 to 12 hours

This syrup is great for suppressing dry, tickly coughs and clearing mucus. Take 2 teaspoons up to six times daily or give ½ teaspoon to children under 10 (remember to avoid giving honey to babies under the age of 1). You can use the prepared honey or garlic from the previous recipes for this.

1 medium white onion, chopped
Raw honey, as needed
5 garlic cloves, chopped (optional)
Small handful of fresh thyme or oregano leaves (optional)

1. Place the onion in a jar and add enough honey to cover it. Add the garlic and/or herbs if desired.
2. Transfer to the fridge to chill for at least 8 hours or overnight. The honey will pull out all the potent juices from the onion and create a syrup.
3. Store in the fridge for up to 1 month and shake well before each use.

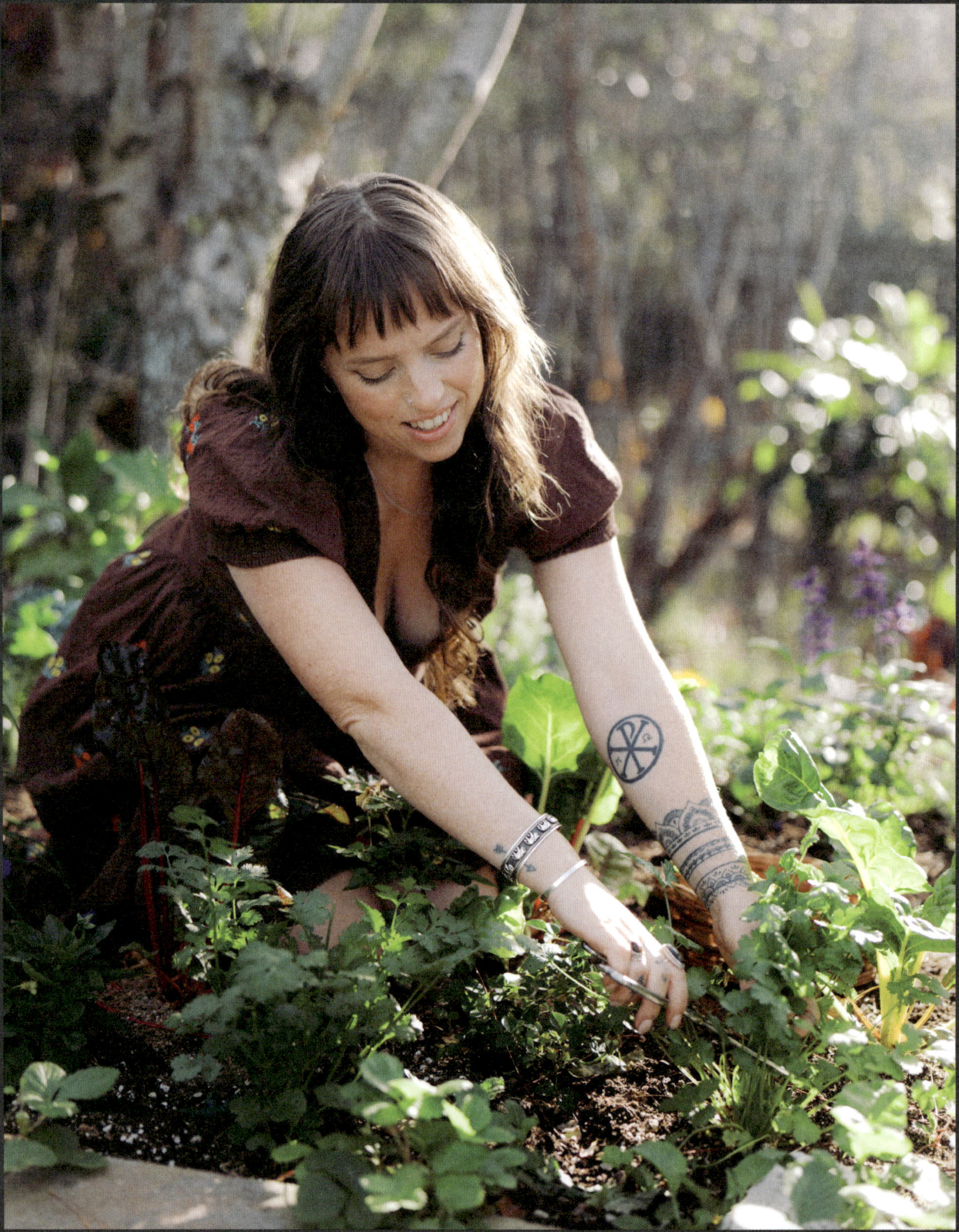

COMMON KITCHEN REMEDIES

FINALLY, I LEAVE YOU with my collection of food and food-adjacent items that you should collect or make and keep on hand for common ailments.

- **HONEY:** Highly antibacterial. Healing for burns, cuts, ulcers, and infected wounds.
- **COCONUT OIL:** Antiviral, antifungal, antimicrobial, antibacterial, and anti-inflammatory. Good for eczema, rashes, fungal infections, nicks and small cuts, dandruff, sunburn, and lice.
- **BAKING SODA:** Neutralizes acid and heartburn. Make into a paste for drawing out bites and stings. Add to a bath for sunburn and rashes.
- **CAYENNE PEPPER:** Stops bleeding. Use topically on cuts or take pills internally. Fast acting pain relief and anti-inflammatory.
- **OATS:** Skin-soothing in baths, facemasks, and poultices. Calming for the nerves in a tea.
- **OLIVE OIL:** Anti-inflammatory, antioxidant. Moisturizing; soothes minor burns, irritation, and ulcers when used topically. Digestive aid, stool softener, gut soother.
- **LAVENDER ESSENTIAL OIL:** Topical use only for bug bites, minor cuts, itching and irritation. Sleep support and calming when used as aromatherapy in a diffuser, in a steamy bath, or on a pillow.
- **PEPPERMINT TEA:** Digestive relief for nausea, gas, bloating, constipation, congestion, and tension headaches.
- **CHAMOMILE TEA:** Calming for nerves and anxiety. Sedative for strong sleep support.
- **FERMENTED GARLIC:** Antimicrobial, antibacterial, antiviral. Use for immune support and heart health, and for acute illnesses like colds, flu, and mild infections.
- **ELDERBERRY TINCTURE:** For immune support and acute cold and flu recovery.
- **FIRE CIDER:** For gut health, day to day wellness, immune health, coughs, colds, and fevers.

REFERENCES

Azizah, Nabilah Sekar, et al. "Sweet Basil (Ocimum basilicum L.)—a Review of Its Botany, Phytochemistry, Pharmacological Activities, and Biotechnological Development." *Plants* 12, no. 24 (2023): 4148. https://doi.org/10.3390/plants12244148.

Brighten, Jolene. "Seed Cycling for Hormone Balance." *Dr. Jolene Brighten*, January 9, 2019. https://drbrighten.com/seed-cycling-for-hormone-balance/.

Chavda, Vivek P., et al. "Inflammation: The Cause of All Diseases." *Cells* 13, no. 22 (2024): 1906. https://doi.org/10.3390/cells13221906.

Chen, Liping, et al. "Beetroot as a Functional Food with Huge Health Benefits: Antioxidant, Antitumor, Physical Function, and Chronic Metabolomics Activity." *Food Science & Nutrition* 9, no. 11 (2021): 6406–6420. https://doi.org/10.1002/fsn3.2577.

Chevallier, Andrew. *Natural Health Encyclopedia of Herbal Medicine.* DK Pub. Inc., 2000.

Cleveland Clinic. "Your Fiber Intake: What's the Right Amount?" *Cleveland Clinic*, April 30, 2025. https://health.clevelandclinic.org/how-much-fiber-per-day.

Crane, Paul K., et al. "Glucose Levels and Risk of Dementia." *New England Journal of Medicine* 369, no. 6 (2013): 540–548. https://doi.org/10.1056/nejmoa1215740.

Domínguez-López, Inés, et al. "Effects of Dietary Phytoestrogens on Hormones throughout a Human Lifespan: A Review." *Nutrients* 12, no. 8 (2020): 2456. https://doi.org/10.3390/nu12082456.

Easley, Thomas, and Steven H. Horne. *The Modern Herbal Dispensatory: A Medicine-Making Guide.* North Atlantic Books, 2016.

ElGhannam, Mai, et al. "Eugenol; Effective Anthelmintic Compound against Foodborne Parasite Trichinella Spiralis Muscle Larvae and Adult." *Pathogens* 12, no. 1 (2023): 127. https://doi.org/10.3390/pathogens12010127.

Halbreich, Uriel, et al. "The Prevalence, Impairment, Impact, and Burden of Premenstrual Dysphoric Disorder (PMS/PMDD)." *Psychoneuroendocrinology* 28, no. 3 (2003): 1–23. https://doi.org/10.1016/s0306-4530(03)00098-2.

Hartvig, Kirsten. *Healing Spices: 50 Wonderful Spices, and How to Use Them in Health-Giving Foods and Drinks.* Nourish, 2016.

Ketchem, Justin M., et al. "Male Sex Hormones, Aging, and Inflammation." *Biogerontology* 24, no. 1 (2023): 1–25. https://doi.org/10.1007/s10522-022-10002-1.

LeWine, Howard E. "Understanding the Stress Response." *Harvard Health*, April 3, 2024. https://www.health.harvard.edu/staying-healthy/understanding-the-stress-response.

Li, Zhi-hui, et al. "Effects of Regular Breakfast Habits on Metabolic and Cardiovascular Diseases." *Medicine* 100, no. 44 (2021): e27629. https://doi.org/10.1097/md.0000000000027629.

Lutter, Chessa K., et al. "The Potential of a Simple Egg to Improve Maternal and Child Nutrition." *Maternal & Child Nutrition* 14 (2018): e12678. https://doi.org/10.1111/mcn.12678.

Ma, Xiao, et al. "Excessive Intake of Sugar: An Accomplice of Inflammation." *Frontiers in Immunology* 13 (2022). https://doi.org/10.3389/fimmu.2022.988481.

Moritz, Bettina, et al. "The Role of Vitamin C in Stress-Related Disorders." *The Journal of Nutritional Biochemistry* 85 (2020): 108459. https://doi.org/10.1016/j.jnutbio.2020.108459.

Mott, Nicholas. "What Makes Us Human? Cooking, Study Says." *National Geographic*, October 26, 2012. https://www.nationalgeographic.com/animals/article/121026-human-cooking-evolution-raw-food-health-science.

Nam, Su Youn, et al. "The Effect of Abdominal Visceral Fat, Circulating Inflammatory Cytokines, and Leptin Levels on Reflux Esophagitis." *Journal of Neurogastroenterology and Motility* 21, no. 2 (2015): 247–254. https://doi.org/10.5056/jnm14114.

O'Keefe, Stephen J. "The Association between Dietary Fibre Deficiency and High-Income Lifestyle-Associated Diseases: Burkitt's Hypothesis Revisited." *The Lancet Gastroenterology & Hepatology* 4, no. 12 (2019): 984–996. https://doi.org/10.1016/S2468-1253(19)30257-2.

Patak, P., et al. "Vitamin C Is an Important Cofactor for Both Adrenal Cortex and Adrenal Medulla." *Endocrine Research* 30, no. 4 (2004): 871–875. https://doi.org/10.1081/erc-200044126.

Paudel, Devendra, et al. "A Review of Health-Beneficial Properties of Oats." *Foods* 10, no. 11 (2021): 2591. https://doi.org/10.3390/foods10112591.

Pickering, Gisèle, et al. "Magnesium Status and Stress: The Vicious Circle Concept Revisited." *Nutrients* 12, no. 12 (2020): 3672.

Rahman, Khalid, and Gordon M. Lowe. "Garlic and Cardiovascular Disease: A Critical Review." *The Journal of Nutrition* 136, no. 3 Suppl. (2006): 736S–740S. https://doi.org/10.1093/jn/136.3.736S.

Rasheed, Naveed, et al. "Effectiveness of Combined Seeds (Pumpkin, Sunflower, Sesame, Flaxseed): As Adjacent Therapy to Treat Polycystic Ovary Syndrome in Females." *Food Science & Nutrition* 11, no. 6 (2023). https://doi.org/10.1002/fsn3.3328.

Robbins, Morley M., et al. *Cure Your Fatigue: How Balancing 3 Minerals and 1 Protein Is the Solution That You're Looking For.* Gatekeeper Press, 2021.

Rojas, Joselyn, et al. "Polycystic Ovary Syndrome, Insulin Resistance, and Obesity: Navigating the Pathophysiologic Labyrinth." *International Journal of Reproductive Medicine* 2014 (2014): 1–17. https://doi.org/10.1155/2014/719050.

Sirotkin, Alexander V. "The Effect of Dietary Oat Consumption and Its Constituents on Fat Storage and Obesity." *Physiological Research* (2023): S157–S163. https://doi.org/10.33549/physiolres.934957.

Vitti, Alisa. *WomanCode: Perfect Your Cycle, Amplify Your Fertility, Supercharge Your Sex Drive, and Become a Power Source.* Hay House, 2013.

Weed, Susun S. *Wise Woman Herbal for the Childbearing Year.* Ash Tree Publishing, 1985.

Witbracht, Megan, et al. "Female Breakfast Skippers Display a Disrupted Cortisol Rhythm and Elevated Blood Pressure." *Physiology & Behavior* 140 (2015): 215–221. https://doi.org/10.1016/j.physbeh.2014.12.044.

Yang, Bowen, et al. "Association of Skipping Breakfast with Metabolic Syndrome and Its Components: A Systematic Review and Meta-Analysis of Observational Studies." *Nutrients* 17, no. 19 (2025): 3155. https://doi.org/10.3390/nu17193155.

INDEX

N

O

P

Q

R

S

Q

R

S

ACKNOWLEDGMENTS

Thank you to everyone who made this dream book
a reality. It was truly a team effort.

To Kandreas, who put everything aside to support me during the last two years, and for all the cups of coffee and late-night encouragement.

Thank you, Kensa and Zimri, for inspiring me every day.

To my parents, who have always believed in me more than I have believed in myself, and all of my family for their love.

To Beth, for your cooking skills; to Josiah, for your patience; and to Johnny, for your safe space.

Thank you to my editor, Olivia, who deserves far more credit than she will get. She made this book a reality and turned my coal lumps into diamonds. We did it, you briny babe.

Thank you, for reading this book. Thank you for your curiosity and trust. I hope this book gives you inspiration and encouragement to keep learning and experimenting. I hope it becomes dog-eared and stained, and you put your own notes and adjustments in the margins. I hope it helps you rediscover the magic a little bit.

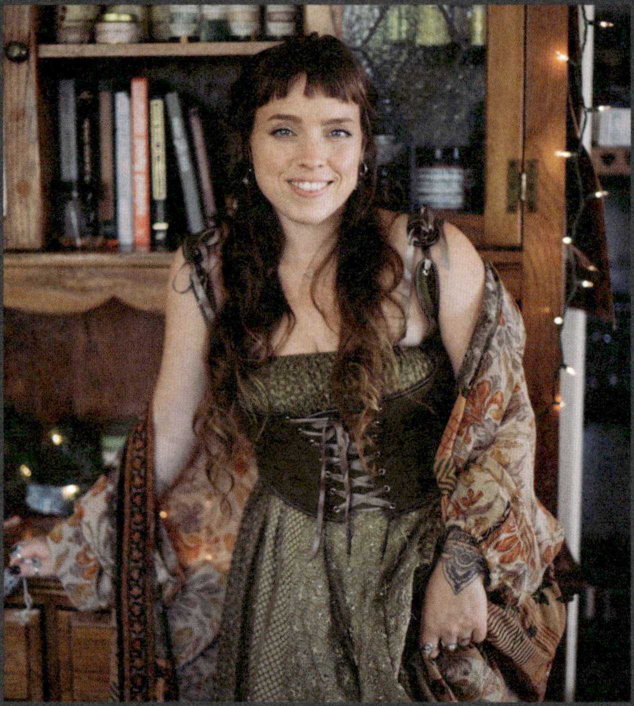

ABOUT THE AUTHOR

REBEKAH "EBBY" MOYER is a content creator, artist, and third-generation nutrition fanatic. She grew up in Cornwall, England, reading *Brambly Hedge*, picking wild elderflowers, and taking tinctures from the local herbalist. Her world-traveling foodie family inspired her love of flavor and cooking, and her kombucha-brewing mom sparked her interest in food's healing "magic." For the past 10 years, she has pursued her curiosity about holistic nutrition through independent study and all the teaching she can access, and she shares that journey on her social media channels. Through sharing, she hopes to encourage others in their health journeys and show that anyone can learn if they know where to look. She makes simple, nourishing meals using accessible, whole-food ingredients and home remedies for common ailments, and seeks to find the magic in every day while raising two rambunctious boys with her husband, Kandreas.